S0-BBP-445

General anesthesia in dental practice

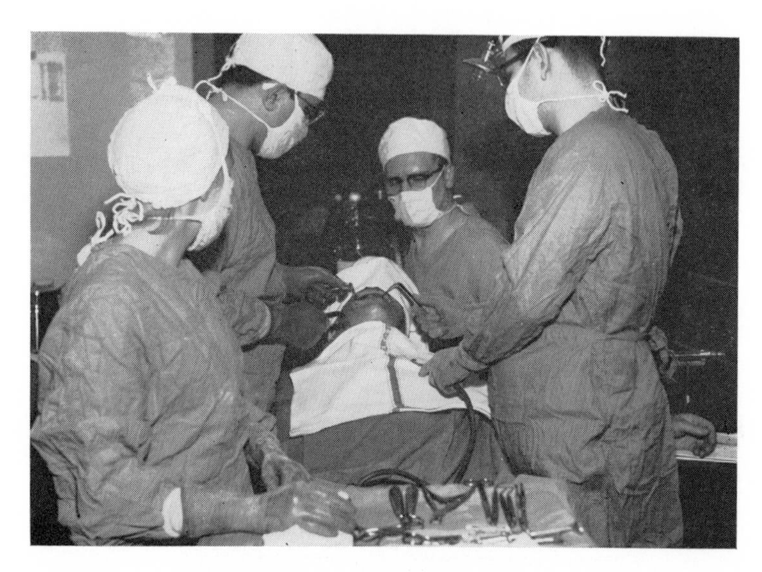

General anesthesia for dental surgery.
Note operating team: anesthetist, surgeon, assistant, and instrument nurse.

General anesthesia in dental practice

LEONARD M. MONHEIM, B.S., M.S., D.D.S.

Professor and Head, Department of Anesthesia,
University of Pittsburgh School of Dentistry;
Professor of Pharmacology,
University of Pittsburgh School of Dentistry;
Clinical Associate Professor, Department of Anesthesiology,
University of Pittsburgh School of Medicine;
Professor, Graduate Faculty (Dentistry), University of Pittsburgh;
Senior Staff Anesthesiologist,
Presbyterian-University Hospital, Pittsburgh, Pa.;
Consultant Staff, Magee-Women's Hospital,
Eye and Ear Hospital, Children's Hospital, and
Veterans Administration Hospital,
Pittsburgh, Pa.

Third edition

With 123 illustrations

The C. V. Mosby Company

Saint Louis 1968

Third edition

Printed in the United States of America

Library of Congress Catalog Card Number 68-21526

Distributed in Great Britain by Henry Kimpton, London

Dedicated to

GEORGE J. THOMAS, M.D.

Teacher, Counselor, Friend

Contributors

ALBERT J. FISHER, M.D.

Former Clinical Instructor in Anesthesiology, University of Pittsburgh School of Medicine, Pittsburgh, Pa.; former Associate Director, Department of Anesthesiology, Presbyterian-University and Woman's Hospitals; present Director of Anesthesiology, Prince George's Hospital, Cheverly, Md.

NEAL A. HARPER, D.D.S., LL.B., M.S.

Brigadier General, Dental Corps, United States Army, Retired; Professor, College of Dentistry, Ohio State University, Columbus, Ohio; Member, Ohio Bar Association; University, Columbus, Ohio; Member, Ohio Bar Association; former Assistant Chief, Army Dental Corps, Office of the Surgeon General and Chief of Dental Service, Walter Reed Army Hospital, Washington, D. C.; former Professor of Military Science and Tactics (Dental), Ohio State University, Columbus, Ohio

JOSEPH H. MARCY, M.D.

Clinical Associate Professor in Anesthesiology, University of Pittsburgh School of Medicine, Pittsburgh, Pa.; Director, Department of Anesthesia, Children's Hospital, Pittsburgh, Pa.

GEORGE J. THOMAS, M.D.

Professor Emeritus, Section of Anesthesiology, University of Pittsburgh School of Medicine, Pittsburgh, Pa.; former Director, Department of Anesthesia, St. Francis General and Medical Center Hospitals, Pittsburgh, Pa.

Foreword

This book, devoted to general anesthesia in dental practice, is authored by a dentist who limits his professional practice to this specialty. Practical application of general anesthesia had its birth in dentistry, and the modern concept of this art and science is presented by Dr. Monheim. The importance of this information is demonstrated by the hundreds of patients who require general anesthesia in dentistry daily.

The need for this book arises from innovations in drugs and techniques. Its scope makes it desirable for use in any teaching program. Most of the teaching of special methods in anesthesia is confined to lectures and demonstations. Attention to these word-of-mouth lectures is given by Dr. Monheim, and several techniques especially relating to anesthesia for dental operations are included. In addition to its use as a textbook in graduate and undergraduate anesthesia courses in dentistry, it should be used daily as a reference by specialists administering anesthesia for dental patients.

Morgan L. Allison, D.D.S.
Professor and Head, Department
of Anesthesia and Oral Surgery,
Ohio State University College of Dentistry

Preface to third edition

My original intent, when writing the first edition, was to prepare a text that would stress my philosophy as well as the fundamental aspects of general anesthesia in dentistry. I hoped that such a book would elevate the standards of general anesthesia as practiced by dentists. It is my belief that the original intent has been accomplished, and thus the fundamental aspects remain the same. However, because of the introduction and acceptance of newer drugs, some concepts have changed; I trust that the third edition of this text adequately discusses these drugs and the manner in which previously accepted concepts have been altered. These important additions and alterations to the field of anesthesia, plus a satisfactory acceptance of the first two editions, have made the third necessary.

I would again like to thank Dr. Albert J. Fisher, Dr. Neal A. Harper, and Dr. George J. Thomas for their contributions. I would especially like to thank Dr. Joseph H. Marcy, not only for the chapter that he contributed, but also for his willingness to discuss and offer suggestions concerning other areas of the book. I wish to express my thanks to Dr. Leroy Harris for his suggestions and to Miss Janet Koncsol, secretary of the Anesthesiology Department of the Presbyterian-University Hospital, for her help in the preparation of this third edition. Also, my thanks to my wife, Marion, for editing the manuscript.

Leonard M. Monheim

Preface to first edition

This book is, in reality, a compilation of lectures on general anesthesia given to the senior and graduate students at the University of Pittsburgh School of Dentistry for a period of over twenty years. The original idea to organize the lectures in pamphlet form was inaugurated over five years ago by a graduate student, Dr. Kenneth Tessler of San Francisco, when he encouraged me to have the lectures mimeographed and given to the students. The lectures, with the help of Dr. Tessler, were mimeographed and used not only for teaching but also for refresher courses before many dental groups. The interest in these lectures demonstrated a desire on the part of the dentist for a more basic understanding of general anesthesia.

As material was added over the years, it was decided that it would be advantageous to expand the contents into book form as a ready source of basic information for the dental student and dentist interested in general anesthesia. There seemed to be a particular need for such a text which would make available to the dentist information on the anatomy and physiology of respiration, circulation, and the nervous system; physics, as applied to anesthesia; the pharmacology of the anesthetic agents and associated drugs; general information dealing with the phases, stages, and signs of anesthesia; methods of administration; the airway; complications and emergencies; preanesthetic evaluation; preoperative preparation and postoperative care of patients; operating room hazards; pediatric anesthesia; medicolegal considerations; and the armamentarium used.

Included is a chapter on the technical aspects of anesthesia, although it is my belief that, while much basic information can be gathered from a variety of reading sources, the actual techniques of administration of anesthetics can be developed and improved only by practical clinical experience under proper supervision. For this reason I do not intend this text to be a primer for the administration of anesthetics for dental patients, but only a ready source of background information. I hope that any dentist undertaking the administration of general anesthesia will devote sufficient time, preferably one year in formal training, to the technical aspects of anesthesia.

In addition to Dr. Tessler, I wish to express my sincere gratitude to Dr. James Breen, Dr. Charles Buttermore, Dr. Wilbur Dickman, Dr. David Ford, Dr. Ralph Fredal, Dr. David Lyons, Dr. Alonzo E. McDonald, Dr. Leonard Rafalko, Dr. Harold Robins, Dr. Donald Shearer, Dr. Charles Stoner, Dr. Roberto Valdeavellano, and especially to Dr. Theodore Century, Dr. Edward N. Cole, Dr. Walter F. Dorer, and Dr. M. Page Snead, all graduate students in anesthesia at the University of Pittsburgh School of Dentistry, for their tireless efforts toward the writing of this book.

I am deeply grateful to Miss Marjorie Kolb, nurse anesthesist, Presbyterian-University and Woman's Hospitals, who spent many hours taking dictation. I am appreciative to my wife, Marion, for the time spent organizing material; to Mrs. Florence Strang, my secretary, for her excellent typing of the manuscript; and to Mr. Tuckerman Day of Concord, Mass., for his thorough editorial services.

The chapters contributed by Dr. Albert J. Fisher, Gen. Neal A. Harper, Dr. Joseph H. Marcy, and Dr. George J. Thomas are indeed an asset to the book. I am grateful to Dr. Sidney S. Spatz, Dr. Harold J. Zubrow, and Dr. Stuart N. Kline of Pittsburgh for the willing use of their office facilities, and to Dr. Joseph Haller of Altoona, Pa., for several photographs that appear in this book.

I am indebted to Mr. Albert Levin, director of medical illustration, University of Pittsburgh School of Medicine; to Mr. Nicholas M. Graver for the excellent photography; to Miss Margaret Croup, medical illustrator, University of Pittsburgh School of Medicine; and to Mr. Thomas Gmitter for the excellent drawings and sketches.

To all those who helped in any way during the preparation of this volume, I am deeply grateful.

Leonard M. Monheim
Pittsburgh, Pa.

Contents

General anesthesia in dental practice

Chapter 1

Anatomy and physiology of respiration

Respiration as interpreted today refers to the gaseous exchange between the cells of the body and the atmosphere. It is no longer interpreted as meaning simply the inspiratory and expiratory phases. Therefore, we must be concerned not only with the exchange of gases between the external atmosphere and the alveoli of the lungs but also with their passage from the alveoli of the lungs into the bloodstream, their transportation to the cells, and the exchange of gases between the bloodstream and the cells.

The respiratory system may be divided into two distinct parts: the *external respiration,* which deals with the exchange of gases between the atmosphere and the bloodstream by way of the alveoli of the lungs, and the *internal respiration,* which deals with the exchange of gases between the bloodstream and the cells.

External respiration (Fig. 1-1)

1. The *conducting portion,* which consists of the nasal and oral passages, the pharynx, larynx, trachea, and bronchi, plays no part in the actual diffusion of gases into the bloodstream other than as a means of communication with the alveoli of the lungs. It is commonly referred to, therefore, as the anatomical dead space.
2. The *ventilating portion,* which consists of the actual functional unit of the lung, namely, the air sac, or lung alveolus, is connected to the conducting portion by a single bronchiole. In this intricate pattern of tissues the contained air is separated from capillary blood by two thin endothelial membranes, one forming

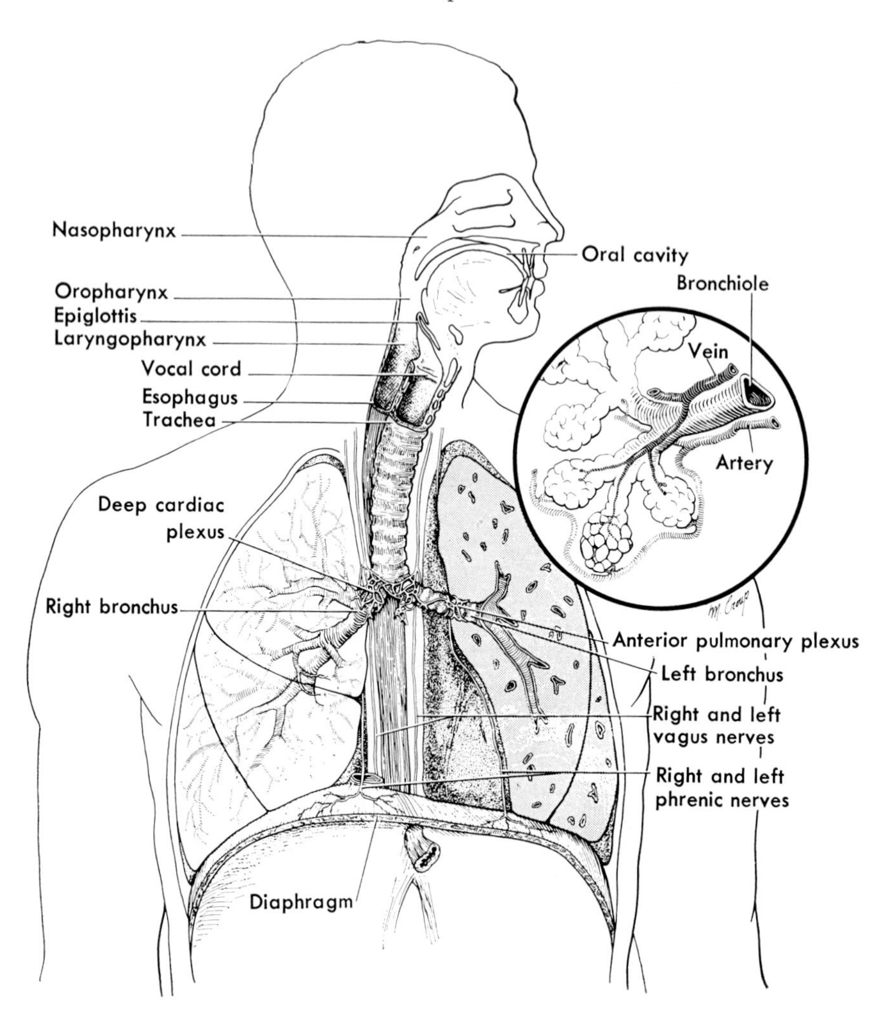

Fig. 1-1. External respiration.

the wall of the capillary and the other the lining of the alveolus. The oxygen and carbon dioxide passing from the lung alveoli to the bloodstream and from the bloodstream into the lung alveoli must diffuse through this dual membrane.

Internal respiration

1. The *transportation portion* consists of the blood plasma and the red cells. The gases that are transported in the bloodstream from

the alveoli of the lungs to the tissue cells are carred in solution in the plasma or in chemical combination within the red cells. The transportation of gases from the tissue cells to the alveoli of the lungs is accomplished in a like manner.

2. The *intracellular respiration* consists of the interchange of gases (carbon dioxide and oxygen) between the bloodstream and the tissue cells.

ANATOMY OF THE RESPIRATORY TRACT

The architecture of the respiratory system is closely correlated with its functions.

Nasal cavity. The nasal cavity is divided into left and right fossae by a central partition called the septum. The septum may be distorted toward one side or the other, and one should bear this in mind when inserting a nasal tube. The anterior openings of the fossae are the nostrils, or nares. The posterior openings into the nasal pharynx are called posterior nares, or choanae. The nasal cavities are separated from the oral cavity by the palate and maxillae and from the cranial cavity by the horizontal plate of the ethmoid. Under normal conditions breathing is accomplished through the nasal cavities.

The entire fossa is lined with mucous membrane that is richly supplied with blood vessels. The epithelial lining of the mucosa is highly specialized, being covered by ciliated columnar epithelium in which goblet cells are interspaced. The endings of the olfactory nerve lie in the mucosa in the region above the superior turbinate.

The paranasal sinuses, or accessory sinuses of the nose, are the frontal, ethmoidal, sphenoidal, and maxillary. These sinuses are lined with ciliated columnar epithelium that is continuous with the lining of the nasal cavities.

Blood is supplied to the nasal cavity by the external and internal maxillary arteries, which are branches of the external carotid. Branches of the internal carotid arteries also furnish blood to the nasal cavity. The olfactory (first), trigeminal (fifth), and facial (seventh) cranial nerves innervate this area.

Oral cavity. The oral cavity consists mainly of the lips, the maxillary and mandibular arches (with or without teeth), the tongue, the checks, and the hard and soft palates.

Pharynx. The pharynx is a musculomembranous tube 12 to 14 cm. in length, extending from the base of the skull above to the esophagus below. The posterior wall rests against the bodies of the cervical vertebrae. The pharynx has openings through which connection is established with the nose, ears, mouth, larynx, and esophagus. The pharynx is divided accordingly into three partitions: nasopharynx, oropharynx, and laryngeal pharynx. The soft palate separates the nasopharynx from the oropharynx. It is a membranous sheet containing muscle and covered with mucous membrane that is attached to the base of the hard palate.

The nasopharynx is that portion of the pharynx which lies behind the posterior nares and above the soft palate. On each lateral wall is the opening of the auditory, or eustachian, tube, which connects with the cavity of the middle ear. The mucosa of the vault of the nasal pharynx contains much lymphoid tissue, which constitutes the pharyngeal tonsils, or adenoids.

The oropharynx extends from the soft palate above to the level of the hyoid bone below. It opens into the mouth at the glossopalatine arch. The palatine tonsils lie on both sides between the two palatine arches.

The laryngeal pharynx lies posterior to the larynx and below the level of the hyoid bone. It communicates anteriorly with the larynx.

Muscles. The muscles of the pharynx are the constrictor muscles and the stylopharyngeus muscles. The constrictor muscles contract in a downward direction, whereas the stylopharyngeus muscles increase the transverse diameter of the pharynx. The mucous lining of the nasopharynx is ciliated columnar epithelium similar to that found in nasal cavities, whereas the mucous lining of the oral and laryngeal pharynx is of stratified squamous epithelium.

Nerve and blood supply. The nerve supply for the pharynx is from the glossopharyngeal nerve, the vagus nerve, and the sympathetic nervous system. The blood supply is from the external carotid artery.

Larynx. The larynx or voice box is placed between the base of the tongue and the trachea. It forms a prominence in the midline of the upper neck, where it lies close to the surface, covered only by skin and fascia. In the adult male the larynx lies anteriorly to the third, fourth,

Table 1-1. Comparison of dimensions of larynx of male and female after puberty

Dimension	*Male*	*Female*
Length	44 mm.	36 mm.
Transverse diameter	43 mm.	41 mm.
Anteroposterior diameter	36 mm.	26 mm.
Circumference	136 mm.	112 mm.

fifth, and sixth cervical vertebrae. In the female and in children it is slightly higher.

During childhood the larynx of the male and female is equal in size. After puberty, the male larynx is much larger due to increases in all dimensions. A comparison of the dimensions is given in Table 1-1.

The larynx is composed of nine cartilages that are held together by ligaments and small muscles. The rigid cartilaginous walls form a boxlike structure that is broad superiorly and dwindles inferiorly to a narrow cylinder that is continuous with the trachea.

The cartilages of the larynx are divided into three single cartilages and three paired cartilages.

Single cartilages

1. Thyroid cartilage. The largest cartilage of the larynx is made up of two laminae fused at an angle to form a shield-shaped structure, the laryngeal prominence, or Adam's apple.
2. Cricoid cartilage. This cartilage is below the thyroid cartilage and forms the lower limit of the larynx. It is shaped like a signet ring, with the wider portion at the back.
3. Epiglottis. This is the last of the unpaired cartilages and is a thin, leaf-shaped structure attached to the thyroid cartilage at the junction of the two laminae. It projects upward behind the root of the tongue and in front of the opening to the larynx.

Paired cartilages

1. Arytenoid cartilages. These are small, pyramid-shaped cartilages attached to the upper border of the cricoid cartilage.
2. Corniculate cartilages. These are two small, elastic cartilages that articulate with the arytenoid cartilages, serving to prolong the arytenoids backward and medially.
3. Cuneiform cartilages. These two small, rodlike cartilages are located in the aryepiglottic folds, just anterior to the corniculate cartilages.

Muscles. The muscles of the larynx are eight in number; five are the muscles of the vocal cords and rima glottidis, and three are connected with the epiglottis.

Muscles of vocal cords and rima glottidis

1. Cricothyroid. This muscle tenses and elongates the cords by drawing up the arch of the cricoid cartilage and increasing the distance between the vocal processes and the angle of the thyroid cartilage.

2. Cricoarytenoideus posticus. This muscle widens the rima glottidis by rotating the arytenoid cartilages outward and separating the vocal folds attached to them.
3. Cricoarytenoideus lateralis. This muscle approximates the cords by rotating the arytenoid cartilages inward.
4. Arytenoideus. This muscle approximates the cords by bringing the arytenoid cartilages together, thus reducing the posterior diameter of the glottis.
5. Thyroarytenoideus. This muscle shortens and relaxes the cords by drawing together the arytenoid cartilages and the thyroid cartilage.

Muscles of the epiglottis

1. Thyroepiglottideus
2. Arytenoepiglottideus superior
3. Arytenoepiglottideus inferior

Nerve and blood supply. The arteries are the superior laryngeal and cricothyroid branches of the superior thyroid (a. thyreoidea superior) from the external carotid, and the inferior laryngeal branch of the inferior thyroid (a. thyreoidea inferior) from the thyroid plexus.

The veins open into the internal jugular and the innominate veins.

The lymphatics open into glands near the bifurcation of the common carotid artery and into others in front of the cricothyroid membrane.

The nerves of the larynx are the superior and recurrent (inferior) laryngeal branches of the pneumogastric (n. vagus), joined by filaments from the spinal accessory (n. accessorius) and the sympathetic.

The superior laryngeal nerve (n. laryngeus superior) is the nerve of sensation. It enters the larynx through a hole in the thyrohyoid membrane and supplies the mucous membrane and the cricothyroid and arytenoideus muscles. It has two branches—the external and the internal laryngeal.

The recurrent laryngeal nerve (n. laryngeus inferior) is the motor nerve. It winds from before backward, around the subclavian artery on the right side and around the arch of the aorta on the left side, and is distributed to all the laryngeal muscles except the cricothyroid and arytenoideus, giving off in its course cardiac, esophageal, tracheal, and pharyngeal filaments, and finally joining with the superior laryngeal nerve.

Interior. The interior of the larynx presents a cavity that is divided into two parts by the inward projection of the true vocal cords. The superior part, sometimes called the vestibule, is broad and triangular;

the inferior part of the cavity is at first elliptical and lower down is circular, becoming continuous with the tube of the trachea.

The glottis, or rima glottidis, is a narrow fissure of varying width between the inferior vocal cords, formed by the projection into the cavity of the larynx of these cords and the thyroarytenoideus muscle. Its greatest length is less than an inch, and its greatest breadth about half an inch.

The superior, or false, vocal cords (plicae ventriculares) contain the superior thyroarytenoid ligaments; they extend from the angle of the thyroid cartilage around to the anterior surfaces of the arytenoids and consist of two folds of mucous membrane, each having a free crescentic margin.

The inferior, or true, vocal cords (plicae vocales) contain the inferior thyroarytenoid ligaments and extend from the angle of the thyroid cartilage around to the anterior angles of the bases of the arytenoids. They consist of two thin layers of mucous membrane covering the ligaments named, each having the thyroarytenoideus muscle external and parallel to it.

The ventricle (ventriculus laryngis) consists of an oblong fossa on each side of the larynx, between the true and false vocal cords, communicating with the sacculus laryngis by a narrow opening.

Trachea. The trachea is a cartilaginous and membranous tube about 10 to 11 cm. (4½ inches) in length and about 2.5 cm. (1 inch) in diameter. It lies in front of the esophagus and extends from the larynx on the level of the sixth cervical vertebra to opposite the fourth or fifth thoracic vertebra, where it divides into a right and left bronchus. The walls of the trachea are strengthened and rendered more rigid by twenty C-shaped rings of cartilage. The rings are incomplete posteriorly where they come in contact with the esophagus. Like the larynx, the trachea is lined with mucous membrane of ciliated epithelium.

Nerve and blood supply. The nerves of the trachea are derived from fibers of the cranial autonomic (vagus or tenth cranial) nerves and of the sympathetic trunk. Stimulation of the cranial autonomic nerves contracts the muscular tissues and increases secretion. Stimulation of the sympathetic nerves causes relaxation of the muscular tissues and checks secretion.

The blood supply of the trachea is primarily from the inferior thyroid arteries, with the veins ending in the thyroid venous plexus.

Bronchi. The bronchi are two continuations of the trachea, both composed of incomplete circles of cartilage joined together by fibrous tissue and smooth muscle. The mucous membrane lining is similar to and continuous with that of the trachea. The right bronchus is shorter (2.5 cm. in length), wider, and more nearly vertical or continuous with the trachea; whereas the left bronchus is longer (about 5 cm. in length), narrower, and more nearly horizontal. The right and left main bronchi in turn divide into a great number of smaller branches called bronchioles.

The bronchi resemble the trachea in structure, but as the bronchial tubes divide and subdivide, their walls become thinner, the cartilage and fibrous tissue disappear, and the finer tubes are composed of only a thin layer of muscular and elastic tissues lined by ciliated epithelium. Each bronchiole terminates in an enlargement called the atrium (infundibulum). From each atrium there is a series of alveoli, or air cells. The walls of the alveoli consist of a thin film of elastic tissue lined internally with a single layer of flat cells.

Lungs. The lungs are cone-shaped structures located in the thoracic cavity and separated by the contents of the mediastinum. The outer surfaces are convex to fit into a concave cavity, whereas the base is concave to fit over the convexity of the diaphragm. The apex of the lungs extends from 2 to 4 cm. above the level of the sternal end of the first rib. The right lung is larger, heavier, and broader and is divided into three lobes. The left lung is smaller and narrower, with the front border deeply indented (position of the heart), and is divided into two lobes.

The lungs themselves are porous, spongy organs consisting of bronchial tubes, atria, alveoli, blood vessels, lymphatics, and nerves held together by connective tissue. The walls of the alveoli consist of a single layer of epithelial cells on a thin layer of connective tissue, which is richly supplied with capillaries.

Nerve and blood supply. The nerve supply to the lungs is from the vagus nerve and the sympathetic (third, fourth, and fifth thoracic) plexus. Afferent vagal fibers pass from the lung alveoli to the respiratory center. Efferent vagal fibers cause contraction of the bronchial musculature. Sympathetic fibers produce relaxation. The mediastinal pleura, the costal pleura, and the diaphragmatic pleura receive motor fibers from the phrenic nerve and sensory fibers from the intercostal nerves.

Blood for aeration is supplied by the pulmonary arteries and veins, with a plexus of capillaries around each alveoli. The bronchial artery supplies the lung substance.

PHYSIOLOGY OF RESPIRATION

Mechanics of respiration. The mechanics of respiration involve the variations in pressures within the thoracic cage and lungs as compared to the external atmosphere. The pressure within the thoracic cage of the resting adult averages from 3 to 5 mm. Hg. This negative pressure area tends to draw the parietal pleura away from the visceral pleura, which maintains the lungs in an inflated state. As the thorax enlarges, the negative intrathoracic pressure is increased to 5 or even 10 mm. Hg. This further increases the pull of the parietal pleura against the visceral pleura, creating a negative pressure (2 mm. Hg) within the lungs and allowing air to rush into the negative pressure area from the external atmosphere until the pressure is equalized.

The inspiratory effort may be divided into four phases:

1. Contraction of the diaphragm and intercostal muscles, which is due to nervous impulses.
2. Enlargement of the thoracic cage in all directions, which is due to the contraction of these muscles.
3. Enlargement of the thoracic cage, which increases the intrapleural negative pressure, forcing the lungs to increase their internal volume capacity, and thus produces a temporary increase in intrapulmonic negative pressure.
4. Since the lungs are connected to the external atmosphere by the conducting portion of the external respiratory system, the air from the external atmosphere enters the lungs until the intrapulmonic and atmospheric pressures are equalized.

Following each normal inspiratory effort there is an expiratory phase, or the act by which a portion of the air is expelled from the lungs. This phase can also be divided into four distinct steps:

1. There is relaxation of the diaphragm and intercostal muscles.
2. The intrathoracic dimensions are reduced by relaxation of the respiratory muscles.
3. Reduction of the intrathoracic dimensions creates an increased pressure upon the intrapleural surfaces, thus raising the pressure within the lungs themselves.
4. Since the lungs are connected to the external atmosphere by the conducting portion of the external respiratory apparatus, the intrapulmonic gases are forced into the external atmosphere until the intrapulmonic and atmospheric pressures are equalized.

As can be seen from the previous explanation, the inspiratory and expiratory phases, while primarily under neural and chemical control, are fundamentally dependent upon the variances of pressure within the intrapulmonic space and the atmospheric air. The intrapulmonic pressure must be less than the atmospheric pressure to induce inspiration. The intrapulmonic pressure will be equal to the atmospheric pressure at the end of the inspiratory effort and will rise above atmospheric pressure during expiration. At the end of expiration and before the initiating of a new inspiratory phase, the intrapulmonic pressure will again be equal to the atmospheric pressure.

In addition to the intrapulmonic pressure, the intrathoracic pressures play an important part in the respiratory cycle. It is the increase in the intrathoracic negative pressure created by an increase in thoracic dimensions that permits varying of the intrapulmonic pressures. The intrapleural pressures are negative throughout the respiratory cycle, varying only in the degree of negativity.

Control of respiration. Respiration is adjusted to serve definite body needs: (1) to supply oxygen to the body cells, (2) to adequately eliminate carbon dioxide, (3) to aid in regulating hydrogen ion concentration in the blood, and (4) to aid in maintaining normal body temperature.

As previously stated, the control of respiration (Fig. 1-2) is neural, chemical, and, to a degree, voluntary. This control must be so coordinated that the changing requirements of the body are met constantly. The necessary changes in pulmonary ventilation are regulated by a complex respiratory center situated in the reticular formation of the caudal medulla. This center is composed of both inspiratory and expiratory portions, which though bilateral, functions as units. In addition to the inspiratory and expiratory centers, which are subdivisions of the respiratory center, there is a pneumotaxic center located in the upper pons. This center periodically inhibits the inspiratory center, giving it a rhythmic pattern of inspiration, expiration, rest, and inspiration again the renew the cycle. The nervous control enables respiration to meet the changing requirements of the body, while the chemical control maintains adequate respiratory ventilation as an aid or supplement to the nervous control. Voluntary control, although limited, does enable a person to vary the respiratory pattern to accomplish such maneuvers as whistling and singing, which require an alteration in respiration.

Neural control. Inspiration is initiated by stimulation and activation of the muscles of respiration by impulses from the inspiratory center. These impulses are discharged through descending pathways to the motor neurons in the dorsal area of the cervical spinal cord and eventually through the phrenic nerves to the diaphragm and the intercostal nerves to the intercostal muscles. During normal breathing, the diaphragm and the external intercostal muscles are the only muscles actively involved. In order that pulmonary ventilation be increased as required under varying circumstances, other auxiliary muscles, as

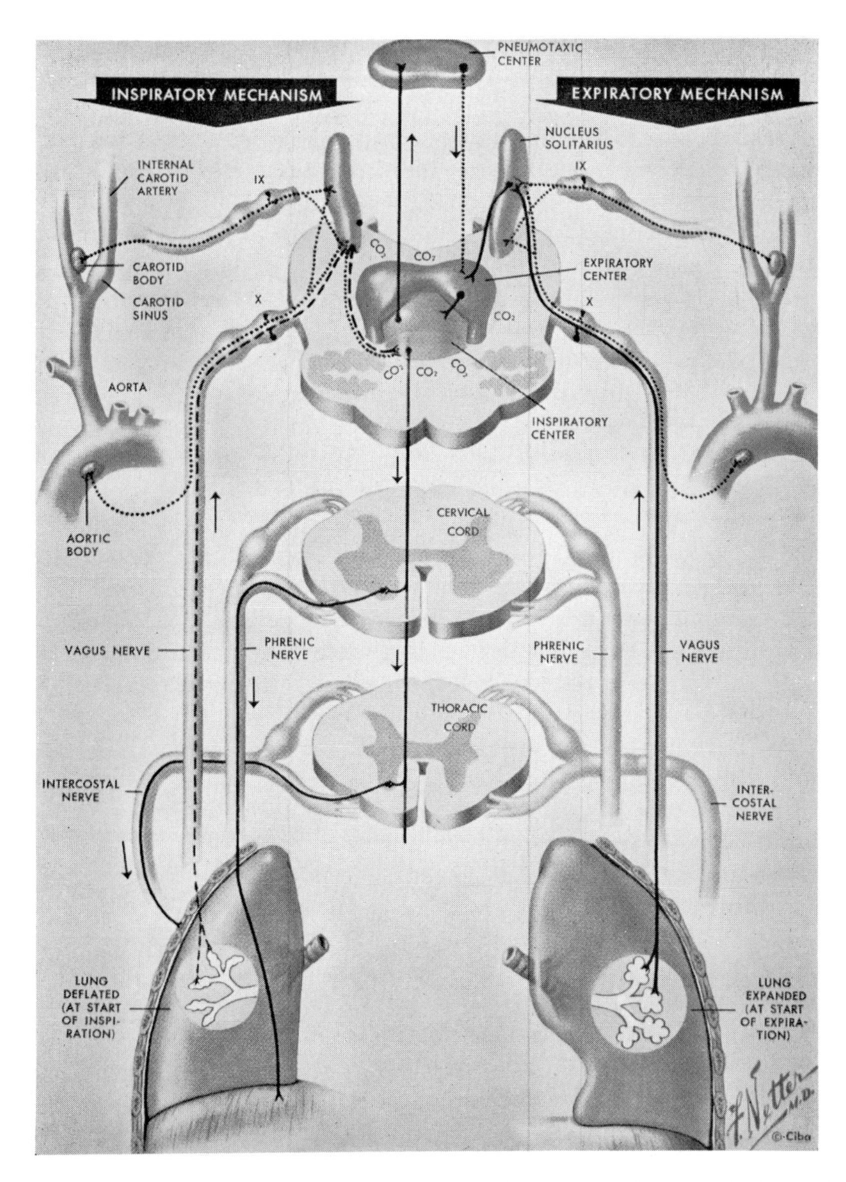

Fig. 1-2. Control of respiration. (Courtesy The Ciba Collection of Medical Illustrations, Volume 1.)

well as more forceful contractions of the diaphragm and intercostal muscles, are brought into play.

During inspiration as the lungs are inflated, stretch receptors located in the alveoli of the lungs are stimulated, sending afferent impulses by way of the vagus nerve to the brainstem, where they exert an inhibitory action to stop further inspiration (Hering-Breuer reflex). As previously stated, inhibitory impulses from the pneumotaxic center are relayed also to the inspiratory center, along with those from the stretch receptors, to terminate the inspiratory effort and impart rhythmicity to the respiratory cycle.

To increase pulmonary ventilation, other muscles, such as the trapezius, rhomboids, sternocleidomastoids, scalene, pectoralis major and minor, levatores costarum, and serratus posterior and anterior, are brought into play. The bronchial tree, which elongates and dilates to a small degree during normal inspiration, increases its elongation and dilation to accommodate the increase in lung ventilation.

Reflex control. Reflex control of respiration is regulated by neural mechanisms and is important in that the respiratory cycle may be affected by reflexes arising anywhere in the body. These occasional reflexes may be initiated by unexpected severe pain, causing sudden, forceful inspiration and in some cases laryngospasm. Intense emotion may quicken the respiratory rate, whereas sudden experience of extreme cold may produce apnea. These reflex experiences may be varied and will depend upon the degree of stimuli they create. The efferent pathways for these reflexes are the phrenic and intercostal nerves, since they are the eventual path for all such reflexes.

The following are the important reflexes that play a factor in controlling respirations:

Hering-Breuer reflex. The Hering-Breuer reflex is important in maintaining rhythmic inspiration and expiration. Afferent impulses, as a result of the action of the stretch receptors in the alveoli of the lungs, are transmitted by way of the vagus nerve to the central nervous system, causing inhibition of the inspiratory center and thus terminating the inspiratory effort.

Chemoreceptors. Chemoreceptors are cells composing the carotid and aortic bodies located at the bifurcation of the common carotid artery into the external and internal carotids and in the walls of the arch of the aorta. These chemoreceptors are the body's only effective mechanism for producing an effective increase in respiratory minute volume to overcome a lack of carbon dioxide stimulation. Reflexes from the carotid and aortic bodies are carried to the respiratory centers by way of afferent fibers of the ninth and tenth cranial nerves.

These afferent reflexes constitute the body's first reaction to decreased oxygen tension in the blood.

The chemoreceptors are usually stimulated when the arterial oxygen falls below 92% saturation. An increase in body temperature and in acidity and certain drugs also stimulate the chemoreceptors. The result of this stimulation is an increase in the depth of respiration rather than in the rate.

When respirations are maintained primarily by stimuli from the chemoreceptors, the sudden inspiration of 100% oxygen will result in temporary apnea since the inhalations of oxygen remove the stimuli of the chemoreceptors. This apnea will persist, however, only until a sufficient carbon dioxide level is built up in the circulation to trigger the respiratory center.

Pressoreceptors. The pressoreceptors are actually sinus formations located at the bifurcation of the internal and external common carotids and in the arch of the aorta. The stretching of the involved vessels (carotids and aorta) brought on by a rise in pressure so affects the sinuses of the pressoreceptors as to create impulses that are transmitted to the expiratory portion of the respiratory center, inhibiting respirations and decreasing the respiratory rate and depth. On the other hand, a sudden fall in arterial blood pressure may stimulate the respirations markedly.

Peripheral reflexes. Afferent fibers transmitting impulses from the periphery may affect the respiratory center markedly. As a rule, severe peripheral pain may cause an increase in respirations, whereas visceral pain may cause a decrease in respirations. As previously stated, sudden changes in temperature may create pronounced changes in the respiratory pattern.

Chemical control. Neural control is not the only factor responsible for the fundamental rhythm of the respiratory cycle; it is the carbon dioxide level that initiates the primary discharge from the respiratory center. Chemical control maintains a guiding influence over neural mechanisms of respiration and overcomes any voluntary effort to alter the respiratory pattern drastically.

The respiratory center is extremely sensitive to carbon dioxide tension in the arterial blood. A minute increase above normal stimulates the respiratory center, which results in an increased rate and depth of respiration. A decrease in carbon dioxide tension in the arterial blood may, if sufficient, produce apnea, which will persist until the arterial carbon dioxide tension again reaches a sufficient level to trigger the inspiratory effort. Pulmonary ventilation, altered as it is by variations in arterial carbon dioxide tension, is a prime factor in the maintenance of acid-base balance of the body. When the carbon dioxide level is increased, the increased pulmonary ventilation reduces the carbon dioxide content of the arterial blood, whereas a lowered carbon dioxide level will result in a decreased pulmonary ventilation, allowing the carbon dioxide tension to increase.

Oxygen tension has a minor effect upon the respiratory center. An increase in oxygen tension in the arterial blood has practically no effect upon ventilation. A decrease in oxygen tension will, if sufficient, eventually depress the respiratory center, since a lack of oxygen always depresses nervous tissue but never stimulates it. Any increase in pulmonary ventilation due to oxygen decrease is initiated through the mechanism of the carotid body, and then only if the respiratory center is sufficiently oxygenated to respond to the stimulation.

In severe respiratory depression caused by lack of oxygen or by anesthetic agents, neither carbon dioxide nor drugs (stimulants) will produce a sufficient response from the respiratory center to initiate an inspiratory effort. It is necessary that such patients be ventilated artificially so that adequate oxygenation can be maintained, thus enabling the respiratory center to respond eventually to carbon dioxide levels and reflex stimuli.

Voluntary control. Voluntary control of pulmonary ventilation is possible only within certain limits as controlled by chemical variations. It is possible to hyperventilate with oxygen and thus to increase the voluntary duration of apnea. Also, the ability to alter the respiratory pattern voluntarily enables a person to sing, whistle, shout, hum, or perform other maneuvers. Voluntary control is managed by impulses from the motor cortex to the respiratory center and will be affected only inso far as chemical control permits. The variations in voluntary control may be increased greatly by training and practice or decreased by disease.

Conduction portion of external respiratory system. The conducting portion of the external respiratory system consists of the nasal and oral passages, the nasopharynx, the oropharynx, the laryngopharynx, the larynx, the trachea, and the bronchial tree. This portion serves primarily as a connection between the alveoli of the lungs and the external atmosphere. The conducting portion itself has an average capacity of 150 ml. of air and plays no part in the actual diffusion of gases into the bloodstream. In other words, there is no interchange of carbon dioxide and oxygen between the conducting portion of the external respiratory system and the bloodstream. Since this conducting portion plays no part in the actual exchange, it is referred to as anatomical dead space. The gases within this space must be moved in and out with each inspiratory and expiratory effort to effect replacement of gases within the alveoli of the lungs adequate for efficient ventilation.

It is within the conducting portion that practically all respiratory obstructions occur. They are most likely to happen in the area of the larynx, where an obstruction may be caused by a spasm of the vocal cords or a partial impediment at the glottal opening. Foreign bodies in the pharynx or relaxation of pharyngeal muscles may also tend to interfere with the free passage of gases along the conducting portion of the external respiration. A narrowing of the bronchioles (bronchial spasm) may have the same effect.

Artificial airways, oropharyngeal, nasopharyngeal, orotracheal, or nasotracheal, are employed to overcome obstructions, either partial or complete, of the conducting system. Tracheotomy into the conducting system is performed also to offer a more satisfactory passage of gases. The maintenance of a patent conducting system is extremely important for successful management of anesthesia.

Ventilating portion of external respiratory system. The ventilating portion of the external respiratory system is concerned primarily with the interchange of gases between the alveoli of the lungs and the bloodstream. This interchange takes place through the alveolocapillary membrane. The rate of diffusion of the involved gases through this membrane is regulated by the gradient ratio of partial pressures of the gases involved and the physical condition of the alveolocapillary membrane.

The ventilating portion is composed of many lung alveoli, each of which is supplied by a single bronchiole. It is the air within the terminal alveoli that regulates the tension of the gases in the arterial blood, since this is the only area in which the gaseous exchange between the lung and bloodstream can be carried out. The average volume of air within the alveoli of the lungs is approximately 3,000 ml.

As the thoracic cage expands, producing an increase in the intrathoracic negative pressure, the lungs in turn increase in capacity. This increase produces an intrapulmonic pressure that is negative as compared to the atmospheric pressure. The first air to enter the increased alveolar spaces is the dead space air from the conducting portion of the external respiratory system. This is followed by additional gases from the atmosphere. During normal breathing, the alteration of gases within the alveoli just compensates for the gaseous exchange taking place between the alveolar air and the pulmonary bloodstream. This alteration of gases will depend upon the amplitude of breathing. During forced ventilation more gases will be taken into the alveolar sacs, whereas if respiration were depressed markedly, the exchange of gases would be decreased until, if the total volume of inspired air were reduced to the volume of the anatomical dead space, very little if any alveolar ventilation would take place.

The gaseous interchange between the alveolar air sacs depends entirely on the physical processes of diffusion created by the difference in the partial pressures of the carbon dioxide and oxygen in the blood and in the alveolar air. The pulmonary tissues play no active part in this exchange and thus ordinarily cannot of themselves increase the diffusion. However, disease of the membrane may reduce the speed and capacity of the diffusion.

The speed of the gaseous exchange between the alveoli of the lungs and the bloodstream will depend on (1) the gradient ratio of pressure difference, (2) the solubility of the gases in blood, or (3) the physical properties of the membrane.

The rate of diffusion may be decreased by (1) pulmonary edema, (2) disease processes within the lungs, or (3) reduced partial pressures of the gases involved.

The total area of the functioning surface of the lungs is approximately 60 to 70 sq. m., whereas the total surface area of the pulmonary capillaries is approximately 40 sq. m. There is approximately 60 ml. of blood in the pulmonary capillaries at any given time. This situation is that of an extremely fine stream of blood, equivalent to the red corpuscles in single file, that comes in contact with the alveolar air.

The oxygen tension in the alveolar air is approximately 100 mm. Hg, whereas in venous blood it is approximately 40 mm. Hg, making a pressure difference of approximately 60 mm. Hg. The carbon dioxide tension in the alveoli of the lungs is approximately 40 mm. Hg, whereas in the venous blood it is approximately 46 mm. Hg.

The pressure difference between the alveolar oxygen and oxygen in the venous blood is approximately 60 mm. Hg, as compared to approximately 6 mm. Hg between the alveolar carbon dioxide and the venous blood. Although the pressure gradient of carbon dioxide (6 mm.) is only one tenth that of oxygen (60 mm.), carbon dioxide is about thirty times as soluble as oxygen, and therefore carbon dioxide, despite its low pressure gradient, diffuses from the bloodstream into the alveolar air more rapidly than the oxygen diffuses from the alveolar air into the bloodstream.

Transportation portion of internal respiratory system. Once the external respiration has completed its function of getting the gases from the external atmosphere into the bloodstream and from the bloodstream into the external atmosphere, the next phase of respiration comes into play, that is, transportation of oxygen to the tissue cells and return of the carbon dioxide.

Oxygen transport. Oxygen is carried in the bloodstream in chemical combination with the red cells as oxyhemoglobin and in simple physical solution in the plasma. The total amount of oxygen in arterial blood is about 20 ml. per 100 ml. of blood. Of this amount, 19+ ml. are carried as oxyhemoglobin in chemical combination with the red cells, and 0.3 ml. is carried in physical solution in the plasma.

Hemoglobin readily combines with oxygen to form a loose chemical combination in the ratio of 1 mol of oxygen to 1 mol of hemoglobin.

$$O_2 + Hb \underset{\leftarrow}{\overset{\rightarrow}{\rightarrow}} HbO_2$$

The arterial oxygen content varies from person to person, depending upon the hemoglobin content. The average hemoglobin content is 15 grams per 100 ml., and 1 gram of hemoglobin when fully saturated will combine with 1.34 ml. of oxygen.

In the venous blood that passes through the capillaries of the lungs, the carbon dioxide tension is higher and the oxygen tension is lower than that of alveolar air. This enables the carbon dioxide to diffuse into the alveoli of the lungs and the oxygen to diffuse into the bloodstream, where it is taken up by the red cells and the plasma in the aforementioned ratio. As the carbon dioxide diffuses out of the bloodstream, the acidity is lowered, thus creating a greater affinity of the hemoglobin in the red cells for oxygen. The oxygen is then transported to the tissues in arterial blood at an oxygen tension of 100 mm. Hg.

Since the arterial blood reaches the capillaries of the tissues with an oxygen tension of 100 mm. Hg and the oxygen tension in the tissues is usually about 35 mm. Hg, the oxygen, due to the gradient ratio of pressures, readily passes from the arterial blood into the tissues until the oxygen tension falls to about 40 mm. Hg. The blood enters the venous circulation with an oxygen content of about 14 ml. per 100 ml. It is evident, therefore, that if the arterial blood contains 19 ml. of oxygen per 100 ml. of blood and the venous blood contains 14 ml. per 100 ml. of blood, the difference of 5 ml. is given up to the tissues.

Carbon dioxide transport. The total amount of carbon dioxide in 100 ml. of venous blood is approximately 55 to 60 ml. It is carried in four ways:

1. As sodium bicarbonate ($NaHCO_3$) in the plasma (approximately 45 to 50 ml. per 100 ml. of venous blood)

2. Combined with the hemoglobin to form carbaminohemoglobin compounds (approximately 10 ml. per 100 ml. of venous blood)
3. In physical solution in the plasma carbonic acid (approximately 2.5 ml. per 100 ml. of venous blood)
4. As potassium bicarbonate ($KHCO_3$) in the red cells (approximately 2 ml. per 100 ml. of venous blood).

The volume of carbon dioxide in venous blood varies according to the activity of a person, with the total content rising to 65 ml. during strenuous exercise. For every mol of oxygen utilized by the tissues, 0.82 mol of carbon dioxide is produced. This carbon dioxide then diffuses into the bloodstream approximately thirty times faster than oxygen as soluble carbon dioxide. The carbon dioxide dissolves in water to form carbonic acid. While this reaction is usually a slow one, the presence of carbonic anhydrase, an enzyme, acts as a catalyst and markedly increases the speed of the reaction. The plasma contains approximately 80 to 85% of the carbon dioxide carried in the bloodstream, whereas approximately 15 to 20% is carried in the red cells. However, the reaction of carbon dioxide plus water to form carbonic acid takes place much more slowly in the plasma than in the red cells, owing to the presence of carbonic anhydrase in the red cells. When carbon dioxide enters the blood from the tissues, there is at first a small increase of carbonic acid in the plasma and a correspondingly larger increase of carbonic acid in the red cells. This is due to the presence of the carbonic anhydrase in the red cell.

The carbonic acid reacts with hemoglobin to form bicarbonate. This reaction takes place primarily in the red cells rather than in the plasma. As the carbonate concentration (HCO_3) of the cell is increased, it diffuses into the plasma, while at the same time an equal amount of chloride diffuses from the plasma into the red cells. This maneuver is called the chloride shift and is significant in that without this exchange practically the entire uptake of carbon dioxide in the form of bicarbonate would be in the red cells, and the transportation of carbon dioxide in the bloodstream would be much reduced. However, because of this ionic shift, the carbon dioxide that has been converted into bicarbonate primarily in the red cells can be transferred readily to the plasma to form sodium bicarbonate and greatly increase the capacity of the blood to carry carbon dioxide. This bicarbonate in the plasma serves three functions: (1) It is the prime means of carrying carbon dioxide in the blood. (2) It maintains the alkalinity of the plasma. (3) It forms the alkali reserve that acts as a buffer to neutralize acid substances entering the bloodstream.

While the total content of carbon dioxide in venous blood is approximately 60 ml. per 100 ml. of blood at a tension of 46 mm. Hg, the carbon dioxide content in arterial blood is 45 to 55 ml. per 100 ml. of blood at a tension of approximately 40 mm. Hg. This indicates that 5 to 15 ml. of carbon dioxide per 100 ml. of blood are taken up from the tissues, depending upon the activity of the person. It has been shown that 0.8 mol of carbon dioxide can be taken up from the tissues and transformed into potassium carbonate for every molecule of oxygen used.

Intracellular respiration. The final stage of respiration is the exchange of carbon dioxide and oxygen between the capillaries and the tissue cells. This is the ultimate function of the respiration, that is, to get oxygen to the cells and to remove the carbon dioxide.

When the arterial blood reaches the meta-arterioles and capillaries where the exchange takes place, it will be carrying approximately 1.34 ml. of oxygen per gram of hemoglobin. Each 100 ml. of arterial blood will be carrying approximately 0.3 ml. of oxygen in solution in the plasma and about 19+ ml. in combination with the hemoglobin as oxyhemoglobin. The oxygen tension in the arterial blood will be about 100 mm. Hg, which is considerably greater than that in the tissues, approximately 35 mm. Hg. This readily allows the oxygen to diffuse from the capillaries into the tissues because of the gradient ratio of oxygen tension favorable to this maneuver.

The oxygen tension in any particular tissue at a given time is dependent upon (1) the activity of the tissue and its subsequent utilization of oxygen, (2) the volume and tension in the arterial blood, and (3) the rate of blood flow through the tissues.

The amount of oxygen extracted from the arterial blood by any given tissue will be directly dependent upon these factors as well. Very active tissues may extract practically all of the oxygen brought to them in the arterial blood. It is quite possible that in extremely active tissue the oxygen tension may approximate zero, which results in a steep oxygen pressure gradient between the arterial blood and the tissues and permits a rapid diffusion of oxygen from the blood into the tissues. The oxygen tension may then fall to as low as 30 mm. Hg, converting arterial blood into venous blood.

During the tissues' period of activity and utilization of oxygen, carbon dioxide is produced, creating a carbon dioxide tension of 46 mm. Hg in the tissues as compared to 40 mm. Hg tension in the blood. Even though this difference may seem small as compared to oxygen, the speed of diffusion of carbon dioxide, which is thirty times that of oxygen, permits the rapid diffusion of the carbon dioxide from the tissues into the bloodstream. As the carbon dioxide diffuses into the bloodstream and consequently increases the carbon dioxide tension in the blood, the rate of dissociation of the oxyhemoglobin is increased, which causes more oxygen to be released into the plasma and into the tissues. Therefore, it is evident that the amount of oxygen given up by the arterial blood to any particular tissue will depend not only on the gradient ratio of oxygen tensions but also on the amount of carbon dioxide diffusing into the bloodstream, which aids further in the dissociation of oxyhemoglobin and makes more oxygen available to the plasma for diffusion into the tissues.

As previously stated, the carbon dioxide diffuses into the plasma and then into the red cells, where, by the action of the enzyme carbonic anhydrase, it is converted into bicarbonate, some of which diffuses back into the plasma to react with the sodium chloride.

$CO_2 + H_2O \rightarrow H\,HCO_3$ (with enzyme carbonic anhydrase in red cells)
$HCO_3 + NaCl \rightarrow NaHCO_3 + CL$ (plasma)
$H + Hb \rightarrow HHb$ (red cells)

As the bicarbonate, as shown in the formulas, is formed within the red cells, it diffuses out of the cells into the plasma, leaving the cells positively charged. As the bicarbonate reacts with the sodium chloride in the plasma, chloride is released and diffuses into the red cells to maintain the electrical neutrality.

This reaction, or chloride shift, occurs because the membrane of the red cells is permeable only to the anions, bicarbonate and chloride. This shift enables the blood to increase markedly the carbon dioxide–carrying properties of the plasma, and thus it is evident that, as the blood gives up oxygen, its efficiency as a carrier of carbon dioxide is increased.

The arterial blood (oxygen 100 mm. Hg, carbon dioxide 40 mm. Hg), having given up oxygen and taken on carbon dioxide from the tissues (oxygen 35 mm. Hg, carbon dioxide 46 mm. Hg), is transformed into venous blood (oxygen tension 40 mm. Hg, carbon dioxide tension 46 mm. Hg). The venous blood is returned to the right atrium and then to the right ventricle, from where it is propelled into the pulmonary artery and into the lungs to be reconverted into arterial blood by the ventilating portion of the external respiratory system.

PHYSIOLOGY OF RESPIRATION WITH SPECIAL REFERENCE TO ANESTHESIA

The previous discussion on the physiology of respiration are singularly important to any person administering general anesthesia, since variations of the respiratory pattern occur during anesthesia. These deviations account for the respiratory signs of anesthesia. It is essential also that the variations in the respiratory pattern be observed closely so that the patient may be assured adequate ventilation and oxygenation.

The respiratory signs of anesthesia are brought about primarily by the depressing effect of the anesthetic agents upon the respiratory center, which makes it less sensitive to stimulation (from carbon dioxide in the blood and reflex stimuli). This reduces the force and number of impulses transmitted to the diaphragm and intercostal muscles and results in a depression of external respiration, with reduced pulmonary ventilation.

Anesthetic agents in general alter both the threshold and sensitivity of the respiratory center to carbon dioxide in the blood. With reduced sensitivity and a corresponding reduction in pulmonary ventilation, an accumulation of carbon dioxide may occur before oxygen deficiency is in evidence. A rise in arterial carbon dioxide tension may occur with the administration of Pentothal, cyclopropane, or Avertin or when large doses of morphine and Demerol are used. The muscle relaxants may cause respiratory acidosis if the ventilation is not augmented. Seemingly effortless respirations under anesthesia may be misleading and allow carbon dioxide to build up to depressing levels. If and when the respiratory center is depressed, as it may be under anesthesia, the excess carbon dioxide will not produce the expected increased respiratory ventilation.

In some instances a decrease in ventilation may occur secondary to reduced sensitivity of the respiratory center. In these patients the respiratory center, because of hypoxia or toxicity to drugs, may not respond to the stimulation of the carbon dioxide in the blood or to nervous stimulation from the chemoreceptors.

Some factors that may create hypoxia sufficient to affect the sensitivity of the respiratory center are cardiac insufficiency, anemia, hypotension, arteriosclerosis, and pulmonary insufficiency.

The toxicity of disease may reduce the sensitivity of the respiratory center; certain depressant drugs (anesthetic agents) also may have a similar effect, rendering normal carbon dioxide levels or other stimuli to the respiratory center ineffectual.

Certain factors may have a definite effect upon the ventilating portion of the external respiratory system. These factors may come about either by mechanical interference with ventilation or by interference with the nervous control of respiration pharmacologically.

Mechanical factors

Position and its effect on vital capacity
  Sitting, 100% of normal

Supine, 91% of normal
Prone, 90% of normal
Lateral, 88 to 90% of normal
Kidney, 85% of normal
Trendelenburg, 85% of normal
Lithotomy, 82% of normal
Obstructed airway
Increased dead space
Abdominal distention
External abdominal pressure
External pressure on chest by assistant or straps

While oxygen has no direct stimulating affect upon the respiratory center, a deficiency of oxygen (hypoxia) may so depress the respiratory center as to render it insensitive to normal stimulating mechanisms. Therefore, when anesthesia is induced, it is essential to maintain adequate oxygenation so that the respiratory center may not be affected adversely and be unable to respond to normal stimuli.

Some combinations of anesthetic agents are severe respiratory depressants. When these combinations are used, the ventilation must be augmented adequately, or, if apnea has occurred, external respiration must be controlled to assure an adequate oxygen uptake and an efficient elimination of carbon dioxide.

In the normal conscious patient the average respiratory rate is 12 to 18 per minute. The average tidal air is 500 ml. The normal respiratory movement consists of an active inspiratory phase quickly followed by a passive expiratory phase. A slight pause follows the expiratory phase before another active inspiration. This pattern is typical during anesthesia unless altered by mechanical, pharmacological, or biochemical stimuli. When these various stimuli affect the normal respiratory pattern, variations in pulmonary ventilation result. These variations may affect the tidal volume, the rate, the rhythm, or the character of respiration.

Any interference with pulmonary ventilation eventually will have a definite effect on the transportation or diffusion portion of the internal respiration system.

RÉSUMÉ OF IMPORTANT DATA RELATIVE TO RESPIRATION

Purpose of respiration

1. To supply oxygen to the body cells
2. To eliminate carbon dioxide adequately

3. As an aid in regulating hydrogen ion concentration in the blood
4. As an aid in maintaining normal body temperature

Control of respiration

1. Neural
   a. Reflex
      (1) Hering-Breuer
      (2) Chemoreceptors
      (3) Pressoreceptors
      (4) Peripheral
2. Chemical
3. Voluntary

Rate of respiration

1. Infant, 30 per minute
2. Child, 20 to 24 per minute
3. Adult, 12 to 18 per minute

Tidal air

1. Infant, 75 to 125 ml.
2. Child, 200 to 250 ml.
3. Adult, 450 to 500 ml.

Percentage of gases in inspired, alveolar, and expired air

	Inspired	*Alveolar*	*Expired*
Oxygen	20.96	14.2	16.3
Carbon dioxide	0.04	5.5	4.0
Nitrogen	79.00	80.3	79.7

Partial pressure of gases and vapors in inspired, alveolar, and expired air at 760 mm. Hg

	Inspired	*Alveolar*	*Expired*
Oxygen	158.2	101.0	116.2
Carbon dioxide	0.3	40.0	28.5
Nitrogen	596.5	572.0	568.3
Water vapor	5.0	47.0	47.0

Volumes percent and pressures of oxygen in arterial and venous blood

Oxygen	*Vol. %*	*Pressure*
Arterial blood	19.0	100 mm. Hg
Venous blood	12.5	40 mm. Hg

Volumes percent and pressures of carbon dioxide in arterial and venous blood

Carbon dioxide	*Vol. %*	*Pressure*
Arterial blood	50.00	40 mm. Hg
Venous blood	56.00	46 mm. Hg

Comparative diffusion rates of carbon dioxide and oxygen

Carbon dioxide diffuses thirty times more readily than does oxygen and therefore diffuses more rapidly at lower pressures.

Tensions of oxygen and carbon dioxide in tissue fluid

Carbon dioxide	46 mm. Hg
Oxygen	25-35 mm. Hg

Carriage of oxygen in the bloodstream

Oxygen is carried in the blood in chemical combination with the red cells as oxyhemoglobin (19 ml. per 100 ml. of blood) and in simple physical solution in the plasma (0.3 ml. per 100 ml.). One gram of hemoglobin can carry 1.34 ml. of oxygen.

Carriage of carbon dioxide in the bloodstream

Carbon dioxide is carried in the bloodstream in four ways:

1. As sodium bicarbonate in the plasma (approximately 45 ml. per 100 ml. of venous blood)
2. Combined with hemoglobin to form carbaminohemoglobin compounds (approximately 10 ml. per 100 ml. of venous blood)
3. As bicarbonate in physical solution in the plasma (approximately 2.5 ml. per 100 ml. of venous blood)
4. As potassium bicarbonate in the red cells (approximately 2 ml. per 100 ml. of venous blood)

Effects of increased carbon dioxide tension on respiration

An increase in carbon dioxide tension results in augmentation of both rate and depth of respiration.

1. 5% carbon dioxide increases the ventilatory volume fourfold.
2. 10% carbon dioxide increases the ventilatory volume tenfold.
3. Carbon dioxide concentration in excess of 10% is intolerable to the patient.
4. 30% will produce anesthesia.
5. 40% carbon dioxide will depress the respiratory center markedly.

Effect of increased oxygen tension on respiration

1. An increase of oxygen tension causes a reduction in pulmonary ventilation in proportion to the decrease of carbon dioxide tension in the bloodstream.
2. At atmospheric pressures increased oxygen tension produces no change in pulmonary ventilation.

Effect of reduced oxygen tension on respiration

Reduced oxygen tension produces no change in pulmonary ventilation until the arterial oxygen falls below 92% saturation. Then respiratory centers are stimulated by afferent fibers from chemoreceptors. This is the only respiratory stimulation created by decreased oxygen tension in the blood.

Buffers in the blood, arranged in pairs

1. Sodium bicarbonate and carbonic acid
2. Sodium basic phosphate and sodium acid phosphate

Table 1-2. Standardized terms versus some previous terms*

Standardized term	*Definition*	*Previous term*
Inspiratory reserve volume (3.3 liters)	Maximal volume that can be inspired from end-tidal inspiration	Complemental air Complementary air Complemental air minus tidal air Inspiratory capacity minus tidal volume
Tidal volume (0.5 liters)	Volume of gas inspired or expired during each respiratory cycle	Tidal air
Expiratory reserve volume (2.2 liters)	Maximal volume that can be expired from resting expiratory level	Supplemental air Reserve air
Residual volume (1.2 liters)	Volume of gas in lungs at end of maximal expiration	Residual air Residual capacity
Inspiratory capacity (3.8 liters)	Maximal volume that can be inspired from resting expiratory level	Complemental air Complementary air
Functional residual capacity (2.2 liters)	Volume of gas in lungs at resting expiratory level	Functional residual air Equilibrium capacity Midcapacity Normal capacity
Vital capacity (5 liters)	Maximal volume that can be expired after maximal inspiration	Vital capacity
Total lung capacity (6 liters)	Volume of gas in lungs at end of maximal inspiration	Total lung volume

*From Comroe, J. H., Jr.: The lung, Chicago, 1956, The Year Book Medical Publishers, Inc.

3. Alkali protein and acid protein
4. Oxyhemoglobin (alkali) and reduced hemoglobin (acid)

One can add three hundred times more acid to blood than to water before the pH changes in equal amounts, because of the buffering action of the blood.

Normal pH of blood

The normal pH of blood is 7.2 to 7.4.

Respiratory acidosis

Respiratory acidosis is a compensatory increase in plasma bicarbonate initiated by any condition causing hypoventilation (emphysema, paralysis of respiration, deep anesthesia, etc.).

Respiratory alkalosis

Respiratory alkalosis is a compensatory decrease in plasma bicarbonate initiated by any condition causing hyperventilation (extreme elevations of temperature, lesions of the central nervous system, cardiac anoxia, controlled respirations, etc.). Both changes are attempts to restore the carbonic acid-sodium bicarbonate ratio and prevent a change in blood pH.

Standardized terms vs. some previous terms (Table 1-2)

Chapter 2

Anatomy and physiology of circulation

Albert J. Fisher, M.D.

A knowledge of the anatomy and physiology of circulation is essential for any dentist who undertakes the study of anesthesia. The circulation composes the transportation system for respiration and is instrumental in completing the ventilating phase of external respiration and the diffusion phase of internal respiration.

A knowledge of the physiology of circulation is necessary in order to evaluate a patient prior to the administration of a general anesthetic and also to evaluate the patient constantly during anesthesia.

The anatomy and physiology of circulation will be discussed insofar as they concern the dentist administering general anesthesia. Undoubtedly, the medical anesthesiologist would pursue the subject much more thoroughly. It is thus reasonable to believe that the advice of a medical consultant, either anesthesiologist or internist, would be sought concerning patients who exhibit cardiovascular disease of any marked degree.

ANATOMY OF CIRCULATION

Circulation is defined as movement in a regular or circular course. This takes place in the body by definite connecting structures.

The connecting structures that form the circulatory system are the heart, arteries, arterioles, capillaries, venules, and veins.

The heart

The heart is the central organ of the circulatory system. It is situated in the thorax, with about two thirds of it to the left and one third to the right of the midline. It is conoidal in shape, and its broad upper end is directed backward and to the right. The apex is directed downward, forward, and to the left. The heart is positioned obliquely in the chest, with the base almost in front of the apex. The average weight of the heart is 250 grams in the female and 300 grams in the male.

The heart is divided into four chambers by partitions, called septa. These chambers are the right and left atria (auricles) and the right and left ventricles. The atria are separated by the interauricular septum and the ventricles by the interventricular septum. The right and left atria are separated from the right and left ventricles by their respective atrioventricular septa. Under normal conditions, the right and left sides of the heart do not communicate directly with one another, so that, with the exception of the conductive system and blood supply, the heart could actually exist as two separate units.

The division of the four cavities is marked on the external surface of the heart by grooves named for their contiguous cavities—the atrioventricular groove transversely and the interventricular groove longitudinally.

The heart itself is enclosed in a two-layered membranous sac called the pericardium. The visceral layer (epicardium) is thin and closely adherent to the heart. The parietal layer is fibrous; it is attached to the diaphragm below and covers the vessels emerging from the heart above. Between these two layers is the pericardial cavity, which normally contains a small amount of fluid to reduce friction between the layers during movements of the heart.

The pericardium is usually considered to be the outermost layer of the heart. The middle layer is the myocardium.

The myocardium is composed of bands of interlocked muscle fibers. Cardiac muscle is a third type of muscle fiber and is highly specialized. Whereas in other parts of the body we find striated voluntary and smooth involuntary muscle fibers, cardiac muscle is striated and involuntary. The striations of cardiac muscle are longitudinal as well as transverse, and the sarcolemmous sheaths of the cardiac fibers are not well defined, so that the fibers form a continuous multinucleated sheet over which an impulse may spread in any direction without interruption. The muscle of the atrium is thinner than that of the ventricle, and the wall of the left ventricle is about three times as thick as that of the right ventricle.

The innermost layer of the heart is the endocardium. This is a smooth serous membrane that is continuous with the lining of the blood vessels. The endocardium assists in the formation of the valves. The valves are triangular leaves of delicate membrane formed by the doubling of the endocardium and attached by their bases to a fibrous ring surrounding the atrial and ventricular orifices. Near the base of these valves, the two layers of epithelium are separated by a small amount of connective tissue. The valves of the heart are so placed as to separate the ventricular and atrial cavities from one another and also to separate the chambers from the great vessels leading from the heart. The valves are five in number.

The *tricuspid valve* is situated at the right atrioventricular opening. It is composed of three irregularly shaped flaps, or cusps, whence the name tricuspid. The pointed ends of the flaps are attached by cords (chordae tendinae) to little muscular pillars (papillary muscles) that arise from the wall of the ventricle. This valve permits blood flow from the right atrium to the right ventricle and in turn prevents regurgitation of blood back into the right atrium. The *bicuspid mitral valve* is composed of two flaps and serves the same purpose as the tricuspid valve. However, its location is at the opening between the left atrium and left ventricle. It too is provided with chordae tendinae and papillary muscles. The *pulmonic semilunar valves* permit flow from the right ventricle into the pulmonary artery. The *aortic semilunar valves* permit blood flow from the left ventricle into the aorta. The *inferior vena cava valve* prevents the return flow of blood into the inferior vena cava.

These semilunar valves—both pulmonic and aortic—consist of three half-moon-shaped pockets, each pocket being attached by its convex border to the inside of the artery, where it joins the ventricle while its other border projects into the interior of the vessel. Small nodular bodies (corpora arantii) are attached to the center of the free edge of each pocket.

These valves offer no resistance to the passage of blood from the heart into the arteries. Once this is accomplished, backflow of blood fills the cusps, closing them and forming a barrier between the heart chamber and arteries. The corpora arantii help make this closure complete.

Each chamber of the heart has several openings into it, some of which have been mentioned already.

Following is a brief summary of the openings into the various chambers of the heart.

Openings into right atrium

1. Superior vena cava, carrying venous blood from the head and upper extremities

2. Inferior vena cava, carrying venous blood from the trunk and lower extremities
3. Coronary sinus, carrying blood from the heart itself
4. Veins of Thebesius, carrying venous blood from the heart muscle
5. Tricuspid valve, opening between the right atrium and right ventricle

Openings in right ventricle

1. Tricuspid valve, opening between the right atrium and right ventricle
2. Semilunar valve, between the right ventricle and pulmonary artery
3. Veins of Thebesius, carrying venous blood from the heart muscle

Openings in left atrium

1. Four openings, carrying oxygenated blood from the lungs
2. Bicuspid valve (mitral), between the left atrium and left ventricle

Openings in left ventricle

1. Bicuspid valve, between the left atrium and left ventricle
2. Veins of Thebesius, carrying venous blood from the heart muscle
3. Aortic semilunar valve, between the left ventricle and aorta.

Blood supply. The heart is supplied with blood by the right and left coronary arteries, which originate from the aortic sinuses (sinuses of Valsalva). These sinuses are located just beyond the attachment of the aortic semilunar valves. They are, therefore, the first branches of the aorta. After supplying the heart itself, the blood is drained into the right auricle by the coronary sinus. A number of smaller veins and veins of Thebesius also return blood to the right atrium, as well as to the left and right ventricles. About 60% of the blood is returned from the coronary system by the coronary sinus. Collateral circulation is furnished to the heart also by anastomosis between the atrial branches of the coronaries and vessels in the pericardium (from the internal mammary arteries) and channels around openings of the great vessels from the bronchial artery.

Innervation. The heart is supplied by both sympathetic and parasympathetic autonomic nerve fibers.

Parasympathetic. The cardioinhibitory center lies within the dorsal nucleus of the vagus nerve, which is located in the floor of the fourth ventricle. The cardiac fibers leave the main trunks of the vagus nerve in the neck and enter the cardiac plexuses. Most of the postganglionic fibers of the right vagus nerve terminate in the vicinity of the sinoatrial (S-A) node; most of the fibers from the left vagus nerve terminate in the atrioventricular (A-V) node. There is some overlapping of this innervation, however.

Sympathetic. The sympathetic, or augmentor, nerves to the heart arise from the lateral horn cells of the spinal cord in the upper five thoracic segments and from the superior, middle, and inferior cervical ganglia. Fibers from the cervical ganglia pass through the corresponding cardiac nerves, whereas those from the thoracic ganglia pass through thoracic nerves to the heart via the cardiac plexuses. The control of this sympathetic activity is probably from some point of higher nervous center. The exact location of this center is unknown, but it is commonly accepted that there is a medullary center. Here again, the fibers from the right side are distributed primarily to the S-A node and from the left side to the A-V node and the bundle of His.

Nervous conduction in the heart itself. The heart itself contains several structures that have to do with the conduction of nervous impulses. These are the sinoatrial node, the atrioventricular node, the bundle of His, and the Purkinje system.

Sinoatrial node. The S-A node lies embedded in the muscle of the right atrium. It is located just in front of the opening of the superior vena cava and extends ¾ inch downward; it has a special blood supply. Its minute structure is of a neuromuscular nature, consisting of striated spindle-shaped muscle fibers arranged in a plexiform manner, embedded in connective tissue, and intermingled with a small number of ganglion cells and nerve fibers.

Atrioventricular node. The A-V node lies in the right atrium at the lower part of the interatrial septum; it is anterior to the opening of the coronary sinus and above the septal leaf of the right A-V valve. Microscopically it resembles the S-A node.

The S-A node and the A-V node are not connected by any special tissue, being separated by atrial tissue.

A-V bundle, bundle branches, and Purkinje system. A bundle of muscular tissue, described by His, runs a short course from its origin at the A-V node, passing over the septal leaf of the tricuspid valve to the upper part of the interventricular septum. At this point the bundle divides into a right and left branch, each going to its separate ventricle. These branches pass beneath the endothelium and give branches to the papillary muscles. The strands continue under the endothelial lining and form delicate subendothelial interlacement.

The cells comprising the ventricular branches and terminal arborizations of the system take on special features, differing from those of the bundle stem and A-V node. These were described by Purkinje and are known by his name. Further investigation by Abramson and associates showed that the Purkinje system not only consists of subendothelial fibers but also penetrates deeply into the ventricular muscle.

The blood vessels

The heart is the central and most important organ of the circulatory system. However, there are many other parts of this system, which, although less spectacular in nature, carry no little degree of importance. Included are the blood vessels, which may be listed in the following manner: arteries, arterioles, capillaries, venules, and veins.

With the exception of the capillaries, the walls of all of the blood vessels are three layered. The histological makeup of these walls varies with the type and location of the vessel. The walls comprise three laryers: the tunica adventita, or outer layer, composed of varying amounts of connective tissue; the tunica media, or middle layer, made up of smooth muscle and elastic fibers; and the tunica intima, or inner layer, consisting of an inner lining of endothelial cells.

Arteries. The arteries are made to withstand great amounts of pressure. The largest of these are the aorta and pulmonary arteries. The large arteries, such as those just mentioned, have thick walls containing an abundance of elastic tissue and are relatively poor in muscle fibers. This allows for a greater amount of distensibility in order to accommodate the great amount of pressure present with the systolic thrust of the heart.

The medium-sized arteries are relatively rich in muscle fibers and have a smaller amount of elastic tissue, and the small arteries are still richer in smooth muscle fibers.

The walls of the larger arteries are supplied by minute vessels (vasa vasorum) that penetrate the outer and middle coats. They are also furnished with nerves.

In tracing the vessels peripherally from the heart, we find that the arteries divide into smaller and smaller vessels until a minute vessel, the arteriole, is formed. These vessels vary in size, but the average outside diameter is about 0.2 mm. The walls of the arterioles are relatively thick, being composed of almost pure muscle tissue lined by an endothelial lining, and are surrounded by a scanty adventitia of connective tissue. They are also supplied with excitor and inhibitor nerves. These arterioles form a sphincter system for the circulation. They gradually lose their connective tissue and muscle coat and continue on as endothelial tubes, the capillaries. It is at this point that the various exchanges between blood and body tissues take place. These capillaries are from 8 to 12 mμ in diameter and about 1 mm. in length. The capillaries form a plexus with one another and connect the arterial and venous systems. The venous ends of these capillaries join to form the smallest veins or venules. These in turn coalesce to form larger veins. This process continues, repeatedly forming veins of larger caliber until the formation of the two main venous trunks, the superior and inferior venae cavae, which in turn pour the return from the entire venous system into the right atrium.

The walls of the veins are much thinner than those of the arteries, the tunica media being only a fraction of the thickness of the corresponding artery. Here the tunica media is composed of a relatively small amount of muscle tissue, a large amount of connective tissue, and a scant amount of elastic tissue. The tunica adventitia may be several times the thickness of the tunica media. Valves, which are present in some of the small veins, are formed by foldings of the tunica intima.

Innervation; vasomotor centers. The blood vessels have both sympathetic and parasympathetic innervations as follows: (1) a constrictor center in the floor of the fourth ventricle at the apex of the ala cinerea, (2) constriction centers at cord level in the lateral cell column with the thoracolumbar outflow, (3) a dilator center lateral to the obex in the medulla, and (4) the hypothalamus and cortex, which exert autonomic and psychic control.

Fibers. The majority of the vasoconstrictor fibers arise in the lateral horn cells of the cord from Th-4 to L-1. The vasoconstrictors to the head and neck are from the plexus investing the blood vessels and from the cervical and cranial nerves.

The vasoconstrictors to the extremities are primarily through mixed spinal nerves, and those to the abdomen and pelvis are through the greater, lesser, and least splanchnic nerves.

The vasoconstrictor fibers to the coronary arteries are from the vagus nerve.

Although the distribution of the vasodilator fibers is about the same as that of the vasoconstrictors, the origin of these fibers is much more diffuse. These impulses emerge from the central nervous system by the following routes: (1) the thoracolumbar outflow, (2) the cranial outflow of the parasympathetic division via the chorda tympani, glossopharyngeal, and vagus nerves, (3) sacral outflow or pelvic nerves, and (4) posterior spinal nerve roots.

Generally speaking, the parasympathetic innervation is usually vasodilator in nature, whereas the sympathetic innervation is usually constrictor.

Divisions of circulation. The circulation is usually divided into two parts: the greater, or systemic, and the lesser, or pulmonary.

Systemic circulation. The systemic circulation comprises all of the circulation from the point of origin at the left ventricle until it reaches the right atrium via the superior and inferior venae cavae. With the contracting force of the left ventricle supplying the motivating force, the blood is forced into the aorta, where it progresses over its arch to send blood to the head and upper extremities and then downward through the descending aorta to supply the organs of the abdomen and lower extremities by way of the arterioles and capillaries. The blood is then collected in the venous system and returned to the right atrium by way of the inferior vena cava (and the superior vena cava from the head and upper extremities). The blood then passes into the right ventricle and lesser circulation.

Among the many important circulations composing the systemic circulation are a few that deserve brief mention here: the coronary, cerebral, renal, and portal.

Coronary circulation. The heart muscle is supplied by the right and left coronary arteries, which arise from the aorta just distal to the aortic semilunar valves and pass outward to encircle the base of the heart like a crown. The left coronary artery has two branches: the circumflex branch and the anterior descending branch. The right coronary artery runs in the A-V groove toward the right and ends in several descending branches on the posterior surface of the right ventricle. Intramural branches leave the main coronary vessels to pass directly inward toward the heart chambers and break up into extensive capillary plexuses. The capillaries coalesce to form cardiac veins, which in general correspond to the arteries. These veins communicate with the right atrium through a terminal division called the coronary sinus. Blood is returned to the atria and right ventricle by way of small venous channels (veins of Thebesius) also. As previously mentioned, collateral circulation is provided to the heart by anastomosis between atrial twigs of the coronaries and vessels in the pericardium from the internal mammary arteries and channels around openings of the great vessels from the bronchial artery.

Ventricular muscle possesses a rich capillary bed. For each muscle fiber there is a capillary, in contrast to one capillary for each two skeletal muscle fibers.

About 5% of the total cardiac output is channeled through the coronary arteries.

Cerebral circulation. The innominate artery is a large but short artery that arises as the first branch from the aortic arch. It passes upward and to the right for a short distance and then divides into the right subclavian and right common carotid arteries. The left common carotid artery arises directly from the aorta.

The common carotid arteries pass upward in the neck and divide into the internal and external carotid arteries. At this point of bifurcation of the common carotid is a small sinus, or dilated portion, called the carotid sinus.

The internal carotid artery enters the cranial cavity, where it sends branches to the orbital structures of the eye and to the brain.

The external carotid artery gives off many branches that supply the face and scalp. The main stem of the artery is continued upward in front of the ear as the superficial temporal artery.

The head and neck regions are drained by two large veins, the external and internal jugular veins. The external jugular vein receives blood mainly from the face and scalp, the regions supplied by the external carotid artery. The internal jugular vein receives blood from the brain through the venous sinuses. Blood from the external jugular vein flows into the subclavian vein just before the latter unites with the internal jugular vein to form the innominate vein.

Renal circulation. The only mention of renal circulation to be made here is that adequate function of the kidneys, without which life cannot be sustained for any appreciable period, is dependent upon adequate pressure in the renal vessels. This must be remembered and provided for.

Portal circulation (portal system of veins). The portal system includes all the veins that drain the blood from the abdominal part of the digestive tube (with the exception of the lower part of the rectum) and from the spleen, pancreas, and gallbladder. The blood is conveyed to the liver by way of the portal vein, which ramifies like an artery and ends in capillary-like vessels called sinusoids, from which the blood is returned to the inferior vena cava by the hepatic veins. This, then, is actually the second time that this blood has been part of a capillary-like system, having first been part of the capillary system of the splanchnic (digestive) area. This blood does not play a great part in oxygenation of the liver; the role of the portal veins is rather to bring products of digestion to the liver. The portal vein is formed behind the neck of the pancreas by the junction of the superior mesenteric and splenic veins. It enters into the liver as described, and blood carried by it is returned to the inferior vena cava by way of the hepatic veins.

Pulmonary circulation. Blood is pumped by the right ventricle into the pulmonary artery, branches of which ramify extensively through the lung substance, and the ramifications accompany the respiratory tubes. With each bronchiole is an arteriole. Within the parenchyma, a dense plexus of capillaries is formed about each alveolus; this is the most important point of the pulmonary circulation. At this point an intimate contact between blood and air is provided, and at the same time a transfer of blood from the right to the left side of the heart is established. It is at this site that venous blood of lowered oxygen content becomes arterial or highly oxygenated. These vast plexuses also act as a blood reservoir. Blood is then returned eventually to the left atrium by four pulmonary veins. These are the only veins in the body that normally and consistently carry highly oxygenated blood—actually arterial blood, as it is commonly thought of. The blood then enters the left ventricle and the systemic circulation.

The pulmonary epithelial surface represents about 70 sq. m., which is twenty-five times the skin surface. The pulmonary respiratory surface is 55 sq. m. and the pulmonary capillary surface is 38 sq. m. In the pulmonary circulation there are relatively fewer and less muscular arterioles than in the systemic circulation. The precapillaries are large, the capillaries wide, and the veins short. The total blood in the pulmonary circulations is 400 to 600 ml., or 8 to 10% of the total blood volume, and it can be as high as 20%. The atria and ventricles contract synchronously, so that the same amount of blood ejected into the pulmonary artery must be received into the right ventricle. If the right side consistently puts out more blood than the left side, there will be a backlog in the pulmonary circulation at the expense of the alveolar space and hence diminished vital capacity. Some congestion actually does occur in recumbency.

PHYSIOLOGY OF THE HEART

Physiologically the heart possesses certain characteristics found nowhere else in the body. The first exists in the heart muscle itself, which possesses excitability (contractility), rhythmicity, and conductivity.

Excitability, or contractility. Excitability, or contractility, may be defined as the ability of a tissue to respond to a stimulus. In muscle, this response is a shortening, or contraction, of fibers. This property brings into evidence the first of the laws of the heart—the all-or-none law. This law states that the weakest stimulus capable of causing a contraction will produce a maximum contraction, depending on condition. Conditions that may influence a change in response include the length of the fiber, the hydrogen ion concentration, the inorganic constituents of the fluid bathing the heart, the state of nutrition, temperature, fatigue, and ionic balance.

Length of the fiber. Starling's law of the heart is brought into play here. This law states that the energy set free at each contraction of the heart is a simple function of the length of the fibers comprising its muscle wall: the longer the fiber, the stronger the contraction.

Hydrogen ion concentration. Acids in moderate excess favor relaxation of cardiac muscle. During exercise a large volume of blood is returned to the heart from skeletal muscle; the resulting rise in carbon dioxide favors more complete relaxation of cardiac muscle. The heart accommodates itself to a greater load of venous blood, and as a result there is an increased cardiac output.

Inorganic constituents of fluid bathing the heart. There are three inorganic constituents essential for normal cardiac action: sodium, calcium, and potassium. Sodium has to do with the maintenance of excitability and contractility. Calcium increases the strength of the contraction and prolongs systole. Potassium reduces the strength of the contraction and favors relaxation.

State of nutrition. An adequate state of nutrition must be present for normal cardiac activity. There must first be sufficient pressure to assure adequate coronary flow. The temperature of heart muscle must be between 20° and 40° C., and there must be an adequate supply of oxygen to the cardiac tissue. The oxygen consumption of heart muscle is high, being about 3.24 ml. per gram per hour. The amount of venous blood returning from the cardiac capillary network is much less than that of systemic venous blood.

Rhythmicity. Rhythmicity occurs independently of the central nervous system. The absolute refractory period is the characteristic that enables cardiac muscle to maintain rhythmicity. In ordinary skeletal muscle, the refractory period is short, about 0.01 second, and corresponds to the period elapsing from the receipt of the stimulus until the commencement of contraction. A stimulus applied to the muscle at any time after it has started to contract will cause a second contraction, which is added to the first (summation). A rapid series of stimuli will cause tetanus. This is not true in cardiac muscle, which has a refractory period that lasts throughout contraction. The muscle will not respond to a stimulus regardless of how strong it is as long as its fibers are in a contracted state. This is the *absolute refractory period.* The time interval during which the muscle is relaxing until the point of complete relaxation is the *relative refractory period,* during which excitability is depressed but not abolished. During this period the muscle is gradually regaining its excitability, and while it will respond to a stimulus, this response will be weak or strong, depending upon the part of the refractory period during which it is applied and the strength of the stimulus. Because the muscle must be in some stage of relaxation before accepting a stimulus, it can be seen why it is impossible for cardiac muscle to enter into tetany—which is really a continued state of contraction.

It might be well at this point to explain the mechanism of a premature beat. Let us suppose that there is a normal regular heart rate of 80 beats per minute. There is then a definite time interval between each beat. The origin of the premature beat is usually from some other point than the sinoatrial node. If this stimulus arrives at the heart muscle after the absolute refractory period of the previous beat and before the beginning of the next expected normal beat, it will elicit a response, or beat. When this next normal beat is due to occur, its stimulus will fall in the absolute refractory period of the premature beat, and hence there will be no response. Rather, there will be absence of activity at that point, and there will also be the normal pause before the third normal beat. This normal pause, plus the pause occurring because of the inability of the second normal beat to occur, produces a prolonged pause, called the compensatory pause. This compensatory pause is what is usually heard at the precordium and felt at the pulse, rather than the premature beat itself. These beats may be referred to on physical examination as premature beats, extrasystoles, or dropped beats. The majority of these are premature beats, but their exact identification can be made only by electrocardiography. With premature beats, the total number of beats occurring over a definite period, such as 15 seconds, will be the same as for the previous 15 seconds in a heart beating at a consistent rate.

Conductivity. Conductivity is the ability of the heart, because of its anatomical structure, to respond as a whole when one part is stimulated.

Origin and transmission of the heartbeat. The heartbeat originates in the sinoatrial node, which sets the pace of the heart and is known as the pacemaker. The impulse spreads through the atrial muscle, causing it to contract. This impulse is picked up by the atrioventricular node, is conducted in the A-V bundle down to the right and left bundle branches and into the Purkinje system, and causes the ventricles to contract simultaneously.

In certain conditions, the S-A node does not act as the pacemaker; if this occurs, the beat will originate in the center having the next highest rate of discharge. Here, then, the atrial, or A-V, node will originate the impulse. If there is a complete block between the atria and ventricles, the ventricles will beat at their own inherent rate of about 35 per minute.

Cardiac cycle. The cardiac cycle is a succession of charges occurring in the heart during each beat. The length varies with the heart rate, and with a rate of 70 the cycle lasts six sevenths of a second. Ventricular systole extends from the closure of the A-V valves to the closure of the semilunar valves. It may be divided into two phases:

1. Period of isometric contraction. This is the period in which the fibers contract upon the blood that fills the closed ventricular cavity. The blood is incompressible, and as a result the fibers are unable to shorten. Pressure increases, causing the semilunar valves to open.
2. Ejection period. This period begins when the semilunar valves open and blood is discharged into the aorta and pulmonary artery. The period of maximum ejection extends from the opening of the valves to the attainment of maximum pressure and is followed by a period of reduced ejection.

During each ventricular systole, a blood volume of 70 ml. is forced into the aorta, and about the same amount is forced into the pulmonary artery so that the cardiac output per beat is 140 ml. With a heart rate of 70 ml. per minute, the left ventricular output is 4,900 ml. The total cardiac output is 9,800 ml. per minute.

The volume of blood ejected with each stroke from each ventricle is called the stroke volume. The average stroke volume is 70 ml.—about 60 ml. at rest and a maximum of about 120 ml. during exercise. The difference between output at rest and maximum output is cardiac reserve. The cardiac output is the quantity of blood expelled per unit time.

A brief period elapses between the end of the reduced injection phase and closure of the semilunar valves. This is known as the *protodiastolic* phase.

During the period of isometric relaxation, the ventricles are closed, and although the fibers are relaxing, they remain the same length. This phase is terminated by the opening of the A-V valves. During diastolic inflow the blood flows rapidly into the ventricles from the atria. As the ventricles begin to fill, the blood flow becomes slower; this slower flow is called diastasis.

The atria contract during the dynamic interval and inflow phase and discharge their contents into the ventricles. At the termination of this phase the A-V valves close, the ventricle contracts, and the cycle begins again.

The electrocardiogram is a record of the change of the electrical potential of the cardiac muscle during the cardiac cycle.

Production of heart sounds. The characteristic heart sound in "lub-dub," with the two sounds separated by a short interval and followed by a longer pause. The first sound (lub) is long, soft, and pitched low. It is produced by contraction of the ventricular muscle, closure of the A-V valves, and vibration of the cusps and chordae tendinae as the intraventricular pressure increases. The second sound (dub) is shorter, sharper, and pitched higher. This sound results from closure of the pulmonary and aortic valves.

REGULATION OF HEART ACTION

Demand of the body for blood varies from moment to moment, so that the rate and stroke volume of the heart must be governed accordingly. Conditions causing these changes may be pathological (hemorrhage, shock, hyperthyroidism, fever, certain cardiac arrhythmias) or physiological (muscular exercise, emotional excitement, high environmental temperature, digestion, sleep).

The rate of the heart is an extremely important index of cardiac action. The normal heart rate varies with each person, and to set a normal rate for a human being would be difficult. In the approximation of a normal range, however, a rate above 100 beats per minute is generally considered tachycardia and below 60 beats bradycardia. Cardiac regulation is generally dependent upon three agencies: nervous, chemical, and mechanical.

Nervous control. The nervous control of the heart consists of inhibition and acceleration.

Vagus nerve (cardiac inhibitor). The vagus nerve carries two types of fibers: the chronotropic, which effects a change in cardiac rate; and the dromotropic, which depresses conduction. Stimulation of the vagus may cause (1) decrease in heart rate (chronotropic property), which is most prevalent, (2) diminished force without affecting the rate (inotropic), (3) a heart stoppage, as the result of reduction of irritability in the S-A node and a decrease in conductivity of the A-V bundle (conductivity slowed, dromotropic), and (4) decreased excitability (bathmotropic).

Accelerator action. Nerve fibers to the heart causing cardiac acceleration are sympathetic in origin. The activity of the cardiac centers is reflex, arising from various parts of the body. Reflexes are received at the cardioaccelerator centers and are transmitted to the anterolateral cell column of the spinal cord, whence sympathetic fibers arise, and on to the heart through pathways already described. Sympathetic fibers affect both the atrium and ventricle. All properties and actions of the heart are augmented: (1) rate is increased (systole is shortened more than diastole), (2) contractions are stronger, (3) coronaries are dilated, (4) conduction is enhanced, and (5) excitability is increased.

Some of the more specific reflexes modifying cardiac activity are as follows:

1. Oculocardiac–slowing of the pulse by pressure in the eyeball.
2. Stimulation of nasal branches of vagus–slowing of the pulse.
3. Stimulation of afferent fibers of the pulmonary vagus by irritating vapors, such as those of anesthetics, with reflex slowing of the pulse.
4. Irregularities as a result of abdominal visceral stimulation.
5. Excitation of peripheral nerves–for example, that of the sciatic nerve, which causes acceleration.
6. Afferent endings in the heart itself (Bainbridge effect). An increase in venous return causes an increase in heart rate. This is brought about by the stimulation of vagal receptors beneath the endothelium in the walls of the great veins. The effective stimulus here is distention.

Drugs. The following drugs affect heart action:

Atropine: This drug depresses vagal activity by competing with acetylcholine at the postganglionic nerve ending.

Prostigmin, Pilocarpine, Acetylcholine: All these drugs bring about action similar to vagal stimulation to the heart.

Physicochemical control. Agents that best elicit chemical control of the heart may be divided into the following five categories: (1) temperature, (2) minerals (calcium, potassium, sodium), (3) acid metabolites (carbon dioxide and lactic acid), (4) oxygen, and (5) hormones (epinephrine).

Increase in temperature in the range of 25° to 45° C. accelerates the heart action. Changes in pH and blood ions also greatly influence cardiac activity. Thus, acidity and potassium ions diminish cardiac activity, whereas alkalies and calcium ions augment activity. The blood gases also are important in the regulation of heart action. Carbon dioxide enhances extensibility of cardiac muscle. Small increases slow the heart and increase vagal tone, whereas high increases depress conduction, so that, with a pH of 7, complete block can occur. High oxygen tensions reduce the cardiac rate, and low tensions increase it. High oxygen tensions reduce cardiac output slightly, and very low tensions increase it. Experiments have shown that with mixtures containing 11.6% oxygen a moderate increase in cardiac output occurs, but if the oxygen lack is profound or of long duration, then cardiac muscle suffers and output is reduced. Reduction of oxygen content by 50% produces change in the electrocardiogram that may resemble cardiac infarct. Oxygen lack first produces an increase in heart rate, then extrasystoles, heart block, or other irregularities, and finally heart failure.

In asphyxia (carbon dioxide excess with oxygen lack) at first there is a slowing of the heart. As this condition progresses, the strength of cardiac musculature weakens, the blood pressure falls, and the heart rate increases, becomes irregular, and finally fails.

Mechanical control. Cardial output is directly proportional to inflow. If venous input is enhanced or peripheral resistance increased, then the heart must do more work. This is accomplished by greater stretching of the muscle fibers, with development of increased tension during contraction. At the same time oxygen consumption rises. This is merely an application of Starling's law of the heart.

CONTROL OF THE BLOOD VESSELS

The actions of the blood vessels, just as the cardiac mechanism, are influenced by stimulation of the autonomic nervous system. The walls of the arterioles are composed chiefly of involuntary smooth muscle arranged in circular fashion. These muscle fibers are supplied by two types of nerves, inhibitory and excitatory. Those which cause contraction are vasoconstrictor and are analogous to the cardiac accelerator nerves. Those that cause relaxation are vasodilators and are analogous to the cardiac inhibitors (vagus). Together they are referred to as the vasomotor nerves. The origin of these nerve fibers has been described previously.

General stimulation of the vasomotor elements elicits either a pressor or depressor response. The former is characterized by an increased heart rate, vasocontriction, and increased blood pressure, whereas the depressor response has an opposite effect. A few of the vasomotor reflexes that bring about a pressor or depressor response are as follows:

1. Somatic nerve stimulation, particularly of pain fibers, causes a pressor response, whereas stimuli transmitted over pain and temperature fibers elicit a depressor response.

2. Vagal afferents by way of the aortic nerve from the arch of the aorta, upper thoracic aorta, and coronary and pulmonary vessels are stimulated by a fall in arterial pressure and elicit a pressor response, whereas an increase in pressure will bring about a depressor response.

3. Cortical influences on the medullary centers may cause definite vascular responses. Anticipation of exercise causes constriction of the

splanchnic vessels and dilation in those muscles in which exercise is anticipated.

4. An increase in pressure on the carotid sinus (a slight enlargement at the bifurcation of the common carotid) elicits a general depressor response, whereas a fall in pressure within the sinus elicits a pressor response.

5. When the vessels of the mesentery dilate, the pacinian corpuscles, which lie in close contact with these vessels, pass messages to vasomotor centers that discharge vasoconstrictor impulses to these vessels. In this manner blood is prevented from pooling in the splanchnics. The vessels of the splanchnic area are capable of pooling the blood of the entire body.

6. The Lovén reflex, the term applied to the reaction in which local dilation of vessels accompanies general vasoconstriction, causes a pressor response. When the central end of an afferent nerve to an organ is stimulated while its efferent vasomotor fibers remain intact, a rise in general blood pressure, together with dilation of the vessels of the organ, occurs. In this manner the organ is provided with an increased blood flow during activity.

7. Axon reflexes produce depressor responses. The efferent and afferent limbs of the axon reflex are formed by the branching of a single nerve fiber. A stimulus applied to one branch sets up an impulse that travels centrally to the point of division, from where it is reflected down the other branch to an effector organ. An example of this may be the skin and the underlying vessel. In this type of reaction, dilation of skin vessels is proportional to the pain and inflammation and causes a rise in temperature without central mediation.

Chemical factors influencing control of blood vessels. In the medullary centers carbon dioxide excess or oxygen lack stimulates the constrictor center and increases peripheral vascular tone. In the spinal centers of the anterolateral columns carbon dioxide and hypoxia stimulate the cells and increase vascular tone.

Locally, acids and metabolites, including carbon dioxide, cause dilation of vessels.

Hormones have various effects on blood vessels. Epinephrine and thyroxin cause constriction of some vascular beds (splanchnic and skin) and dilation of others, notably muscle.

Vasopressin causes constriction of arterioles and of capillaries.

CONTROL OF VEINS

Venous pressure is normally low. It is 40 to 110 mm. H_2O in the median basilic vein in the arm and diminishes progressively toward the heart. The only veins giving evidence of nervous supply are the large superficial veins with sympathetic constrictor fibers.

Carbon dioxide dilates veins by local action. The type of nervous stimulus is also a factor in the control of veins. A strong, continuous stimulus elicits a constrictor response, whereas a weak, rhythmic stimulus produces a dilator response, as does mechanical irritation.

SYSTEMIC BLOOD PRESSURE

In traversing the circuit the blood exerts a pressure against the walls of the vessels. This is the arterial blood pressure. This pressure, which is measured in millimeters of mercury, varies greatly in different parts of the body. The pressure falls gradually the farther the blood travels from the heart because it overcomes peripheral resistance. The gradient is steepest in the arterioles—50 to 60 mm. Hg. Pulse pressure is absent in the capillaries, but then gradually appears again and is present as far as the right atrium.

The maximum pressure exerted by the ventricle is the systolic pressure. The point of minimal pressure is the diastolic pressure. One half the sum of these two is the mean pressure. The difference between the two is the pulse pressure.

The diastolic pressure shows the constant load on the vessels, as well as the resistance the ventricle must overcome.

Factors that form normal blood pressure. Five factors combine to form and maintain normal blood pressure: pumping action of the heart, peripheral resistance, quantity of blood in the system, viscosity of the blood, and elasticity of the arterial walls.

Pumping action of the heart. When more blood is forced into an already filled system, it cannot escape at once; therefore, the arterial walls are stretched because of the increased pressure until the velocity of flow from the system (arteriole) can balance it out.

Peripheral resistance. Peripheral resistance involves the arterioles primarily and the capillaries secondarily. Constriction or dilation at this point causes an increased amount of blood to be held or released from the arterial side of the circulation. These vessels exert their greatest influence in the splanchnic area (abdominal vessels). Stimulation of the greater splanchnic nerve causes constriction of the muscles in the walls of the vessels in this area, and consequently a reduction in the outflow from the system occurs. Dilation of the vessels causes the opposite effect. The vessels of the splanchnic area can accommodate all the blood in the body.

Quantity of blood in the system. The system must be overfilled in order to exert pressure. Therefore, conditions such as hemorrhage deplete the system and cause a fall in pressure.

Viscosity of blood. The greater the viscosity of a fluid, the higher will be the pressure required to force it along a tube. Viscosity depends to a degree upon how the parts of a liquid cohere. Blood is five times as viscous as water.

Here again the matter of outflow through the arterioles has to do with pressure. Dilution of blood, as in anemia, decreases viscosity; polycythemia increases it. Carbon dioxide increases viscosity, whereas oxygen decreases it. Therefore, venous blood is more viscous than arterial blood.

Chloroform, morphine, hyperglycemia, hypercalcemia, and acidosis increase viscosity. Increased temperature decreases it.

Elasticity of arterial walls. The elasticity of arterial walls is concerned mainly with the origin and maintenance of diastolic pressure. Below 30 to 40 mm. Hg the walls are not affected. However, normally they are stretched and tend to recoil against the stretching force.

VELOCITY

The velocity at which blood traverses the circuit should not be confused with blood pressure. Velocity is inversely proportional to the cross-sectional area. As a result, the velocity is greatest in the arteries, decreases several hundred times in the capillaries, and increases as large veins are entered. This statement at first seems to be contradictory. However, even though the cross-sectional area of each capillary is small, the combined cross-sectional area of all the capillaries is six to eight hundred times that of the aorta.

In the capillaries, the velocity is extremely slow—with an obvious advantage. It is at this area that internal respiration and the exchange of nutritive materials and water products take place. When the blood reenters the venous side of the circulation, velocity gradually rebuilds. In the aorta, velocity is 400 mm. per second, in the capillary 0.5 mm. per second, and in the vena cava 150 mm. per second. The time required for a cell to pass through the pulmonary and systemic circulations is 23 seconds.

Among many conditions that cause normal variations in arterial blood pressure are the following:

1. Age—there is a gradual increase in pressure to 16 years of age. Pressure then levels off, but a slight increase occurs after the age of 25 or 30 years.
2. Sex—women usually have a slightly lower pressure than men of comparable age.

3. Digestion produces an increase of 5 to 10 mm. Hg in systolic pressure, lasting about 1 hour.
4. Emotions such as fear, excitement, and anger cause a marked rise in systolic pressure.
5. Muscular exercise is accompanied by a pronounced increase in systolic pressure.
6: Posture—diastolic pressure is higher when one stands than when one lies down. Systolic pressure usually remains unchanged.

VENOUS PRESSURE

Just as with arterial blood pressure, certain things combine to maintain venous pressure.

Pumping action of the heart. The energy expended by cardiac contraction provides part of the force for venous pressure. By the time the atrium is reached, this energy is almost completely expended.

Quantity of blood through arterioles in relation to the capacity of the capillaries and veins. Generally, the more blood received from the arterial side, the higher is the pressure in the capillaries and veins. The capillaries and veins are capable of adjusting to the quantity of blood received and thus tend to maintain a constant pressure.

Subatmospheric pressure in the thorax. The negative pressure within the thorax tends to suck the blood from extrathoracic vessels. This action is greatest during inspiration, when intrapleural pressure is lowest. In addition, venous return to the heart is increased during the inspiratory phase due to the increased pressure in the inferior vena cava caused by compression of the abdominal contents when the diaphragm contracts.

It should be mentioned here that, whereas deep inspiration increases venous return to the heart, overinflation of the lungs by controlled positive pressure will decrease venous return. This fact should be remembered when one becomes too ambitious in breathing for a patient during anesthesia.

Massaging action of the muscles. Intermittent pressure brought about on the vessels by muscular contraction milks the blood toward the heart. Backflow is prevented by the valves in the veins.

Above the heart, gravity opposes the flow of blood in the arterial system but aids in the venous return. Below the heart, the reverse is true.

NOTES ON SPECIAL CIRCULATION

Arteriolar-capillary circulation. One arteriole may have several metarterioles, and each of these in turn may have innumerable precapillaries, which are further divided into many capillaries. Only a small number of capillaries are open at any one time; most are closed, but have potential function. The total area of all capillaries is approximately 6,300 sq. m.

Arteriolar constriction arises from sympathetic stimulation. Depending on the degree of stimulation, the flow is regulated and tissue oxygenation is controlled. Mild constriction diminishes blood flow, but extreme constriction may produce true anemia of the tissues and cellular hypoxia. Dilation of arterioles is passive. The passage of blood from an arteriole to a venule requires 1 second. The velocity of blood flow is 0.5 mm. per second in capillaries as compared with 40 cm. per second in the aorta.

Capillaries are controlled by sympathetic innervation and also by an inherent automatic factor that provides the capillary with a property called vasomotion. Capillaries are highly sensitive to local stimuli—nervous, thermal, etc.—and as a result there is a change in the number and size of the capillaries functioning at one time.

Since arterioles and capillaries have the ability to hold or release blood from the arterial side of circulation, it is evident why the arteriolar-capillary circulation can be referred to as the sphincter system of the circulation. It also can be seen how these vessels maintain an arterial circulating volume and why a complete loss of tone in these vessels could be disastrous to adequate circulation.

Capillary blood pressure. At the arterial end of the capillary the pressure is 32 mm. Hg, whereas at the venous end it is 12 mm. Hg. The former is greater than the osmotic pressure of blood, and the latter is less.

Coronary circulation. Oxygen consumption of cardiac muscle is high compared to that of skeletal muscle, the former being 3.24 ml. per gram per hour. Each cardiac muscle fiber has an accompanying arteriole, in contrast to one arteriole for each two skeletal muscle fibers.

About 5% of the total cardiac output is channeled into the coronary arteries. This is 65 to 85 ml. of blood per 100 grams of tissue per minute. The circulation time from the coronary ostia to the right atrium is 8 seconds.

Inflow of blood into the coronaries occurs during diastole and the isometric period of contraction.

Coronary pressure is regulated by the following:

1. Diastolic aortic pressure (after aortic valves are closed).
2. Sympathetic and vagal supply to large branches, mainly vagal fibers to arterioles.

3. Cardiac output influences coronary flow; a rise in output augments flow.
4. Oxygen lack increases flow locally, but anoxemia acting centrally causes constriction of coronary vessels. Decreased oxygen supply accelerates coronary flow, and there is a correlation between myocardial oxygen consumption and coronary flow.
5. Rate of heart—coronary flow occurs chiefly during diastole. Since an increased rate shortens diastole, coronary flow will decrease.
6. Drugs—vasodilators such as xanthenes and epinephrine (200% increase with epinephrine); vasoconstrictors such as certain posterior pituitary extracts.

Pulmonary circulation. The pulmonary circulation is generally referred to as the lesser circulation. The flow in the pulmonary artery is 0.3 m. per second as compared to 0.5 m. per second in the aorta.

Pulmonary circulation time is 11 seconds; during most of this period the blood is traversing the capillary bed.

Blood pressure in the pulmonary artery is 25/8, or about one sixth of systemic pressure.

Total blood in the entire pulmonary circulation is 400 to 600 ml., or about 8 to 10% of total blood volume.

The output of the right side of the heart is equal to that of the left side of the heart. Should the output of the right side exceed that of the left side, there should be a storage of blood in the pulmonary circulation at the expense of vital capacity. Some congestion does occur during recumbency.

As stated previously, deep breathing increases venous return to the heart. Controlled respirations decrease the return to the right atrium and, because of the massaging action on the lungs, increase the output of the left ventricle.

The effect of vasomotor regulation and pressor drugs on pulmonary circulation is negligible.

Cerebral circulation. Circulation in the brain depends on the mean systemic arterial pressure and resistance to blood flow in the brain.

The total amount of blood is limited by the space in the brain; an increased need for oxygen is met by changes in blood flow and by factors of resistance. Blood flow in the brain in young men is 54 ml. of blood per 100 grams of tissue per minute. When systemic pressure falls, there is a fall in cerebral flow. In healthy males, the average value for consumption of cerebral oxygen is 3.3 ml. per 100 grams of tissue per minute.

Carbon dioxide causes dilation of pial vessels, as does increased acidity. Inhalation of 5% carbon dioxide may increase cerebral flow by 75% with a significant decrease in resistance.

Lowering carbon dioxide tension by about 40% may, by hyperventilation, increase resistance by 75%, with an accompanying 35% reduction of blood flow.

CARDIAC ARRHYTHMIAS

In many instances cardiac rhythm deviates from normal, presenting one or more types of cardiac arrhythmia. The significance may be great or minor, depending on the particular type of arrhythmia and the cause. Some of these arrhythmias can be diagnosed by physical means, whereas others can be determined only by electrocardiography. Following is a brief discussion of some of the irregularities.

Stem of bundle. Experimentally, conduction from the atrium to the ventricle may be delayed or blocked by crushing, cutting, or applying a cold stimulus to the A-V bundle. This point in conduction may be similarly affected by disease, and depression or abolition may result. Three degrees of affliction are generally recognized.

Delayed conduction. Delayed conduction is slowed conduction between the atrium and ventricle. All atrial beats reach the ventricle. The condition can be recognized by electrocardiography or tracing of the venous pulse.

Missed beats; partial heart block. When the delayed conduction becomes more advanced, occasionally one of the atrial beats fails to reach the ventricle, resulting in a missed beat. Should this delay become more profound, impulses from the atrium may reach the ventricle in a definite ratio, such as 2 to 1 or 3 to 1, and as a result there is partial heart block.

Complete heart block. When there is a complete barrier between the atrium and ventricle, each beats at its own rate—the atria at about 70 per minute and the ventricles at about 35 per minute. When this occurs, a rhythm called the idioventricular rhythm results. The presence of some abnormality can be detected, but usually an electrocardiogram must be taken to identify it. Complete heart block may be caused by drugs or disease and may be reversible. A persistent heart block may be the result of overactive vagal tone and may be reversed by the administration of atropine.

Stokes-Adams syndrome. This condition is featured by a slow pulse and syncopal attacks or convulsive seizures. In the majority of instances the slowed cardiac action is a result of heart block, and the cerebral symptoms are a direct result of the bradycardia. The prolonged pause between beats causes a reduced blood supply to the cerebral centers (due to the low level to which the diastolic pressure is allowed to drop). Arteriosclerosis of the large arteries, aortic regurgitation, etc. will enhance the effect of the bradycardia. Epinephrine or ephedrine has been used to treat this condition, with some success.

Bundle-branch block; interventricular block. When one of the primary branches is blocked by disease, such as myocardial infarction resulting from coronary occlusion, the impulse reaches the diseased side a fraction of a second after reaching the healthy side. The affected ventricle is activated by the escape of the impulse from the healthy side through the septum. The variation in arrival of impulse causes the ventricles to beat asynchronously. Here again, the condition can be diagnosed only by electrocardiography.

Disturbances in rhythm due to abnormal impulse formation. Certain disturbances in cardiac rhythm may be due to abnormal impulse formation, in which are included the following types of abnormal beats.

Extrasystole, or premature beats. These heartbeats may be caused by stimulation of the cardiac muscle at any time except during its phase of absolute refractoriness. They may be due to organic heart disease, but more often they are not. They may be reflex in origin, from abdominal viscera, or may be due to some intoxication, such as that caused by the administration of digitalis or an ansethetic, the presence of hyperthyroidism, smoking, etc. The site of origin of the beat may be atrium, ventricle, or A-V node.

Ventricular extrasystoles. The premature beat occurs after the normal ventricular beat has recovered from its refractory state. This beat is not preceded by an atrial beat. The impulse does not originate in the upper chamber. This beat is followed by a compensatory pause, unless it occurs early in diastole in a slow-beating heart, at which time no such pause is present. Except in the latter instance these beats are usually premature, but not *extra* in the sense that there is no increase in he number of beats over a set period of time in a heart beating at a constant rate.

Atrial extrasystoles. This impulse arises as some point in the atrium outside the S-A node and is usually followed by a ventricular contraction. In an abnormal atrial contraction, however, there is rarely a long compensatory pause. This is explained by the fact that usually the energy accumulated in the S-A node is created during quiescence of the muscle following a beat and that during the abnormal beat this energy is discharged. Therefore, a definite time interval elapses after the premature beat in order for energy in the S-A node to be created.

Nodal extrasystoles. Extrasystoles may form as a result of formation of impulse in the A-V node or supraventricular part of the stem. Because of the anatomical position of the A-V node, impulses raising therein pass upward and downward to cause simultaneous or nearly simultaneous responses from the atrium and ventricle. Depending on its position of origin on the A-V bundle, the ventricular contraction may actually precede the atrial contraction. This is because the pathway to the ventricle is shorter than that to the atrium.

• • •

Abnormal beats rarely arise in the S-A node. When they do occur, there is complete contraction of the heart, with only a slight disturbance in rhythm.

When extrasystoles occur after each normal beat and are followed by a prolonged pause, the pulse beats appear to be paired. This irregularity is referred to as a pulsus bigeminus, or coupling. It can be identified by auscultation and a great many times by palpation of the radial pulse. In some persons, however, the second of the paired beats is difficult to detect at the radial pulse, and as a result a false rate of the heart is recorded. In any person in whom the radial pulse rate suddenly falls to approximately half its former rate, pulsus bigeminus should be suspected, and the rate should be checked at the apex by auscultation. This irregularity may occur with overdosage of digitalis and is not an infrequent complication during anesthesia because of hypoxia, reflex action, etc.

The presence of an irregularity, be it a premature beat, an extrasystole, or a dropped beat, can be detected by irregularity of the pulse. However, its exact identification is usually made only by electrocardiography. Of these three arrhythmias, premature beat is by far the most prevalent.

Paroxysmal tachycardia. Paroxysmal tachycardia is a condition where in the rate of the heart greatly accelerates for a short or long period without obvious cause. This rate may be from 140 to 250 beats per minute. The onset is sudden and regular and may last from a few seconds to days. A paroxysm longer than 10 days is rare. The attack ceases as abruptly as it began, and a normal rate is resumed almost immediately.

The paroxysm consists of a series of rapidly recurring extrasystoles that completely submerge the physiological rhythm. The site of origin of the extrasystoles, as in the case of single premature beats, may be the atrium, A-V node, bundle stem, or ventricle. The atrial type is most common.

Atrial flutter. Atrial flutter may be pure or impure. The atrium

Table 2-1. Differences between atrial flutter and paroxysmal atrial tachycardia

	Atrial flutter	*Paroxysmal atrial tachycardia*
Rate	250 to 400	Usually 140 to 250
Duration	May be transient, but may be months or years	Rarely over 10 days
Conduction	Ventricle fails to follow rate of atrium; state of relative heart block exists	Ventricle follows atrial rate
Origin	Produced by passage of impulses over one or more circular pathways (circus movement)	Normal beats suppressed and substituted by abnormal beats

beats at rates of 250 to 400 per minute in pure flutter. Rhythm is regular in pure flutter and irregular in impure flutter. Table 2-1 lists the differences between atrial flutter and paroxysmal atrial tachycardia.

In flutter, the atrial walls do not relax completely. Some of the fibers are always in a state of contraction, but they do not all contract together; therefore, both systole and diastole are incomplete. The ventricle rarely keeps pace with the atrium, and as a result of state of relative heart block develops. An atrioventricular rate of 2 to 1, 3 to 1, or 4 to 1 may develop, although it is most frequently 2 to 1. If the ventricle were to respond to each atrial beat, serious circulatory disturbances due to shortened diastole would follow. Here the ventricle would receive a reduced load of blood. The output of the heart would be so greatly reduced that unconsciousness and death might occur.

Atrial fibrillation. In this disorder the atrial muscle is the seat of incomplete contractions, which recur at a frequency of 400 to 600 per minute. The contractions are so rapid and incomplete that the atrium looks as though it were quivering; the separate contractions are indistinguishable from one another. The atrium is never emptied of blood. Atrial fibrillation is the most common of the serious cardiac irregularities. It occurs most frequently in mitral heart disease and thyrotoxicosis and is rarely present in the absence of myocardial disease.

Because of the refractory period of ventricular muscle, only a relatively few beats pass from the atrium to the ventricle. Although the rate of the arterial pulse may be normal or slow, it usually ranges from

100 to 150. The manner in which beats do reach the ventricle is bizarre, and as a result the pulse is totally irregular as to rate, rhythm, and quality. So weak are some of the ventricular beats that the impulse does not reach the arterial pulse, and as a result the rate at the apex is faster than that at the radial pulse. This difference is called a pulse deficit. With treatment, this deficit can be reduced.

Ventricular fibrillation. The ventricles may enter into a state of rapid, tremulous, ineffectual contractions similar to those of atrial fibrillation, This may be due to a condition of coronary occlusion, drug intoxication, electrocution, or any condition causing hypoxia of the heart muscle. The effects of ventricular fibrillation point out the differing importance of the two musculatures in regard to the dynamics of circulation. The ventricle must provide the propulsive force for circulation, and since this force is absent in fibrillation, circulation ends and death ensues within a few minutes.

Pulsus alternans. Pulsus alternans is a condition in which alternate strong and weak ventricular contractions eject large and small volumes of blood into the aorta. There is usually no change in the interval between beats felt at the arterial pulse. Pulsus alternans cannot be detected by palpation of the pulse, but it can be revealed on the sphygmogram. The variations in the strength of the pulse are too slight to be perceptible. This condition can be detected by use of a blood pressure armlet. The pressure in the armlet is raised gradually, and at a certain level the weaker beats are suppressed and the stronger ones are let through. The pulse at the wrist is then about one half the ordinary rate. The pressure difference during the weaker beats may be as much as 25 mm. Hg less than during the stronger beats, but usually the difference is from 5 to 10 mm. Hg.

Persistent alternation of the heartbeat in the presence of slow or normal pulse is usually indicative of grave myocardial disease. It may occur at more rapid rates, such as in atrial fibrillation and paroxysmal tachycardia, but it is then usually of lesser significance.

Irregularities due to variations in vagal tone. Some irregularities in cardiac rhythm are due to variations in vagal tone.

Sinus arrhythmia. In sinus arrhythmia rhythmical variations in the rate of the whole heart occur synchronously with respiration. The condition is due to alterations in the strength of the influence of the vagus nerve on the S-A node (pacemaker) as a result of respiratory excursions. The heart rate increases toward the end of inspiration and slows toward the end of expiration. This irregularity is typical of youth; it is extremely common in children and may be considered physiological. It is abolished by the administration of atropine and by increases in heart rate such as occur during exercise, with fever, etc. but is enhanced by deep breathing.

Phasic irregularity. Phasic irregularity is a slowing of the heart rate for a few seconds, independent of respiration. The manner of production is unknown, but the irregularity sometimes occurs during convalescence from acute fevers and as a result of overdosage of digitalis. It, too, is abolished by the administration of atropine.

Sinus bradycardia. Sinus bradycardia is persistent slowing of the heart due to the influence of increased vagal tone on the S-A node. The rate may be as slow as 40 per minute. Apparently, this type of bradycardia is normal in healthy persons, especially athletes.

Sinoatrial block. In sinoatrial block the whole heart misses a beat, either regularly or irregularly. The block may be abolished by the administration of atropine and may be produced by stimulation of the vagus nerve; therefore, it is probably due to action of that nerve on the S-A node. It may result from the administration of digitalis.

Atrioventricular block. In atrioventricular block there is defective conduction between the atrium and ventricle due to heightened vagal tone. The block is abolished by the administration of atropine.

Gallop rhythms. In certain cardiac conditions, three distinct sounds, producing a ryhthm similar to the gallop or canter of a horse, are heard. In the presystolic type two sounds are heard in rapid succession, followed by a third sound. In the early diastolic type the abnormal sound follows shortly upon the second sound. Sometimes the extra sound is merely an intensification of the third sound that occurs in some normal subjects and may follow strenuous muscular exercise.

In some instances, gallop rhythm is associated with cardiac failure and is then usually indicative of severe myocardial damage.

A middiastolic type of gallop rhythm also may be heard.

Summary

Ausculation of the heart and palpation of the pulse may furnish a highly useful index of cardiac activity. As can be seen, a great many of these cardiac irregularities cannot be identified by physical examination, but many of them can be detected. The important factor, therefore, is the ability to detect the deviation from normal. The pulse has three characteristics: rate (per unit time), rhythm (regularity), and quality (strength). Any deviation in the degree of these characteristics should be detected and explained, especially if they occur during anesthesia. It becomes imperative, then, that one be fully familiar with the sound of a normal heart and the feel of a normal pulse if an abnormality is to be detected. It almost goes without mentioning that one must know the characteristic of a patient's pulse, heart sounds, and blood pressure before anesthesia is begun.

COMPOSITION OF BLOOD

Blood, with all its constituents, is referred to as whole blood and is divided into the following components:

Cells

1. Red corpuscles (erythrocytes)
2. White corpuscles (leukocytes)
3. Platelets (thrombocytes)

Plasma

1. Water, 91 to 92%
2. Solids, 7 to 9%
    a. Proteins (7%): serum albumin, serum globulin, and fibrinogen
    b. Inorganic constituents (0.9%): sodium, calcium, potassium, magnesium, phosphorus, iodine, iron, copper, etc.
    c. Organic constituents (other than a and d): nonprotein nitrogenous substances (urea, uric acid, xanthene, hypoxanthine, creatine and creatinine, ammonia, and amino acids), neutral fats, phospholipids, cholesterol, and glucose
    d. Internal secretions, antibodies, and various enzymes

The specific gravity of blood is 1.050 to 1.060. It is five or six times as viscous as water.

Plasma has a specific gravity of 1.027 (depending on the concentration of protein) and constitutes about 54% of the volume of blood. The normal pH is 7.39 to 7.44; limits compatible with life are 6.8 to 7.8. It might be well to note some of the many functions of the proteins.

Fibrinogen is essential for the clotting of blood. All three proteins serve to maintain the osmotic pressure of blood. Albumin exerts the greatest influence here. The proteins give a certain viscosity to the blood and therefore enter into the maintenance of blood pressure. They aid in regulating acid-base balance; the globulin and fibrinogen fractions also influence the red cells to adhere and form clumps, or rouleaux, thereby adding stability to the blood. The proteins are essential for the formation of substances used to nourish tissue cells; they form immune substances (antibodies) and also act as a reserve of protein for the body to use during fasting or other need.

Cells. The total cells comprise about 46% of the volume of human blood.

Red blood cells. The red blood cell, or erythrocyte, is disk-shaped and nonnucleated. It has a mean diameter of 7.2μ and is about 2.2μ thick near the circumference and about 1μ thick near the center. There is considerable variation in the size of both the largest and smallest red cells in normal blood and in the size of any one cell during its circulation.

Erythrocytes are manufactured by bone marrow and have an approximate life-span of 125 days. These cells are usually destroyed by simple wear and tear and disintegrate in the bloodstream or are ingested by the macrophages of the spleen.

The main function of the red cell, the transportation of oxygen, is accomplished by hemoglobin, which composes 80 to 90% of the total solid in the cell. Hemoglobin is a combination of iron porphyrin and globin protein. Transportation of carbon dioxide is also furnished by the red cell.

A red cell that is normal in size and hemoglobin content is called normocytic and normochromic. In abnormal conditions, the cells may be microcytic, macrocytic, hypochromic, or hyperchromic.

In its transport by the red cell, oxygen enters into chemical combination with the iron of the hemoglobin molecule to form oxyhemoglobin. A remarkable feature of this combination is the readiness with which the gas is released from combination when its tension in the surrounding medium is reduced. Hemoglobin from which the oxygen has dissociated is called reduced hemoglobin. The relationship between the partial pressure of oxygen and the percentage saturation of the hemoglobin with the gas—that is, the proportion of oxyhemoglobin to reduced hemoglobin—can be shown in the form of a curve, the oxygen dissociation curve (Fig. 2-1).

Certain features of this curve demonstrate important physiological considerations. As shown, with the partial pressure of oxygen in arterial blood (97 mm. Hg) the hemoglobin is already nearly 98% saturated with the gas. Exposing the hemoglobin to a higher oxygen tension, therefore, will cause but a small increase in the total quantity of oxygen taken up by the blood. To gain even 2 to 3% the oxygen pressure would need to be raised to over 300 mm. Hg.

The flattening out of the upper part of the curve means that relatively little reduction in the percentage saturation of the hemoglobin occurs until the oxgen pressure falls to about one half its normal value. At pressures above 60 mm. Hg relatively wide variations in alveolar oxygen pressure can occur, with minimal changes in the total oxygen load of the blood. At an oxygen tension of 70 mm. Hg the hemoglobin is still about 90% saturated. The slope of the lower part of the

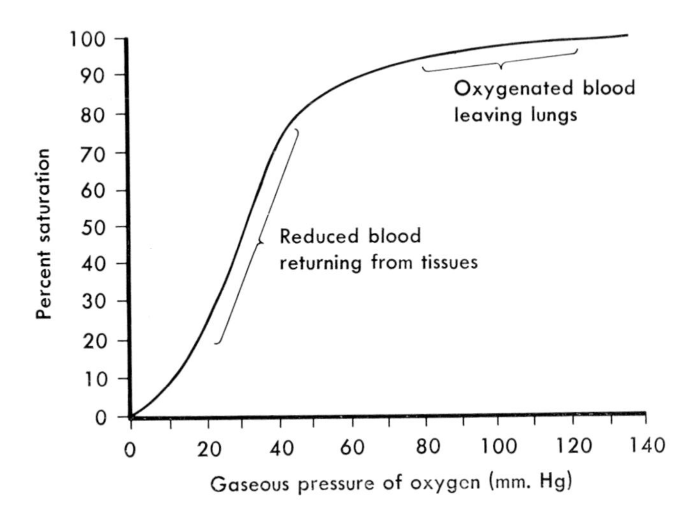

Fig. 2-1. The oxygen dissociation curve.

curve is such that a given fall in oxygen pressure causes a much greater desaturation of the hemoglobin. Because of the action of hemoglobin and oxygen, a maximum uptake of oxygen in the lungs is favored as long as the oxygen pressure is above 80 mm. Hg, and a rapid release of gas is favored at the pressures that prevail in the tissues.

A change in the reaction of the blood toward the acid side causes the curve to flatten toward the right—the affinity of hemoglobin for oxygen is reduced. Carbon dioxide and lactic acid liberated during tissue activity will exert this effect, which was discovered by Bohr and is called the Bohr effect. Temperature exerts a similar effect on the dissociation curve.

White blood cells. The white blood cells, or leukocytes, are of several varieties. The two main types are agranulocytes, which have an unlobulated nucleus and no granules in the cytoplasm, and the granulocytes, which have a nucleus possessing two or more lobes and granules in the cytoplasm.

Agranulocytes

1. Small lymphocytes, about 8μ in diameter, constitute 20 to 25% of the total number of white cells in the blood and are the most common cell found in the lymph. They are manufactured by the spleen and lymph nodes and are destroyed by dissolution in lymphoid tissue and blood to supply serum globulin.

2. Large lymphocytes are about 12μ in diameter. They are virtually confined to lymphoid tissue.
3. Monocytes, 10 to 15μ in diameter, constitute 5 to 7% of the white cells. They are manufactured by the spleen and bone marrow and are actively motile and phagocytic.

Granulocytes

1. Eosinophils constitute 2 to 4% of the white cells, at most. Their function is not completely understood.
2. Basophils constitute up to 0.15% of the white cells. Their function is not known.
3. Neutrophils, 10 to 12μ in diameter, constitute 65 to 70% or more of the total white cells. Together with the monocytes, they constitue the most important element the body possesses for defense agains microorganisms that invade the blood. They are motile and phagocytic.

The change in number and percentage of the various white blood cells is highly indicative in many disease conditions. For example, an appreciable rise in the total number of white cells generally suggests infection. If this rise is predominantly neutrophilic, the infection is acute, whereas chronic infection is usually accompanied by a rise in lymphocytes.

LYMPH AND TISSUE FLUID

Still another system concerned with the circulation of body fluids is the lymphatic system.

The lymphatic system commences peripherally as a network of delicate vessels (capillaries) that drain the tissue spaces of the various organs and tissues and ultimately enter the innominate vein at the junction of the subclavian and left internal jugular veins on the left and the right subclavian vein on the right. The system is a closed one, its vessels being formed by complete walls of endothelial cells. The capillaries of the lymphatic system have a diameter of 30 to 60μ and do not show an increase and decrease in size, as do the blood capillaries. The walls of the lymph capillaries are much more permeable than those of the blood capillaries. The arrangement of the lymph vessels resembles the arrangement of the veins, with deep and superficial vessels. Valves are numerous. There are many sets of communications between the deep and superficial lymphatic vessels; however, they are not as numerous as the communications in the venous system. Blockage of these vessels results in edema of the part distal to the blockage. Small nodes are interposed along the pathways of the vessels at various strategic points and act to stop the spread of infection or foreign material in the lymphatic channels. In addition to these small lymph nodes, there are other areas of lymphatic tissue, such as the spleen, tonsils, thymus, and Peyer's patches. Lymph tissue is actually modified connective tissue and lymphocytes. The cutaneous lymph vessels are so numerous that a skin puncture virtually penetrate the walls of these vessels.

The lymph of the tissue spaces and that of the subcutaneous vessels are similar; both resemble plasma.

Formation of lymph. Water comprises about 70% of the body weight –50% within the cells, 4.5% in the plasma, and 15.5% in the lymph and the serous cavities of the body. The formation of lymph is governed by filtration pressure and protein osmotic pressure. A gradation in concentration of the products of metabolism exists between the cells, tissue fluid, and blood. The filtration pressure or hydrostatic pressure tends to force fluid out through the capillary membrane, whereas the osmotic pressure (set up by proteins) acts to draw fluid into the capillary. Osmotic and hydrostatic pressures are exerted at both the venous and arterial ends of the capillary (by the blood). These pressures are also present in the tissue spaces at both the arterial and venous ends of the capillary (exerted by tissue fluid). When these opposing pressures are expended, a pressure called the effective pressure results.

If at the arterial end of the capillary the blood hydrostatic pressure is 30 mm. Hg and the blood osmotic pressure is 25 mm. Hg, the effective pressure wil be 5 mm. Hg, which favors the formation of lymph. At this same point, the tissues exert a constant hydrostatic pressure of 8 mm. Hg and a protein osmotic pressure of 10 mm. Hg. In the tissues the effective force will be 2 mm. Hg, which favors the formation of lymph. As a result, the effective pressure of both the blood and the tissues will be 7 mm. Hg, which favors the formation of lymph at the arterial end of the capillary.

At the venous end of the capillary, the hydrostatic pressure of the blood has fallen to about 15 mm. Hg while the protein osmotic pressure is relatively constant at about 25 mm. Hg, with the resultant pressure of 10 mm. Hg favoring filtration into the capillary. Meanwhile, since the pressure in the tissue spaces remains relatively the same, the resultant effective pressure will be 8 mm. Hg, which favors filtration into the capillary. This 8 mm. Hg is the difference between the force of 10 mm. Hg, which favors filtration into the capillary and the force of 2 mm. Hg exerted by the tissue fluids, which favors filtration out of the capillary.

Flow is maintained chiefly by the difference in pressure at the two ends of the system. Pressure is high in the capillaries and low in the large ducts. Respiratory activity and muscular contraction aid in the movement of lymph.

An increase in the flow of lymph may result from a number of conditions, including increased capillary pressure due to venous obstruction, increased capillary permeability caused by toxic agents such as poisons, or histamines or by hypoxia, or formation of hypertonic solutions. When any pathological condition results in an upset of the inward and outward flow of exudate (that is, when adsorption exceeds transudation) or in an obstruction in the lymphatic channels, edema develops.

FLUID BALANCE

The functioning cells of the body live in an environment of fluids that furnish the cells with nutrition and convey waste products of metabolism to the organs of excretion. This fluid medium which surrounds the cells produces the internal environment within which the body functions. Normal body mechanisms depend upon the maintenance of this internal environment, or fluid balance.

The total amount of water in the body varies from person to person, but as a rule it is about 60 to 70% of the body weight. The fluid content is divided between two body compartments: the intracellular compartments (50% of body weight) and the extracellular compartment (20% of body weight). The extracellular compartment is subdivided into interstitial fluid (15% of body weight) and blood plasma (5% of body weight).

Within the body fluids are electrolytes, substances which when placed in water dissociate into charged particles called ions. When positively charged, the ions are called cations, and when negatively charged, they are called anions.

The cations are sodium, potassium, calcium, and magnesium. The anions are chlorine, phosyphate, and bicarbonate, as well as organic acids and proteins. Glucose and urea are also found in blood serum, but since they have no electrical charges and do not dissociate into charged particles, they are not electrolytes.

Intracellular fluid. The intracellular fluid contains potassium, magnesium, and sodium as cations (fixed bases) and phosphate, sulfate, bicarbonate, and protein as anions (acid ions). The intracellular fluid also contains other organic compounds such as glycogen and amino acids. Potassium appears to be the most important intracellular cation.

Extracellular fluid. The extracellular fluid consists of the interstitial fluid and the blood plasma, both of which seem to be identical in chemical structure. This fluid contains sodium, potassium, calcium, and magnesium as cations (fixed bases) and chlorides, bicarbonate, phosphate, sulfate, organic acid, and protein as anions (acid ions). Except for the protein, the same electrolytes in similar proportions are found in both the interstitial and intravascular fluids.

Second only to oxygen is the need for fluid in the function of cells. The cells themselves hold the greater part of the fluid (water) in a colloidal and bound state. The free or available fluid functions in the circulating system to transport food to the cells and to enable the kidneys to remove waste products.

Water is lost from the body by perspiration, respiration, defecation, and urination. The water lost by perspiration may be considerable. Urinary output must be adequate to remove the nitrogenous waste products (chiefly urea) of cellular metabolism. Minerals, mostly sodium chloride, are excreted simultaneously in direct ratio to the excreted fluids and urea.

Vomiting, diarrhea, hemorrhage, and other fluid-depleting conditions may cause an abnormal loss of water and electrolytes. It is impractical to separate fluid balance totally from electrolyte balance because neither water nor electrolytes can be lost independently of the other. However, the proportion in which they are lost may vary.

Under ordinary circumstances a person will take in by normal processes (food and drink) an excess of fluids and electrolytes daily. Excesses are excreted, and a normal balance is maintained, with no reserve to be called upon in case of abnormal losses. This may produce a disturbance in fluid and electrolyte balance, but since there may be a shift of fluid and electrolytes, these early losses may not be demonstrable immediately.

The various body compartments (intracellular, interstitial, intravascular) have a different osmotic pressure that governs the rapid and continuous passage of fluid from one compartment to another.

After oxygen, fluid, and electrolytes, the most critical requirement for the maintenance of life and normal metabolism is dextrose. A sudden, marked drop in blood sugar (hypoglycemia) may produce extreme nervous disturbances and convulsions. Continuation of the condition may produce death. The dextrose content of the blood is normally maintained at close to 100 mg. per 100 ml. Any amount in excess of immediate needs is converted to glycogen under the influence of insulin and stored in the liver. The glycogen in the liver is reconverted to dextrose and released into the bloodstream as the need arises. It is important to remember that storage of glycogen is limited; it has been

***Table* 2-2.** Daily water gain and loss in average healthy adult

Intake	
Fluid	1,000 to 1,500 ml.
Water in solid food	700 ml.
Oxidation of food	300 ml.
Total	2,000 to 2,500 ml.
Output	
Urine	1,000 to 1,500 ml.
Feces	150 ml.
Skin	500 ml.
Lungs	350 ml.
Total	2,000 to 2,500 ml.

estimated that the maximum storage of glycogen will supply caloric needs for only about 13 hours.

The fluid intake should be about 2,500 ml. daily. This should adequately cover the obligatory loss of fluids by perspiration and respiration and at the same time permit a renal excretion of about 1,100 ml. of urine. Fluid intake is of concern to the dentist for the following reason. If a patient is eating and drinking normally, he should have no difficulty in maintaining normal fluid balances. If oral intake is not possible or adequate, the patient should be given intravenous supplements, with medical consultation. The daily water gain and loss in the average healthy adult are itemized in Table 2-2.

As can be seen in Table 2-2, in health the production of urine equals the amount of fluid ingested. If, however, the patient does not take any solid food during a 24-hour period, an extra 1,000 ml. must be given to maintain the fluid balance.

EFFECTS OF DEPLETION OF BODY FLUID

Water depletion. The progressive effects of deprivation of water on the patient are as follows:

1. The patient is deprived of water.
2. Water continues to be lost through the skin, lungs, and kidneys.
3. Increased reabsorption of water in the kidney tubules leads to a reduction in normal urinary volume.
4. Water lost is drawn from the extracellular fluid, which becomes hypertonic.
5. Water is drawn into extracellular fluid from intracellular fluid.

6. There is urinary excretion of sodium and chlorine to maintain tonicity.
7. Potassium ions pass from cells and are excreted in the urine.
8. Continuing deprivation of water leads to a decreased volume of blood plasma and hemoconcentration.
9. Diminished blood flow through the kidneys and cellular desiccation result.
10. In the last stages there is a rise in the amount of sodium, chlorine and potassium in the plasma.
11. Death occurs when 40% of body water is lost (approximately 17 liters in a man weighing 70 kg.).

The proper treatment is to supply water in excess of electrolytes, for, if isotonic saline solution is given, the water will continue to be lost through the skin and lungs, and cellular desication will progress.

Acid-base balance. Acidosis and alkalosis are clinical terms that often are used incorrectly to mean bodily states in which an abnormal concentration of hydrogen ions in the blood, producing certain signs and symptoms, occurs.

The term pH (hydrogen ion concentration) is used ordinarily to indicate the degree of acidity or alkalinity, as well as the chemical solution, of blood.

Water is very slightly ionized, with a hydrogen concentration of 7 to 10. The hydroxyl ion concentration is, however, also 7 to 10. Since these concentrations are equal (though slight), the solution is neutral.

Since in any ionized solution, regardless of its acidity or alkalinity, the product of hydrogen and hydroxyl ions is a constant, the concentration of hydrogen ions bears a reciprocal relationship with that of the hydroxyl ions. Either one or the other, therefore, can be used as a measure of the acidity or alkalinity of the solution. The hydrogen ion concentration is the one used more frequently.

For simplication, the concentrations of hydrogen ions are expressed in logarithms. Therefore, the term pH may be defined as the negative logarithm of the hydrogen ion concentration.

$$pH = -\log (H)$$

The pH of water and hence electrical neutrality is 7. Acidic solutions will have a pH below 7, and the pH of alkaline solutions will be greater than 7.

The pH of plasma is slightly alkaline at 7.4 and ordinarily varies very little from this point. The narrow range of variation is maintained through three different mechanisms: the kidneys, the buffer system of the blood, and the respiratory control of carbon dioxide.

Acidosis, strictly speaking, should be defined as a condition in which the bicarbonate of plasma is decreased below the normal level (Van Slyke). It refers only to the reduced quantity of bicarbonate in plasma, and in the truest sense it should not be used to describe a decreaes in pH, although in practice the lowered pH is a consequence of acidosis.

Alkalosis is the reverse—an increase in the bicarbonate of plasma.

Four conditions of altered acid-base balance may occur:

1. *Metabolic acidosis* (primarily alkali deficit or simply acidosis), in which the plasma bicarbonate (alkali reserve, carbon dioxide combining power) is reduced. Although by definition reduction in the pH of blood does not occur, in practice it is reduced. Compensation will occur by increased minute volume of respiration, which will tend to eliminate carbon dioxide in an attempt to bring it down to a level that will restore the 20 to 1 ratio. The kidneys will excrete excess acids.

Clinical conditions in which metabolic acidosis commonly occur are diabetes, starvation, ingestion of acidifying salts, and infantile diarrhea. It also occurs as a result of strenuous or excessive exercise.

2. *Metabolic alkalosis* (primary alkali excess or simply alkalosis), in which the plasma bicarbonate is increased. The blood pH will, if anything, be increased. Compensation will occur by decreased minute volume of respiration in order that enough carbon dioxide may be retained to match the increased plasma bicarbonate. Here again there is an attempt to retain a 20 to 1 ratio of bicarbonate to carbonic acid, although at increased values.

Clinical conditions in which metabolic alkalosis may occur are vomiting and hypertrophic pyloric stenosis.

3. So-called *respiratory acidosis* (primary carbon dioxide excess), in which the pH of the blood is decreased. There is no immediate change in the plasma bicarbonate, but as compensation occurs, the plasma bicarbonate, that is, the carbon dioxide combining power, tends to *rise* in order to restore the 20 to 1 relationship. Since the carbon dioxide combining power is *increased,* in contradistinction to metabolic acidosis, a laboratory test, alone, to determine carbon dioxide excess will not give the diagnosis.

Clinical conditions in which there is primary carbon dioxide excess include pulmonary diseases in which interference with the elimination of carbon dioxide occurs, instances in which concentrations of carbon dioxide are breathed, and diminished pulmonary ventilation such as occurs during anesthesia or from morphine poisoning.

4. So-called *respiratory alkalosis* (primary carbon dioxide deficit), in which the blood pH is increased. As compensation occurs, the plasma bicarbonate, or carbon dioxide combining power, tends to fall.

(Note: In metabolic alkalosis, the carbon dioxide combining power is increased.)

Clinical conditions involving primary carbon dioxide deficit include hyperventilation syndromes, salicylate poisoning, some forms of meningitis and encephalitis in which respiration is increased, hyperpyrexia, and hysteria.

Plasma electrolytes. The plasma electrolytes may be measured in either milligrams per 100 ml. or preferably in milliequivalents per liter. If the latter system is used, the interaction of the electrolytes of the plasma may be understood more clearly.

Definitions

Mol: a gram-molecular weight that is the amount in grams of a substance equal to its molecular weight

Atomic weight of sodium	= 23
Atomic weight of chloride	= 35
Molecular weight of sodium chloride	= 58
(i.e., 1 mol of sodium chloride	= 58 grams)

Molar solution: 1 mol dissolved in 1 liter solution

58 grams of sodium chloride dissolved in 1 liter of solution

Equivalent: atomic weight divided by valence. If the atom is monovalent, the terms are synonymous. If the atom is divalent, the equivalent weight is one half the atomic weight.

Atomic weight of sodium = 23	Equivalent weight = 23
Atomic weight of calcium = 40	Equivalent weight = 20

One equivalent weight of a substance will react completely with one equivalent weight of another substance since, although the atoms may be of different weight, the number of atoms in each substance is the same.

Milliequivalent: one one-thousandth of an equivalent. This is the term commonly used in clinical medicine. The plasma electrolytes contain 155 milliequivalents of cations and an equal number of anions.

Sodium (Na)	142	Bicarbonate (HCO_3)	27
Potassium (K)	5	Chloride (Cl)	103
Calcium (Ca)	5	Phosphate (HPO_4)	2
Magnesium (Mg)	3	Sulfate (CO_4)	1
		Organic acid	6
		Protein	16
Total	155	Total	155

Table 2-3. Effects of various agents on circulation

Drug	*Effect on myocardium*	*Effect on conductive system of heart*	*Effect on vascular bed, arterioles, or blood pressure*
Procaine	Depressed by intravenous dose; no effect during regional anesthesia	Rate decreased at first, then tachycardia noted	No effect during regional anesthesia; intravenous doses dilate due to direct action on smooth muscle; constriction in toxic doses
Pontocaine	Same as above, but ten times more potent	Same as above, but ten times more potent	Same as above, but ten times more potent
Xylocaine	Same as above, but two times more potent; has vasoconstrictor action on vascular bed	Same as above, but two times more potent; has vasoconstrictor action on vascular bed	Same as above, but two times more potent; has vasoconstrictor action on vascular bed
Pronestyl (procaine amide)	Depresses excitability of all cardiac muscle	Causes bradycardia; large doses produce bundle-branch block and ventricular tachycardia	Lowers blood pressure
Curare	No significant effect	Does not prevent arrhythmias; no effect on ECG	No significant effect with therapeutic doses, but blood pressure may fall
Succinylcholine	No effect	Curarizing doses do not change heart rate; high doses may cause tachycardia	Blood pressure unchanged; high dose may raise blood pressure
Digitalis	Increases tonus, excitability, contractility, and refractory phase of cardiac muscle	Heartbeats are slower but more powerful; conduction slowed through bundle of His	Blood pressure generally unchanged; toxic dose may raise blood pressure

Oxygen (deficiency)	Depresses	Rate increased at first with increased minute output; slowing later; then irregularities due to functional changes in conductive system	Blood vessels dilated by anoxemia; constricted by excess oxygen tension
Epinephrine	Stimulates; increases output	Increases rate	Constricts
Levophed	No notable stimulating effect	Increases cardiac output	Increases peripheral resistance
Ephedrine	Stimulates; increases output	Increases rate	Constricts
Neo-Synephrine	Stimulates; increases output	Increases rate	Constricts
Cobefrin	Same as epinephrine, but less potent	Same as epinephrine	Constricts
Wyamine (mephentermine)	Stimulates; increases output	Does not initiate ventricular fibrillation in cyclopropane anesthesia	Increases peripheral resistance
Aramine (metaraminol)	Similar to ephedrine but more potent; stimulates, but large doses depress	Rate quickened, sometimes slowed; occasional arrhythmias	Vascular bed constricted
Physostigmine (eserine)	Depresses cardiac muscular excitability	Generally slows rate and converts irregular rhythm to regular	Blood pressure rises by strong vasoconstriction; peripheral vessels dilate
Neostigmine (Prostigmin)	Depresses cardiac muscular excitability	Antagonizes supraventricular tachycardias; decreases rate	Blood pressure rises by strong vasoconstriction; peripheral vessels dilate

Continued.

Table 2-3. *Effects of various agents on circulation—cont'd*

Drug	*Effect on myocardium*	*Effect on conductive system of heart*	*Effect on vascular bed, arterioles, on blood pressure*
Carbon dioxide	Output increased by moderate amounts	If pH lowered, arrhythmias result	Peripheral vessels dilate
Nitrous oxide	Not affected; depression in severe anoxia	Rate unaffected; bradycardia with anoxia	Not changed; increased with hypoxia at first, then blood pressure falls in severe hypoxia
Ethylene	Not affected; depression in severe hypoxia	No change in rhythm; hypoxia causes bradycardia and arrhythmias	Not affected; stimulated by mild hypoxia
Cyclopropane	No significant effect in Stages I, II, and III of anesthesia; depressed in Stage IV	Rate decreased; bradycardia common; arrhythmias may occur at any time, but more commonly with deep anesthesia	Little change; blood pressure may be elevated in deeper planes
Ethyl ether	No effect	Rate increased during induction, normal during maintenance; occasional arrhythmias	Unchanged; may be mildly depressed; skin vessels dilate; depressed in Stage IV of anesthesia
Vinethene	No effect	Rate may be slightly increased or decreased	No change; dilation in deep anesthesia

Chloroform	Depressed in deeper planes of anesthesia	High blood levels may cause asystole; use with epinephrine causes arrhythmias	Little change in upper planes of anesthesia; vasodilation in deeper planes
Trichloroethylene	No effect	Irregularities common; arrhythmias caused by increased vagal tone; can cause ventricular tachycardia; enhanced by epinephrine	No significant deviations
Ethyl chloride	Depressed directly	Primary decrease in rate followed by increase; cardiac output decreased; ventricular fibrillation may occur early; arrhythmias enhanced by epinephrine	No affected; peripheral vasodilation in deep planes of anesthesia from depression of vasomotor center
Pentothal (thiopental sodium)	Not affected; depressed by massive dose	Rate increased; arrhythmias not common with adequate oxygenation; does not sensitize heart to epinephrine	Blood pressure may fall during induction and deep hypnosis; normal during maintenance
Nembutal and Seconal	No effect; depressed by massive dose	Rate unchanged during hypnosia or sedation; tachycardias and arrhythmias with massive doses; does not sensitize heart to epinephrine	No significant effect; massive doses cause hypotension

EFFECTS OF VARIOUS AGENTS ON CIRCULATION

Table 2-3 shows the effects of various general anesthetic agents, anticholinesterase drugs, muscle relaxants, local anesthetic agents, digitalis, sympathomimetic agents, carbon dioxide, and oxygen want on the myocardium, directly, on the specific tissues of the heart, and on the peripheral vascular bed.

Chapter 3

Anatomy and physiology of the nervous system

The nervous system is of vital interest to the anesthetist since all the drugs administered to obtain anesthesia affect the nervous system to some degree. For this reason anyone interested in general anesthesia should have at least a basic understanding of the anatomy and physiology of the nervous system.

The varied activities and stresses of the body are controlled and organized in respect to each other by the regulation of the chemical constitution of body fluids and by the nervous system. By means of the nervous system, the body is able to maintain a rapid coordination of function of widely separated cells and organs. Not only is the body thus able to regulate its internal functions, but it can also continuously adjust to its external environment.

For the sake of study, the nervous system may be divided into two parts: the central nervous system and the peripheral nervous system.

CENTRAL NERVOUS SYSTEM

The central nervous system consists of the brain and spinal cord. It is the depression of these structures that produces general anesthesia.

Brain (encephalon). The brain, which is located within the cranial cavity, is the largest and most complex mass of nervous tissue in the body. In the adult male, it weighs about 1,380 grams and in the female about 1,250 grams. The brain may be subdivided into the following parts.*

---

*From Elliott, H. C.: The nervous system, ed. 2, Philadelphia, 1954, J. B. Lippincott Co.

Brain (Encephalon)	Forebrain (Proencephalon)	End brain (Telencephalon)	Cerebral hemispheres, including corpus striatum, and lamina terminals or rostral end of brainstem
		Interbrain (Diencephalon)	Thalamus, hypothalamus, etc.
	Midbrain (Mesencephalon)	No subdivisions	Colliculi, red nucleus, cerebral peduncles
	Hindbrain (Rhombencephalon)	Cross brain (Metencephalon)	Cerebellum, pons
		Myelencephalon Medulla oblongata bulb	Brainstem caudal to pons

Cerebrum. The cerebrum is the largest part of the brain and fills the whole upper portion of the skull. Its outer surface is composed of gray matter and is called the cortex. The interior of the cerebrum is composed mainly of white matter. Located within the cerebrum are nerve centers that control mental activity such as awareness, intelligence, reason, and memory. The functioning cerebrum permits the interpretation and correlation of various sensations and allows a person a degree of control over certain reflexes and responses to stimuli. Since it is the primary seat of consciousness, its depression is of vital importance to the anesthetist. However, no one area of the cerebrum reacts independently since all portions are connected, and any activity is the result of changes throughout the entire cortex.

The thalamus and the hypothalamus, located within the diencephalon, are important structures within the functional brain. Although there is no general agreement on the exact function of the thalamus, most writers state that certain nuclei are associated with definite sensory systems. Some authorities assert that thalamic activity is intimately related to cortical activity.

The hypothalamus is the correlation center of the autonomic system and thus is involved in both simple and complex activities. It is concerned with the regulation of body temperature, metabolism, fluid balance, and sleep and may even be a factor in personality and moods.

Closely related to the brainstem and deep in each cerebral hemisphere are the basal nuclei (ganglia). The nuclei include the thalamus, hypothalamus, and other structures such as relay stations of the sensory and motor nerve fibers that connect the spinal cord and the brain.

Midbrain. The midbrain, which has no subdivisions, is a short, constricted portion of the base of the brain that connects the pons and cerebellum with the hemispheres of the cerebrum. Functionally, it carries tracts connecting with other parts of the nervous system, such as the corticospinal and sensory pathways. The midbrain evidently dominates and organizes simple reticular activities of the bulb. Fine coordination appears to be located within the midbrain, although its status in this respect is uncertain.

Cerebellum. The cerebellum, which lies behind the pons and medulla and below the cerebrum, occupies the inferior and posterior part of the skull cavity. Its surface consists of gray matter. The activities of the cerebellum in man are below the level of consciousness, and this organ most likely acts as a reflex center. The maintenance of muscular tone, coordination, and equilibrium is a function of the cerebellum.

Pons (varolii). The pons, the bulbous section of the brain, is located between the midbrain and the medulla oblongata. Functionally, the pons acts as a connection between the cerebellum, medulla, and midbrain. Also, within the pons is located the nucleus of the fifth (trigeminal), sixth (abducens), seventh (facial), and eighth (acoustic) cranial nerves.

Medulla oblongata. The medulla oblongata is continuous with the spinal cord and extends from this structure to the lower margin of the pons. The medulla is about 1 inch in length and externally resembles the spinal cord. All the afferent and efferent tracts of the spinal cord are present in the medulla, and all impulses between the spinal cord and the brain must pass through it. Also within the medulla are nerve cells grouped to form nuclei that give rise to the ninth (glossopharyngeal), tenth (vagus), eleventh (accessory), and twelfth (hypoglossal) cranial nerves.

In addition to being the main link between the spinal cord and the brain, the medulla contains the vital nerve centers that control cardiac function, vascoconstriction, and respiration. In addition to these, other reflex functions such as coughing, sneezing, and vomiting are located within the medulla.

Reticular formation system. The brainstem reticular formation system is a part of the central nervous system and is made up of a multisynaptic network of nerve cells and fibers. It is actually the reticular core of the brainstem, and extends through the medulla, pons, and midbrain, with relays in the thalamic and hypothalamic nuclei and the cerebral cortex (Fig. 3-1).

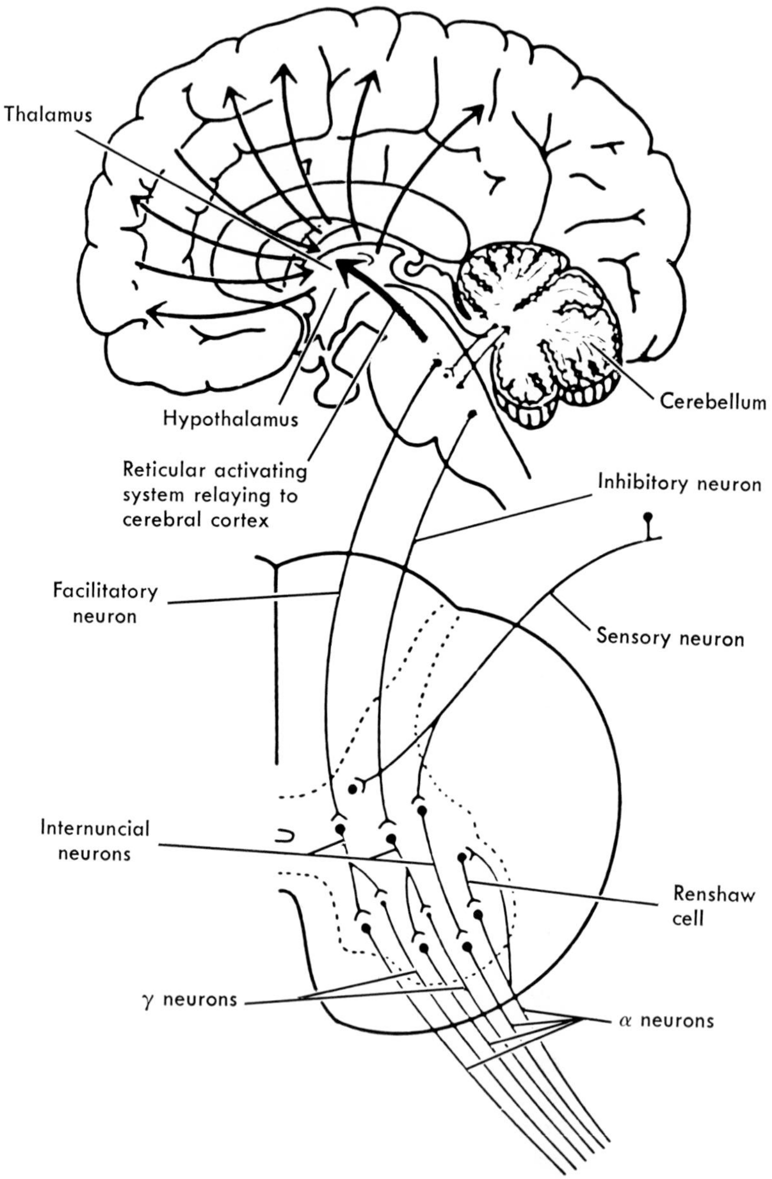

Fig. 3-1. Connections of the brainstem reticular formation system. Stippled area: brainstem reticular formation. (From Wyburn, G. M.: Nervous system, New York, 1963, Academic Press, Inc.)

The reticular formation produces an effect on respiration and circulation, thus indicating the presence or association of respiratory, cardiac, and vasomotor centers. Also worthy of note are the effects of the reticular activating system on the cerebral cortex, whereby an "arousal" mechanism maintains a state of awareness and wakefulness. Although the reticular activating system can be depressed with resulting unconsciousness, it should not be looked upon as the seat of consciousness.

Spinal cord. The spinal cord is contained within the spinal canal of the vertebral column. Superiorly, it is continuous with the medulla oblongata and extends inferiorly to about the level of the first or second lumbar vertebra. It is an important structure for reflex action of the extremities, and included within it are the principal conducting pathways of the higher centers in the cord and brain.

Longitudinal bundles of fibers or spinal cord tracts conduct impulses up and down the spinal canal. Those fibers which arise from lower levels and conduct impulses upward are termed ascending tracts, while those which arise from higher levels and conduct impulses downward are termed descending tracts. Independent tracts perform separate functions, such as transmitting impulses of touch, heat, cold, pain, and movement.

The depression of the central nervous system is responsible for the induction of general anesthesia. Sections of the central nervous system (brain and spinal cord) are paralyzed in an irregular manner in that the medulla is bypassed temporarily by the depressing action of the anesthetic agents as the cerebrum, cerebellum, and spinal cord are affected progressively. In general, anesthetics exert their influence upon the brain and spinal cord from above downward, with paralysis of the spinal nerves following loss of consciousness, special senses, and coordination. Depression and paralysis of the medullary centers of respiration and circulation are the last to occur.

The brain receives a profuse blood supply by way of the internal carotid and veretbral arteries, and although it represents only about 2% of the body weight, it receives about 33% of the output of the left ventricle. This enormous blood supply accounts for the high oxygen consumption of the central nervous system. Anoxia for 10 seconds will produce unconsciousness, whereas anoxia for a period of 4 minutes will, in a vast majority of persons, produce irreversible damage. Periods of hypoxia may produce varying degrees of injury to the central nervous system, resulting in personality changes and other manifestations of damage.

PERIPHERAL NERVOUS SYSTEM

The peripheral portion of the central nervous system is composed primarily of the following: cranial nerves, spinal nerves, and autonomic nervous system.

Cranial nerves. The cranial nerves are attached to the brainstem. Each of them has a nucleus either at its origin or at its termination within the central nervous system, and each nucleus is connected with the cerebral cortex. The cranial nerves differ from the spinal nerves in that some are entirely motor, some entirely sensory, and some both sensory and motor (sensorimotor).

Although the cranial nerves are conventionally numbered as twelve pairs, the optic nerve is not a true nerve, while the olfactory is a group of small bundles. However, the traditional listing is as follows:

I. Olfactory	Not a true nerve, but a fiber tract of the brain.
II. Optic	Also not a true nerve, but a fiber tract of the brain.
III. Oculomotor	Has motor branches to all the ocular muscles except the lateral rectus and superior oblique; also parasympathetic fibers to the sphincter of the pupil and to the ciliary muscle.
IV. Trochlear	Innervates the superior oblique muscle, which rotates the eyeball inward and downward.
V. Trigeminal	The primary sensory nerve of the face and head (tongue and teeth); some motor fibers run to the muscles of mastication.
VI. Abducens	Rotates the eyeball outward by supplying the two heads of the lateral rectus muscle.
VII. Facial	Supplies motor and sensory innervations to the head, face, ears, tongue, and neck.
VIII. Auditory	Controls hearing and equilibrium.
IX. Glossopharyngeal	Supplies sensory and motor innervations to the tongue, tonsils, and pharynx.
X. Vagus	Motor and sensory; has a wider distribution (extending through the neck, thorax, and abdomen) than any other cranial nerve.
XI. Accessory	Purely motor; consists of a cranial and spinal part and is accessory to the vagus nerve.
XII. Hypoglossal	The motor nerve to the muscles of the tongue.

Spinal nerves. There are thirty-one pairs of spinal nerves, divided into five groups. Each group derives its name from the region of the vertebral column from which they emerge. They are cervical (eight pairs), thoracic (twelve pairs), lumbar (five pairs), sacral (five pairs), and coccygeal (one pair).

The spinal nerves are mixed nerves containing both motor and sensory fibers, and each nerve divides into four main trunks after leaving the spinal column: (1) meningeal—to the meninges; (2) dorsal—

to the muscles and skin of the back of the head, neck, and trunk; (3) ventral—to the extremities and body anterior to the spine; and (4) visceral—connecting with sympathetic ganglia and called autonomic nerves.

Sensory nerves conduct impulses toward the central nervous system. These are afferent impulses, and the nerves are composed of afferent fibers. Motor nerves conduct impulses away from the central nervous system (efferent impulses).

This difference in function does not depend upon the properties of the nerve fibers themselves, since, if a nerve is stimulated experimentally anywhere along its length, identical impulses will be conducted in both directions from the point of stimulation. An impulse that travels over an axon contrary to normal direction is called antidromic. This does not normally occur in the body because of anatomical connections of sense organs with sensory nerves and motor nerves with muscles. Also, synaptic junctions between axons, unlike the axons themselves, conduct in one direction only.

A sequence of investigations has demonstrated that chemical substances are formed at synaptic and neural tissue junctions that have excitatory properties resembling those of certain drugs. On the basis of similarities to effects produced by epinephrine and acetylcholine, Dale suggests that fibers which produce such substances at their terminals be called adrenergic and cholinergic, respectively.

In the adrenergic group are most of the postganglionic fibers of the sympathetic nervous system, although there are some exceptions. The cholinergic group contains all the preganglionic fibers of the sympathetic nerves and most of the fibers of the parasympathetic nerves, as well as motor fibers to skeletal muscles.

Since stimulation of sympathetic nerves may augment the action of some organs and inhibit the action of others, it has been postulated that epinephrine or norepinephrine, the neurohumoral agents of the sympathetic system, combine with alpha or beta receptors to produce their effects. The alpha receptors are generally considered to be excitatory whereas the beta receptors are inhibitory.

Acetylcholine is synthesized in cholinergic nerves by the action of the enzyme choline-acetylase. Upon stimulation of the nerve acetylcholine, the neurohumoral agent of the parasympathetic system, is released. Normally, the acetylcholine exists only momentarily at the synapse or motor end plate, being rapidly hydrolyzed by the enzyme cholinesterase. A number of drugs (for example, eserine and neostigmine) act as anticholinesterases, inhibiting the action of cholinesterase and thereby prolonging the action of acetylcholine.

The presence in serum of a nonspecific cholinesterase was demonstrated by Mendel and Rudney. They called it pseudocholinesterase. It differs from true cholinesterase in being capable of hydrolizing noncholine esters (for example, tributyrin) as well as acetylcholine. Pseudocholinesterase is most active when the acetylcholine concentration is high, whereas it has but slight hydrolytic action at the low physiological concentration of acetylcholine at which true cholinesterase is most active.

The cells of origin of the sympathetic division of the autonomic nervous system are situated in the lateral horns of the spinal cord from C-8 or Th-1 to L-2 or L-3. The axons of these cells leave the cord by the corresponding anterior nerve roots and connect with nerve cells in one or another of the outlying ganglia. The fibers arising from the cells of the ganglia are nonmedullated and are called postganglionic. The fibers arising from the spinal cord are medullated and are called preganglionic.

In the parasympathetic system, the cells giving rise to parasympathetic fibers are situated at three different levels in the central nervous system. The axons of these cells leave the central nervous system to connect with ganglion cells lying within or closely related to the innervated organ. The axons of the central cells are called preganglionic. Those of the ganglion are postganglionic.

In order for an impulse to traverse the length of a nerve fiber, a difference of electrical potential must exist. This potential exists since the outer covering of the nerve fiber has a positive charge and the inner surface has a negative charge. When the nerve fiber is in this state, it is said to be polarized. If, however, through the action of some blocking agent, such as a local anesthetic, the nerve membrane is made impervious to electrolytes. The membrane cannot become depolarized and the impulse cannot be conducted beyond that area.

Autonomic nervous system. The autonomic nervous system is concerned with the internal environment of the body. This is in contrast to the rest of the central nervous system, which deals with response to external stimuli. It supplies smooth muscle, cardiac muscle, and glandular tissues throughout the body and thus regulates visceral organs, especially those of circulation, respiration, digestion, excretion, and reproduction. This system functions with a marked degree of independence, and a person normally exerts little direct influence over it. As such, the autonomic centers within the cerebral cortex have little control over the autonomic system. The so-called automatic centers in the cerebral cortex seem to provide for cooperation rather than control.

The hypothalamus, in the diencephalon, is said to be the correlating center of the autonomic system. It supposedly regulates and coordinates the more fragmentary activities of the lower centers in the brain stem and spinal cord. It integrates these activities into harmonious patterns and is thus involved in both simple and complex actions. Autonomic controls are also centered in the cerebellum, medulla, and brain stem, as well as in the thalamus and cortex. The fundamental significance and complete function of all these structures are by no means clear.

Anatomically, the autonomic nervous system might be considered a definite portion of the nervous system. However, physiologically, pathologically, and pharmacologically it acts as a functional unit. The anatomical concept of the autonomic nervous system, therefore, comprises all the nerves, peripheral ganglia, and centers that serve the internal organs.

The autonomic nervous system is divided into two portions: the sympathetic (thoracolumbar) system and the parasympathetic (craniosacral) system.

The sympathetic portion of the autonomic system is derived from the eighth cervical nerve to the twelfth thoracic nerve and the first, second, and third lumbar nerves and thus is termed the thoracolumbar division. The parasympathetic portion is derived from the third, seventh, ninth, and tenth cervical nerves and the second, third, and fourth sacral nerves and thus is termed the craniosacral division.

A REVIEW OF AUTONOMIC DRUGS AND THERAPY

The autonomic nervous system provides for the integration of various body mechanisms in time of stress and corrects changes in the internal environment of the body that might be detrimental to its function. In doing so it attempts to maintain a stable equilibrium, or homeostasis, by which the body is best suited to maintain its functional integrity at optimal conditions.

General anesthesia is a peculiar type of stress in that its end result produces changes in the adaptive mechanisms, as well as in the various body tissue. The suitability of an agent, therefore, depends on its ability to depress higher centers, producing anesthesia and relaxation with minimal change in the autonomic system. It is the relative insensitivity of medullary, respiratory, and vasomotor centers to anesthetic depression that provides the rationale for safe anesthesia.

Various anesthetic agents are similar in that they have a depressant action on the central nervous system. They do not, however, depress the centers in the same manner or order. Supplementary drugs are used because of their selective nature to affect vital functions and improve physical status while maintaining central depression.

To aid the anesthetist in maintaining a correct physiological function and obtaining optimal anesthetic conditions, certain drugs known as the autonomic drugs are available.

A knowledge of the anatomy and function of the various portions of the autonomic system aids in understanding the working of the autonomic drugs and provides a rationale for their actions. Excluding the autonomic centers of the central nervous system, such as the vasopressor and respiratory centers in the medulla and the integration areas of the hypothalamus and cortex, the autonomic nervous system consists of various ganglia and peripheral nerve fibers. These fibers are both afferent and efferent. The afferent fibers are carried into the cerebrospinal axis by the vagus, pelvic, splanchnic, and other autonomic nerves, and their cell bodies lie in the dorsal root ganglia of the spinal nerves and the sensory ganglia of certain cranial nerves. These nerves create a synapse within the central nervous system with nerves which in turn produce a synapse with neurons in the autonomic ganglia located outside the central nervous system, which completes the reflex arc.

On the efferent side, two divisions exist: the sympathetic, or thoracolumbar, and the parasympathetic, or craniosacral. The two systems have distinct physiological and anatomical differences. They are not always antagonists but may have synergistic or dissimilar actions. In the sympathetic nervous system, the preganglionic fibers arise in the spinal cord from Th-1 to L-3, inclusive, and create a synapse with neurons outside the cerebrospinal axis lying in the sympathetic ganglia. Postganglionic neurons innervate the effector organs. An exception, however, is the adrenal medulla (Th-5, Th-6, and Th-7), which is directly innervated by preganglionic fibers.

The parasympathetic innervation is directed through fibers of the third, seventh, ninth, and tenth cranial nerves and the second to fourth sacral nerves. In contrast to the sympathetic system, ganglia are located close to the effector cells, and the ratio of postganglionic to preganglionic fibers is lower. The result of this is that sympathetic stimulation produces a much more diffuse effect than does parasympathetic stimulation.

The sympathetic system is not essential for life, but it does function constantly and increase its outflow during times of stress. The parasympathetic system is concerned with conservation and restoration of energy by such functions as slowing the heart rate, lowering blood pressure, and aiding in alimentation.

The neurohumoral concept of transmission of nerve impulses provides the basis for chemical intervention by drug therapy. Autonomic drugs affect end organs by intervening during the humoral phase of synaptic transmission. They may do so by competing with, inactivating, or destroying the normal enzymatic reactions at the synapse and may also affect the end organ directly.

The autonomic drugs may be divided into groups which, by their action on end organs, are similar or antagonistic to the actions of the sympathetic and parasympathetic nervous systems. The differences in action of the various drugs may be attributed to the fact that they may effect one or more of the individual portions of the system to a greater or lesser extent than others.

These drugs may not act specifically on the end organs of the autonomic nervous system, but because of the integration of the somatic and autonomic nerves within the central nervous system, they also may have somatic effects. Conversely, nerves of the cerebrospinal axis may show autonomic properties. It is not physiologically correct to view the autonomic nervous system as a strictly peripheral network since autonomic reflexes may be elicited from spinal to cortical levels. The former is illustrated in reflex activities produced by temperature changes, whereas the latter is seen in the correlation of somatic and vegetative functions such as those within the scope of emotional activity and conditioned reflexes.

A logical division of the autonomic drugs is to group them by anatomy and those affecting either the sympathetic or parasympathetic system and by principal effects of stimulation and depression. Thus we have (1) sympathomimetic (adrenergic), (2) sympatholytic (adrenergic blocking), (3) parasympathomimetic (cholinergic), and (4) parasympatholytic (cholinergic blocking). Also included in the grouping are the cholinesterase-inhibiting drugs and the ganglionic blocking agents.

Anatomically, adrenergic fibers are autonomic fibers in which impulses cause the appearance of norepinephrine at their termination. Cholinergic fibers carry impulses mediated by acetylcholine. All postganglionic fibers of the sympathetic division are adrenergic, with the exception mentioned on p. 80. All preganglionic fibers of the sympathetic and parasympathetic divisions and postganglionic fibers of the parasympathetic division are cholinergic. Acetylcholine is also associated with impulses by sympathetic nerves to sweat glands and certain vascular beds, splanchnic fibers to the adrenal medulla, and the cerebrospinal motor fibers to skeletal muscle.

Autonomic agents. Autonomic agents are drugs that mimic or oppose the effects of impulses from the autonomic nervous system.

Parasympathomimetic agents. Parasympathomimetic agents may be divided into three groups: the choline esters, the cholinesterase inhibitors, and the naturally occurring cholinergic alkaloids.

Acetylcholine is of interest mainly because of its experimental importance as a natural neurohumoral mediator and because knowledge of its action better enables one to understand other parasympathomimetic agents.

Three distinct actions of acetylcholine may be noted: muscarinic, nicotinic, and curariform. Muscarinic actions are those of the postganglionic cholinergic fibers and may be blocked specifically by atropine. These fibers innervate the visceral autonomic effector organs (smooth and cardiac muscle and exocrine gland cells). Nicotinic actions are seen at the autonomic ganglia and adrenal medulla. The curariform action takes place at the skeletal myoneural junction. It is due to persistent depolarization of the motor end plate and produces paralysis of skeletal muscle. Curariform action may be viewed as a form of nicotinic action because of certain similarities between the autonomic ganglion and the myoneural junction. Thus nicotine and curare block the nicotine actions of acetycholine, nicotine acting mainly on the ganglia and curare on the myoneural junction.

Acetylcholine is produced in neural impulse and acts directly on effector cells to cause depolarization of the postsynaptic membrane. This response is of very short duration due to the rapid hydrolysis by cholinesterase, an enzyme present in blood and tissues.

Pharmacological responses to acetylcholine may vary, owing to antagonistic effects produced by the nicotinic and muscarinic properties. Normally, the muscarinic properties predominate. Peripheral autonomic effects may be counteracted by acetylcholine-induced sympathoadrenal discharge.

The cardiovascular system will respond to intravenous doses with vasodilation, drop in blood pressure, bradycardia, and electrocardiographic irregularities. Therapeutic doses may produce only a slight fall in blood pressure, owing to autonomic compensatory mechanisms and rapid destruction.

Acetylcholine in higher concentrations causes increased smooth muscle tone, peristalsis, and stimulation of secretions. In the exocrine glands, an increase in salivation, lacrimation, and sweating is noted. Bronchospasm and increased secretion may be seen in the bronchial tree.

Other agents similar to acetycholine, but exhibiting greater stability, are utilized in situations in which parasympathetic effects are desired.

The following drugs are utilized because of nicotinic ganglionic, nicotinic neuromuscular, and muscarinic properties.

Methacholine is less readily hydrolyzed by cholinesterase but shows similar properties, with the exception that nicotinic effects are less prominent. It finds its chief use in paroxysmal atrial tachycardia, certain peripheral vascular diseases, and intestinal distention.

Carbachol differs from methocholine in that it is not hydrolyzed by cholinesterase. It also has greater gastrointestinal and urinary effects and cardiac activity than has methacholine.

Urecholine (bethanechol) is not affected by cholinesterase and has little or no nicotinic properties. Its actions are directed mainly to the urinary bladder, gastrointestinal tract, and eyes.

Cholinesterase inhibitors enhance the action of acetylcholine by removing the means for its elimination. *Physostigmine* (eserine) and *neostigmine* (Prostigmin) inhibit cholinesterase by forming a reversible bond with it. They are used in the treatment of glaucoma to reduce intraocular tension by producing miosis, which facilitates reabsorption of aqueous humor. They are also utilized in the treatment of gastrointestinal atony, urinary retention, and myasthenia gravis.

Of special interest is edrophonium (Tensilon). Its curare-antagonizing properties make it useful in curare-induced respiratory depression. Unlike the preceding drugs, its actions on skeletal muscle are more prominent than those on autonomic ganglia or cholinergic visceral receptors. The skeletal muscle effects of this drug seem to be the result of both a direct action on the end plate and its anticholinesterase activity. In practice, edrophonium should not be used if the patient is apneic since it is in itself a blocking agent, and the effect on respiratory exchange is the only means of judging dosage. Untoward effects are chiefly muscarinic in nature, such as visual disturbances, lacrimation, perspiration, mild gastrointestinal stimulation, slight hypotension, and bradycardia.

Pilocarpine is the only drug in the third group that is commonly used clinically. It is highly selective in action, affecting almost entirely cells innervated by postganglionic cholinergic fibers. In other words, its action is entirely muscarinic. It is used therapeutically to produce miosis and promote salivation in the treatment of xerostomia.

Sympathomimetic agents. Many sympathomimetic drugs, varying in intensity, duration, and principal sites of action, are available.

Epinephrine is the standard of comparison for these drugs since it probably is the one that has been studied the most extensively; however, norepinephrine is more important in the neurohumoral conductive mechanisms of the body.

Epinephrine acts directly on effector cells, producing inhibition in some cells and excitation in others. Denervation of effector organs greatly enhances their sensitivity to epinephrine. No specific enzyme that destroys epinephrine exists, and thus its effect is more prolonged than that of acetylcholine. The actions of epinephrine are similar to those produced by stimulation of adrenergic nerves. They include mydriasis of the iris, acceleration of heart rate, increased stroke volume, and arrhythmia. Dilation of coronary vessels, constriction of cutaneous vessels, and dilation of muscle vascular beds occur. Subcutaneous injection causes systolic pressure to rise, but diastolic pressure falls. This rise in pulse pressure is due to increased cardiac output, and the diastrolic drop to the predominance of vasodilation over vasoconstriction in the peripheral circulation.

The bronchial muscle is relaxed, gastrointestinal tone is decreased, and salivary glands are stimulated to produce a sparse but thick mucinous secretion. The blood sugar level is increased by acceleration of glycogenolysis in the liver and muscles. In conventional therapeutic doses epinephrine has little stimulating effect, in contrast to other sympathomimetic amines.

Epinephrine is used clinically in local control of hemorrhage, in the treatment of the congestion of nasal mucosa, and in local anesthesia because of its vasoconstricting effect. It may be used with caution in the treatment of heart block and cardiac arrest due to asystole by direct application to heart muscle. It should not be used in the treatment of shock because of its secondary vasodilating activity. The most dramatic use may be seen in the treatment of asthma and allergic phenomena, where prompt administration may be lifesaving.

Levarterenol (Levophed) is the major pressor amine present in postganglionic adrenergic nerves. Its pharmacological properties are similar to those of epinephrine but have less activity. The chief difference between the two is the rise in diastolic pressure, along with systolic, and the increase in total peripheral resistance. Reflex vagal bradycardia may occur, but arrhythmias are still evident. The hyperglycemia produced is not as marked with epinephrine.

Levarterenol is used as a potent vasopressor in certain types of shock. It is administered as an intravenous drip and may be effective when other vasopressors fail. It is ineffective in the treatment of cardiac arrest and complete heart block and may precipitate ventricular arrhythmias.

Ephedrine differs from epinephrine in that it is effective orally and has a more prolonged action. It also lacks the vasodilator components of epinephrine. Tachyphylaxis is also noted, which is absent with epinephrine. Ephedrine is used clinically in spinal anesthesia because of its prolonged vasopressor action. For this effect it is administered subcutaneously or intravenously with caution. It may be incorporated into the anesthetic agent to prolong and intensify the anesthesia. It is also administered in the treatment of postural hypotension, Stokes-Adams disease, and allergic disorders such as bronchial asthma and hay fever; it is also used as a mydriatic of short duration.

Amphetamine resembles ephedrine in a number of respects, but it has a greater ability to stimulate higher nervous centers. It has an addiction potential, and tolerance may be exhibited. Chief therapeutic actions involve its effects on the central nervous system, and it is useful in the treatment of narcolepsy, parkinsonism, alcoholism, and psychogenic disorders. It is widely used to reduce the appetite in obese persons.

Phenylephrine (Neo-Synephrine) has predominantly cardiovascular actions. Along with the sustained vasopressor effect, a pronounced and consistent bradycardia is noted, which coincides with the rise in diastolic pressure. Cardiac irregularities are noted rarely, and cyclopropane-induced arrhythmias are fewer than with other sympathomimetic amines.

Therapeutic uses include topical application in the treatment of sinusitis, production of mydriasis, and as a vasopressor agent with minimal side effects and absence of tachyphylaxis. This agent is also effective by inhalation in the treatment of bronchial asthma.

Methoxamine (Vasoxyl) is outstanding for its sustained vasopressor action, brought about almost exclusively by increased peripheral resistance. It is used to increase blood pressure without cardiac stimulation and appears to be safely administered during cyclopropane anesthesia.

Mephentermine (Wyamine) is similar to methoxamine in that it has a prolonged duration of action and minor effect on the myocardium. Its principal uses are as a nasal decongestant and for support of blood pressure in hypotensive states.

Metamphetamine (Desoxyn; desoxyephedrine) is quite similar in action to amphetamine, but has slightly less effect on the cardiovascular system and is a more potent central stimulant. It is employed primarily for its central action.

Isoproterenol (Aludrine; Isuprel) is a valuable bronchodilator in the treatment of asthma. It is administered by oral inhalation as an aerosol and is somewhat more active than epinephrine by this route. It is of value in the treatment of status asthmaticus. Side effects are due to action on the myocardium and central nervous system. Intravenous or intramuscular injection produces a marked fall in blood pressure due to vasodilation.

Agents of dissimilar chemical structure used principally as nasal decongestants include, among others, naphazoline (Privine), cyclopentamine (Clopane), tuaminoheptane (Tuamine), and prophylhexedrine (Benedrex).

Autonomic blocking agents. Autonomic blocking agents are drugs that inhibit the transmission of autonomic impulses.

Cholinergic blocking agents (muscarinic-inhibiting). Muscarinic-inhibiting cholinergic blocking agents are drugs that inhibit transmission of nervous impulses at the postganglionic autonomic affector cells.

Postganglionic cholinergic nerves. The autonomic blocking agents are drugs inhibiting structures innervated by postganglionic cholinergic nerves. The naturally occurring belladonna alkaloids, atropine and scopolamine, are representative of this series. Synthetic substitutes have been introduced for specific purposes, but they are not so useful over as wide a range of therapy as the naturally occurring drugs.

Atropine and *scopolamine* exhibit actions on the central nervous system and block the cholinergic-stimulated organs. Therefore, in a general way, the end result may resemble sympathetic stimulation.

Scopolamine is a more effective blocking agent for the iris, ciliary body, and salivary, bronchial, and sweat glands, whereas the action of atropine is more pronounced on the cardiac, intestinal, and bronchial musculatures. Centrally, scopolamine exhibits greater activity; drowsiness, euphoria, amnesia, and sometimes excitement and restlessness occur. Atropine in small doses usually produces mild vagal excitation and respiratory stimulation.

The therapeutic uses of these drugs are varied. In obstetrics, scopolamine combined with a barbiturate or meperidine has been used to obtain amnesia and analgesia. Atropine and scopolamine are useful in preventing laryngospasm during intravenous barbiturate anesthesia. They are also used to reduce salivary and pulmonary secretions and correct bradycardia. In ophthalmology, they find use as mydriatic and cycloplegic agents. Probably the most extensive use of the belladonna alkaloids is in the treatment of gastrointestinal disorders. These drugs and their synthetic counterparts act as antispasmodics and control excess motor activity. Side effects produced include difficulty in vision, dizziness, palpitation, and xerostomia.

The synthetic alkaloids in this series are utilized almost exclusively for their mydriatic or antispasmodic activities.

Cholinergic blocking agents (nicotinic-inhibiting). Nicotinic-inhibiting cholinergic blocking agents are capable of inhibiting neuromuscular transmission.

Drugs inhibiting skeletal muscle and ganglionic blocking agents. These drugs are grouped together because of the similarity of their action. *Curare,* the curariform drugs, and the methoniums act on both the end plates of skeletal muscle and ganglion cells.

Curare (Intocostrin) in its commonly used form—*d*-tubocurarine—and its dimethyl ether (Metubine; Mecostrin) produce elevation of the threshold of the motor end plate to acetylcholine by competing with it. However, they also show mild ganglionic blocking effects and a histamine-like action. They are effectively antagonized by the anticholinesterases. Like other curarizing agents, their principal uses are in general anesthesia as skeletal muscle relaxants and in shock therapy.

Gallamine (Flaxedil) is similar in action to curare, but its duration of action is slightly shorter. It has little ganglionic blocking action and does not cause the release of significant amounts of histamine.

The *methonium* compounds vary from those which produce neuromuscular blockade almost entirely to those which are principally ganglionic blocking agents.

Decamethonium (C-10; Syncurine) is of the former group. Its action is produced by sustained depolarization of the end plate and is not antagonized by the anticholinesterases. The action of C-10 is definitely shorter than the above drugs, and there may be some tachyphylaxis. It is eliminated in the urine unchanged.

Succinylcholine (Anectine; Quelicin) is the most commonly used depolarizing neuromuscular blocking agent. It is similar to C-10 in its action except for its rapid hydrolysis by nonspecific plasma cholinesterase. For this reason, it should be used with caution in the treatment of patients with liver disease or malnutrition. Doses of succinylcholine much larger than required for neuromuscular blockade stimulate and then depress autonomic ganglia. Because succinylcholine hydrolyzes rapidly, the intensity of muscular relaxation may be controlled from moment to moment.

Pentamethonium (C-5), hexamethonium (C-6), Bistrium, Arfonad, and *TEA* are agents that show very little activity on the neuromuscular end plates but are effective blocking agents at both sympathetic and parasympathetic ganglia. It is therefore difficult to predict empirically the actions of various members, since a predominance of either sympathetic or parasympathetic stimuli is involved. These vary with the physiological state of the end organ and may change under different circumstances.

In most organs, one system has predominance over the other, although a balance of stimuli is maintained. C-6 is representative of this group. Its administration may decrease blood pressure and peripheral resistance and produce hypotension. Gastric motility is inhibited, and the pupil is slightly dilated. The effects of administration may be overcome by epinephrine or norepinephrine since peripheral effector cells remain sensitive to autonomic drugs.

C-5 and C-6 are used in the treatment of hypertensive heart disease and peripheral vascular disorders and in surgically controlled hypotension.

Adrenergic blocking agents. Adrenergic blocking agents prevent the effector cells from responding to sympathetic adrenergic nerve impulses and to the epinephrine-type amines. The blocking action takes place at the effector cells and is more effective against circulating agents than against nerve impulses.

Drugs in this group have their principal value as peripheral vasodilating agents in the treatment of peripheral vascular diseases such as Raynaud's disease, and they are of use in surgery for pheochromocytoma since they act to stabilize blood pressure. Their role in the medical control of hypertension is still being evaluated.

Cardiac arrhythmias that occur during the deeper stages of cyclopropane anesthesia may be prevented with these agents, especially in thyrotoxicosis, in which the heart is particularly sensitive to adrenergic stimuli.

Drugs in this group include dibenzyline, the ergot alkaloids, tolazoline (Priscoline), and phentolamine (Regitine). Much remains to be learned about their nature and actions, but they are extremely useful adjuncts in therapy.

Chapter 4

Physics as applied to anesthesia

In the study of anesthesia it is necessary to apply a knowledge of physics since one is constantly dealing with gases under pressure, partial pressure of gases, diffusion of gases, solubility of gases, and so forth. It will therefore be advantageous to review a few basic principles of physics that apply to anesthesia and the anesthetic equipment.

Structure of matter. Molecules of gases may be composed of one or more atoms. There are three structural types of elemental gases: (1) monatomic (helium), (2) diatomic (nitrogen, oxygen, and hydrogen), and (3) triatomic (ozone).

An atom is the smallest quantity of an element that can exist and still retain the chemical properties of the element.

A molecule is a chemical combination of two or more atoms that form a specific chemical substance.

An element is a simple substance that cannot be decomposed by chemical means and that is made up of atoms.

A compound is composed of two or more elements chemically united to form a substance different from the individual elements in its composition.

Molecular movement. The molecules of which matter is composed are in a state of incessant motion, and the magnitude of the movement and the ability of the molecules to alter their position will vary according to whether the substance is in the solid, liquid, or gaseous state.

In the solid state, the molecules do not alter their relative positions and merely oscillate about a fixed point.

In the liquid state, the molecules are mobile and shift their position throughout the whole liquid.

In the gaseous state, at normal temperature and pressure the molecules have a much greater degree of mobility. The speed at which they travel is approximately the same in all three states.

Atomic weight. Atomic weights are relative, being based on the standard of oxygen whose weight is designated as 16. Hydrogen, being sixteen times lighter than oxygen, has an atomic weight of 1. All other atomic weights are calculated by using oxygen as the standard.

Molecular weight. The molecular weight of a substance is the sum of the atomic weights of the element or elements of which it is composed.

Vapors and gases. A gas is any elastic aeriform fluid in which the molecules are separated from one another and so have free paths.

Vapor (from the Latin) signifies steam, gas, or exhalation.

Vapors and gases behave similary in most respects, but certain technical differences may exist. A gas exists at a temperature above the critical temperature; a vapor is a gas existing at about the critical temperature of the liquid from which it is derived. A vapor may be liquefied by pressure without cooling.

Pressure. The pressure of a gas is a measure of the molecular bombardment on each unit area of the wall of its container in unit time. The closer the molecules, the greater are the number that strike each unit area, and therefore the greater is the pressure exerted. At the same temperature and pressure, the same number of molecules of any gas occupy the same volume.

Partial pressure. A single component in a mixture of gases exerts the same force in combination as it would if it existed alone.

Pressure gradient. A gas or vapor passes from a point of higher pressure to a point of lower pressure, the difference being known as the pressure gradient.

For example, during induction of ether the vapor passes from the mask, where the pressure is 30 to 40 mm. Hg, to the alveoli of the lungs, where it is less, to the blood, where it is still less, and then to the tissues, where it is zero. During recovery the reverse takes place.

Vapor pressure. When speaking of a percentage of vapor in air, one refers to its volume. Therefore, a 5% ether vapor in air means that 5% of the volume of the mixture is ether vapor and the remaining 95% is air. A mixture of gases exerts pressure on the walls of its container. The part of this total pressure that is exerted by any one of the vapors—the partial pressure of that vapor—bears the same proportion to the total pressure as the volume of the vapor bears to the volume of the mixture. Thus 5% ether vapor in air at sea level exerts a pressure of 5% of 760 mm. Hg, or 38 mm. Hg. When a liquid at a given temperature is in a closed container, the number of molecules ultimately reentering the liquid becomes exactly equal to the number leaving it. A state of equilibrium is reached; no increase in the vapor occurs. The saturated vapor now above the liquid is the strongest vapor it is possible to have at that particular temperature. At a higher temperature a higher concentration of vapor results. The boiling point of any given liquid is the temperature at which its vapor pressure equals the pressure of the atmosphere.

Density. Density equals mass divided by volume. The density of a gas is usually expressed as the weight in grams of 1 liter of that gas. Then the density in grams per liter of a gas is found by dividing the molecular weight by 22.4.

By using such data as density and specific gravity (see Table 4-1, p. 95) of a liquid anesthetic agent, one can calculate, for instance, the amount of ether vapor produced when a given amount of liquid ether or another liquid agent is volatized.

Vaporization. The molecules in a liquid are in a continuous state of motion. The liquid does not disintegrate because of a strong mutual attraction of the molecules for each other. Some of these molecules in the surface layer move with sufficient speed to overcome the attraction and escape into the surrounding atmosphere. Here they form what is called the vapor of the liquid. This escape increases with an increase in room temperature. In a closed container, evaporation stops when the concentration of the vapor above the liquid reaches a certain value for any given temperature. The process of vaporization entails an expenditure of energy. This loss of energy, which is called the latent heat of vaporization, is defined as the number of calories required to change 1 gram of the liquid into vapor without a change of temperature. Anesthetists prefer to think of the latent heat of vaporization per cubic centimeter of a liquid since they refer to volumes rather than weights of liquids. When oxygen is blown over the surface of ether, the percentage of ether vapor delivered from the bottle depends on the temperature of the liquid and on the time during which each unit volume of oxygen is in contact with the liquid ether. A more practical way of delivering a greater percentage of ether vapor is to bubble the oxygen through the ether, thereby increasing the area of contact between the ether and the oxygen.

Diffusion of gases. Diffusion of gases is a spontaneous attempt to equalize physical states. If a gas exists on either side of a permeable membrane, the direction of its diffusion is determined not by a difference in its amount but by a difference in the partial pressures that it exerts on either side of the membrane. A gas diffuses from a place where it is at a higher partial pressure to one where it is at a lower partial pressure, even though the latter area may contain a larger volume of the gas.

In the alveoli, the percentage of oxygen is 14; the partial pressure this gas exerts, therefore, is 14% of 760 mm. Hg, or 100 mm. Hg. The tension of oxygen in the venous blood in the capillaries of the lungs is 40 mm. Hg. The thin alveolar membrane is readily permeable to oxygen and allows oxygen to diffuse from the place of high partial pressure, the alveoli, to the place where it is at a lower tension, the venous blood. This process of diffusion raises the tension of oxygen in the venous blood, converting it to arterial blood.

Osmosis. Molecules of any fluid pass through thin sheets of a substance called a membrane. Membranes are said to be permeable to the particular molecules they let through. Diffusion, or intermolecular mingling, can take place through a permeable membrane on both sides of which the total pressures are equal. This process should be distinguished from transfer in bulk of the fluid, which is caused by the difference of hydrostatic pressure on either side of the membrane. Some membranes allow only certain substances (molecules) to pass through them, hence the names semipermeable membrane. Osmosis is diffusion of molecules through a semipermeable membrane, such as occurs in the lungs, for example.

Heat. The difference between heat and temperature is that heat can be given to a substance or abstracted from it, whereas temperature is the thermal state of a substance that determines whether it will give heat to, or receive heat from, another substance when brought in contact with it. The unit of heat is the calorie and is defined as the quantity of heat required to raise the temperature of 1 gram of water by 1 degree centigrade. To raise the same weight of different substances through any given range of temperature requires different quantities of heat. The specific heat of a substance is the number of calories required to raise the temperature of 1 gram of that substance by 1 degree centigrade.

Boiling point. When the pressure of a vapor from a liquid exceeds that of air, the liquid boils. The temperature at which this takes place is the boiling point. Various factors affect the boiling point, and thus the boiling point of any liquid may vary with changing conditions. For example, impurities contained within the liquid may alter its boiling point, and pressure will markedly affect the boiling point of a liquid.

While the boiling point of a liquid changes with pressure, there is a temperature above which a liquid substance can exist as a gas only. This is known as the critical temperature.

Specific volume. The volume that 1 gram of any substance—solid, liquid, or gas—occupies under given conditions of temperature and pressure is known as its specific volume. This is inversely proportional to the density. When a given weight of a gas is allowed to expand, its specific volume increases. There are now fewer molecules per cubic centimeter and fewer molecular impacts on each unit area of the walls. The pressure falls. The fall in pressure is proportional to the reduction in the number of molecular impacts on each unit area of the containing vessel and is thus inversely proportional to the increase in the specific volume. This is Boyle's law.

Solution of gases. When a gas is in contact with a liquid, the molecules of the former, in their ceaseless motion, impinge on the surface of the liquid. Some intermingle with the molecules of the liquid and are said to be in solution. The amount of a given gas that dissolves in a liquid is directly proportional to the pressure of the gas on that liquid (Henry's law). The higher the temperature, the less will be the amount of gas that goes into solution. When no further gas dissolves in a liquid, a state of equilibrium exists between the gas over the liquid and the gas dissolved in it. The liquid is said to be fully saturated with the gas at that temperature and pressure. Gasses are carried in blood in two forms—simple solution and chemical combination. In all cases a far greater amount can be carried in chemical combination.

Fluid flow. Fluid flows along a tube only when there is a pressure difference between the two ends. Fluid flows along a uniform tube from a region of high pressure to a region of low pressure. The volume of fluid flowing through a tube of given length varies as the fourth power of the diameter of the tube. The volume flow rate through a straight tube of uniform bore is directly proportional to the pressure gradient within it.

Some fluids flow through a given tube more readily than others. The only intrinsic property of the fluid that influences its flow rate is its viscosity. The coefficient of viscosity of a fluid is the measure of its rate of flow through a tube under standard conditions. The rate of flow of a fluid is inversely proportional to its coefficient of viscosity. Viscosity has the same effect on the laminar flow rate of a gas as it has on that of a liquid. These data can be appied to the rate of flow of gases through endotracheal tubes and the rate of flow of fluids through syringes and needles.

Laminar flow. When a fluid, liquid, or gas streams through a tube, the particles comprising the fluid may move parallel to the walls of the tube. The flow, smooth and orderly, is referred to as laminar flow.

Turbulent flow. If, however, the lines of flow are not parallel to the walls of the tube but are irregular and broken up, the now disorderly flow is called turbulent. When the flow is turbulent, the pressure loss rises approximately with the square of the flow rate.

When the flow rate, in liters per minute, of a given fluid in a given tube exceeds what is known as the critical flow rate, laminar flow is replaced by turbulent flow throughout the whole length of the tube. This critical rate of flow varies directly with the internal diameter of the tube; the larger the diameter, the greater is the volume of fluid that can be made to flow through it in unit time without the occurrence general turbulence. In anesthetic practice, the volume flow rates of inspired gases are below the level that results in general turbulence.

When the flow is laminar, the resistance is mainly dependent on the diameter of the tube, rising sharply as the diameter becomes smaller. The resistance due to local turbulence arises in the regions of constrictions and sharp bends. Breathing tubes and connections, therefore, should have wide lumens and be shaped to avoid local turbulence. When the flow is mainly turbulent, the flow rate of a fluid is influenced much more by its density than by its viscosity.

Resistance. The resistance to the flow of gases of a piece of apparatus is the pressure difference under given conditions between the entry and exit ports of the apparatus. This resistance varies with the volume of gases flowing through it in unit time, and this flow rate must be stated, therefore, when resistance is described.

Fluid flow through orifices. The flow rate of a fluid through an orifice depends on the cross-sectional area of the orifice and the difference in pressure on either side of the orifice. The flow of fluid through an orifice is always partly turbulent. As soon as the flow becomes turbulent, the density of the fluid, rather than the viscosity, plays the important part in determining its volume flow rate. The less the density, the greater will be the volume flow rate for any given pressure difference on either side of the orifice.

Gas laws. Gas laws are principles governing the fundamental behavior of gases.

Avogadro's law (molecular weight of gases). Unit volumes of gases, although dissimilar, contain the same number of molecules at identical temperature and pressure.

Bernoulli's principle. The velocity of an incompressible fluid passing through a tube of varying diameter is increased at constricted portions and reduced at wider portions. The pressure is inverse to the velocity. Hence the theorem: The pressure of a fluid in motion through a tube of varying diameter is least at the narrowest portion, where speed is greatest, and greatest at the widest portion, where speed is least. However, because gases are compressible, they vary somewhat from this theorem.

Boyle's law (pressure of gases). If a volume of gas is halved, the pressure is doubled, and provided the temperature is unchanged, molecular motion stays the same. This law reads: The volume of a gas varies inversely as the pressure varies, provided the temperature remains constant. For example, if a unit volume of gas is reduced to one fourth, the pressure is quadrupled.

Charles's law (expansion of gases). A unit of gas at 0° C. shrinks 1/273 of a unit for each degree below zero and expands 1/273

Table 4-1. Specific gravities and molecular weights of anesthetic gases and vapors

Specific gravity of anesthetic gases (***air equals 1***)	
Ethylene	0.97
Oxygen	1.10
Cyclopropane	1.46
Carbon dioxide	1.50
Nitrous oxide	1.53

Specific gravity of vapors of volatile agents	
Fluroxene	1.13
Methoxyflurane	1.42
Divinyl ether vapor	2.20
Ethyl chloride vapor	2.28
Ether vapor	2.60
Chloroform vapor	4.12
Trichloroethylene vapor	4.53
Fluothane vapor	6.80

1 atmosphere = 14.7 lb. per square inch or 760 mm. Hg
1 pound per square inch of pressure = 51.7 mm. Hg or 70 cm. of water

Molecular weights of anesthetic gases (***air equals 29***)			
Ethylene	28	Divinyl ether	70
Nitrogen	28	Ether	74
Oxygen	32	Chloroform	119
Cyclopropane	42	Fluroxene	126
Carbon dioxide	44	Trichloroethylene	131
Nitrous oxide	44	Methoxyflurane	155
Ethyl chloride	64	Fluothane	197

	Equivalents	
1 cubic foot	7.48 gallons	28.3 liters
1 gallon	3.785 liters	0.132 cubic feet
1 liter	0.264 gallon	0.035 cubic feet

for each degree above zero, provided the pressure remains constant. This law states that the volume of a gas, provided the pressure remains constant, is directly proportional to its absolute temperature.

In practical application these laws are not important when measuring gases with a rough approximation, such as the vital capacity with a spirometer. However, when alkaline reserve is measured in volume of carbon dioxide percent of oxygen content of blood, the exact temperature and pressure at which the volume has been measured must be known.

Dalton's law (partial pressure of gases and vapors). A single component in a mixture of gases exerts the same force in combination as it would if it existed alone. The law states that the sum of the pressures of each gas in mixture equals the total pressure.

For example, in a mixture of 25% carbon dioxide, 25% oxygen, and 50% nitrogen at 760 mm. Hg, the pressure of each is 190, 190, and 380 respectively.

Graham's law (diffusion of gases). The molecules of a gas or vapor passing into space become equally distributed and exert pressure of equal magnitude upon the enclosing vessel. This equalization of molecular concentration of a gas in space is called diffusion. According to this law, the rate of diffusion of one gas compared to another varies inversely as the square root of their molecular weights.

Henry's law (solubility of gases). Molecules of a gas overlying a liquid penetrate into it and dissolve in it until an equilibrium is established. Increasing the pressure increases the diffusion into the liquid. Thus the solubility of a gas into a liquid is dependent on the pressure. This law says that if the temperature remains constant, the quantity (weight, not volume) of a gas that dissolves in liquid varies directly with the pressure of the gas.

This law applies only to gases that do not combine chemically with the solvent and to the solution of anesthetic gases and vapors in the blood.

Physics and the anesthetic agents. The principles of physics apply to the storing, transportation, and use of all the anesthetic agents. For this reason, a basic, fundamental understanding of these principles is most helpful.

The vaporization of the volatile agents is essential for their use. The compressing of gases into cylinders makes possible their storage, transportation, and use.

The entrance of the gases and vapors into the bloodstream depends upon vaporization of the volatile agents, gradient ratios of pressures, and the diffusion of all the inhalation agents, as well as oxygen and carbon dioxide.

The inhalation anesthetic agents, both gases and vapors, are, with two exceptions, chemically inert within the body and are thus carried in simple solution to the capillaries, where again gradient ratios of pressures, osmosis, and diffusion play an important part in their reaching the body cells, where their absorption is dependent upon their solubility.

Although the entrance of oxygen and carbon dioxide into the bloodstream and the cells depends upon the same principles (gradient ratios of pressures and diffusion), the transportation of these two gases within the bloodstream is accomplished by chemical combination with blood constituents, as well as in simple solution, the greater volume by far being carried in chemical combination as compared to that carried in simple solution.

Nitrogen, being completely inert, is carried entirely in simple solution. The inhalation anesthetic agents, being inert and nonreactive within the body, depend to a varying degree upon the displacement and removal of nitrogen for their effectiveness.

Chapter 5

Definition and theories of anesthesia

DEFINITION

General anesthesia may be defined as the controlled reversible irregular paralysis of cells of the central nervous system. It is possible that this paralysis could be due to chemical, electrical, thermal, or physical influences. At present, however, only chemical means are commonly used.

The various media by which general anesthesia may be produced should be controllable to a degree so that the extent of the depression and consequent paralysis of the cells can be regulated. This depression must be reversible, since full recovery is of vital importance.

The word anesthesia is derived from Greek and may be literally interpreted as meaning without sensation. All modalities of sensation, including consciousness, are lost.

When a general anesthetic is administered in sufficient quantities, the central nervous system (Fig. 5-1) is thought to be depressed in the following sequence: (1) cerebrum (cerebral cortex)—memory, judgment, consciousness; (2) cerebellum (basal ganglia)—muscle coordination; (3) spinal cord—motor and sensory impulses; and (4) medullary centers—respiratory and circulatory centers.

The cerebrum, being the most highly developed area of the central nervous system, is the first to be depressed. This produces a loss of memory (amnesia), impairment of judgment, obtunding of the special senses, and finally unconsciousness. The patient will still react, however, to painful stimuli with somewhat coordinated muscular movements.

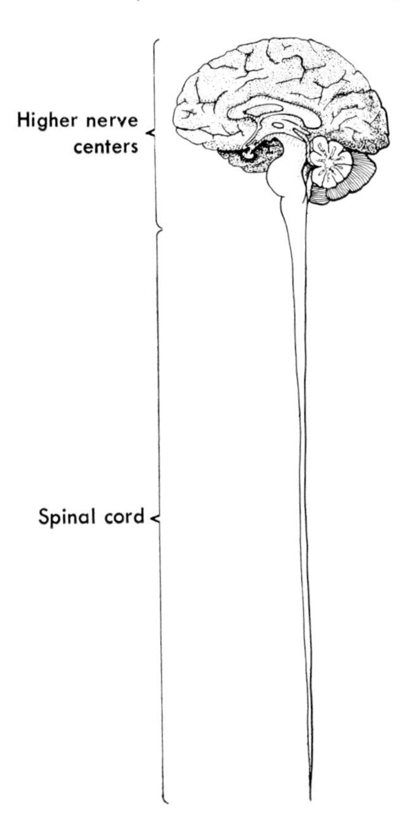

Fig. 5-1. Schematic drawing of central nervous system (brain and spinal cord).

As the cerebellum and basal ganglia are depressed, the patient loses muscle coordination and may exhibit only purposeless movements in response to paintful stimuli. As the amount of anesthetic agent is increased, the irregular descending depression will manifest itself as the medullary centers of respiration and circulation are bypassed and the spinal cord is depressed. The patient has now lost the ability to convey motor and sensory impulses and thus cannot respond to painful stimuli by any muscular movements. Last, the medullary centers are gradually depressed until, if the depression is allowed to continue, respirations and then circulation will cease.

THEORIES OF GENERAL ANESTHESIA

General anesthesia has been used extensively for over one hundred years. The clinical applications of the various drugs are well understood, but the exact mechanism by which they produce the reversible paralysis of the central nervous system defies detection.

An acceptable theory for general anesthesia should explain adequately the cellular depression produced by the general anesthetic agents in common usage. To analyze the many theories or draw rational conclusions from them would be quite impossible. There are at present approximately twenty-five theories of general anesthesia, and many of them are contradictory even though allegedly they have been substantiated by clinical and experimental evidence. Moreover, all the present theories lack confirmation by groups of experimenters over an extended period of time. It can best be stated that at present no one theory has been sufficiently confirmed to be acceptable.

As logical as the irregular descending depression of the higher centers of the central nervous system might seem, newer concepts must cause us to consider the part played by the brain stem reticular activating system in the production of general anesthesia. Specific parts of the reticular system extend through the diencephalon to the cerebral cortex, and are a diffuse network of multisynaptic nerve cells and fibers. The reticular activating system discharges diffusely into the cerebral cortex and maintains cortical activity. It might be assumed that whereas the reticular formation is not the seat of consciousness, it does, by an "arousal" reaction, influence an individual's awareness, alterness, and receptivity. It is said that by a feedback mechanism the cortex may influence the activity of its own arousal system. However, total interruption of the discharges of the reticular formation can result in the loss of consciousness.

It is of interest to list the various theories that have been expounded over the years. While in all probability the list given in Table 5-1 is not complete, it will suffice to show that this has been by no means a neglected subject.

To discuss all these theories would be not only repetitious but also valueless. Therefore, only the more popular theories that tend to explain the cellular action of the chemical agents will be taken up. This presentation will by no means be complete or authoritative but will by necessity be a review of the various theories as previously given by many authors.

Anoxic theories. The many theories using anoxia as their basis were no doubt predicated on the intimate relationship commonly exhibited between the effects of anoxia and those of anesthesia. In effect, they stated that various anesthetic agents inhibit the oxidative processes of the cells of the central nervous system.

Lipid theory. The lipid theory was formulated by Meyer and

Overton in 1899 and 1901 while each worked independently of the other. In its original form the theory stated that there is a parallelism between the oil-water distribution coefficient of an anesthetic agent and its potency. Evidence for this theory has been strengthened by the fact that the lipid-solubility coefficient of anesthetic agents compares favorably with their anesthetic potency.

Surface tension theory. The surface tension theory is based on the ability of the anesthetic agents to lower surface tension, on which their potency depends. This property enables the agents possessing it to interfere with the permeability, polarization, and metabolic processes of the cells.

Adsorption theory. The adsorption theory was based to a great de-

Table 5-1. Theories of anesthesia

Year	*Experimenter*	*Theory*
1847	Bibra and Harless	Displacement
1869	Bernard	Protein coagulation
1880	Spencer	Elective affinity for nervous centers
1882	Binz	Ganglion cell or nerve cell
1885	Dubois	Dehydration
1894	Schleich	Phylogenetic
1899–1901	Meyer and Overton	Lipid solubility
1901	Wright	Neuronal biochemical
1904	Traube	Surface tension
1905	Muller	Neuroglial
1905	Matthews and Brown	Hypoxic
1905	Moore and Roaf	Chemical combination
1906	Gill	Hypoxic
1907	Hober	Colloidal inhibition
1908	Baglioni	Hypoxia
1908	Reicher	Lipid antithesis
1909	Verworn	Oxygen deprivation
1910	Gros	Summation of previous theories
1910	Burker	Lipid solubility-hypoxic
1912	Lillie	Permeability
1912	Quastel	Tissue oxidation
1913	Beutner	Electric potential
1923	Kochman	Dehydration
1930	Lillie, Warburg, and Hillar	Adsorption
1931	Bancroft and Richter	Coagulation
1934	Cloetta	Chemical
1936	Burge	Electrical polarity
1941	Seifritz	Thixotropic setting

gree on the concept of surface tension and assumed that the anesthetic agent thus retarded the adsorption of other substances. The theory was substantiated by the finding that much lower concentrations of an anesthetic agent were necessary to influence the activity of enzymes within the cellular structures that have a large surface than in structure-free fluids.

Cell permeability theory. The cell permeability theory is an extension of the adsorption theory and states that reversible paralysis is produced by a reversible decrease of cell permeability. It is believed that the anesthetic agents affect the permeability of the lipid membranes. According to this theory, the decreased permeability is true only for water and water-soluble substances, whereas permeability for fat-soluble substances seems to be increased.

Coagulation theory. The coagulation theory was the earliest of all the theories of anesthesia and has been revived at intervals since its introduction. According to it, anesthesia is due to a reversible coagulation of proteins. This theory holds true for a limited number of agents.

Dehydration theory. The dehydration theory is based on the assumption that anesthesia is produced by dehydration of the cells of the central nervous system. It supposes that the brain loses some of its water content under anesthesia, particularly ether anesthesia. The theory is supported by meager experimental evidence, and it has been pointed out that on many occasions dehydration causes excitation and not anesthesia.

SUMMARY

In the light of the previous discussion, it seems self-evident that an acceptable theory should explain the properties possessed by the agent that enable it to reach the individual cell and penetrate it. Also, the action of the agent, or its effect on the function of the cell, should be clarified. The first of these can be explained adequately since experimental evidence indicates that moderate water solubility, good lipid solubility, and adsorbability must be present in an anesthetic agent to permit its transportation to the cell and penetration of it. The second question is much more obscure, and as yet no one has sufficiently clarified the actual effect of the agent on the function of the cellular structure of the central nervous system.

Chapter 6

Methods of administration and modes of action

If general anesthesia is to be obtained, the anesthetic agent must be introduced into the body so that it will eventually be absorbed into the bloodstream and thus reach the susceptible areas of the central nervous system. When the agent attains a certain concentration in these areas, it begins to exert its depressant effect on the cells. As the concentration is increased, the depression becomes more pronounced, until unconsciousness and other manifestations of general anesthesia develop.

In addition to a sufficient concentration of the anesthetic agent, two other factors are essential for the production and maintenance of satisfactory general anesthesia: enough oxygen to supply the patient's metabolic needs and an efficient elimination of carbon dioxide.

ROUTES OF ADMINISTRATION

There are various routes by which the anesthetic agent may be introduced into the body. They are inhalation, intravenous, rectal, intramuscular, and intraoral.

The effectiveness of these routes depends on the degree of controllability that they permit. The inhalation and intravenous routes can be more accurately controlled and are thus more widely used for the administration of general anesthesia. The rectal, intramuscular, and intraoral routes offer a rather limited controllability and therefore are used primarily to induce basal narcosis and for premedication.

Inhalation route. In the inhalation route of administration the anesthetic agent is given as a gas, a vapor, or a liquid, vaporized through a mask so that it is eventually taken into the lungs by the tracheobronchial tree. The anesthetic agent is then absorbed from the alveoli of the lungs and is transmitted across the alveolar membrane into the bloodstream. This exchange depends on a gradient ratio of pressures between the concentration of anesthetic in the alveoli of the lungs and that in the bloodstream. When the gradient ratio is higher in the alveoli of the lungs, the exchange is from the lungs into the bloodstream; when it is higher in the bloodstream, the exchange is from the bloodstream into the alveoli of the lungs.

It thus can be seen that when the induction of an anesthetic is begun, its concentration immediately reaches a higher level in the alveoli of the lungs, with the result that the agent readily passes from the alveoli of the lungs into the bloodstream. On the other hand, when the administration is discontinued and the patient is allowed to breathe free oxygen or room air, the concentration of anesthetic agent in the alveoli of the lungs drops precipitously, reducing the pressures, and the exchange is then from the bloodstream to the alveoli of the lungs.

Five different methods of administration may utilize the inhalation route: open drop, semiopen drop, insufflation, semiclosed, and closed.

Open drop method. The open drop method employs a suitable mask (Fig. 6-1) or gauze structure (Fig. 6-2) through which the volatile

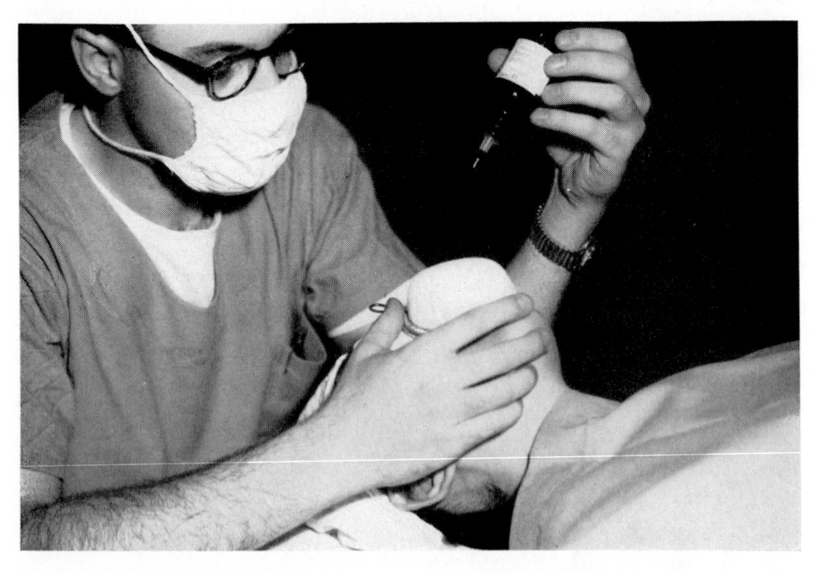

Fig. 6-1. Open drop method, in which a wire mask with a gauze covering is used.

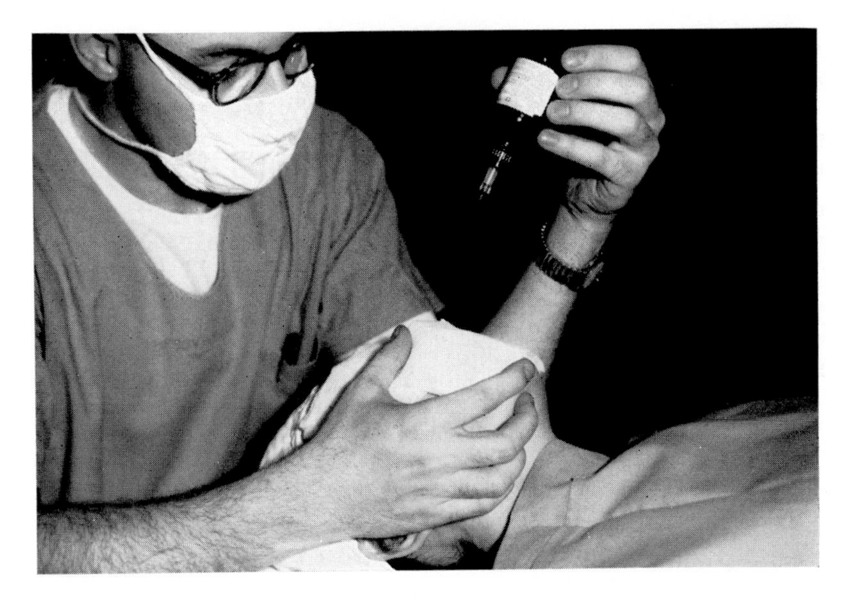

Fig. 6-2. Open drop method, in which layers of 4 × 4 gauze are used.

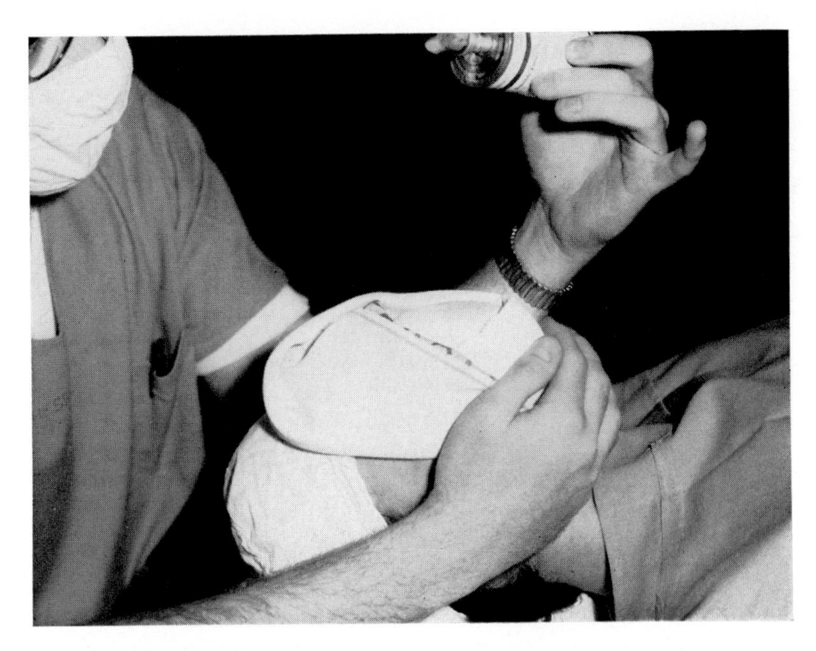

Fig. 6-3. Semiopen drop method; note towel around mask.

anesthetic agent penetrates and vaporizes. No other cloth or confining covering besides that employed to vaporize the anesthetic is used.

Semiopen drop method. The semiopen drop method (Fig. 6-3) is the same as the open drop method, with the exception that a confining wrapper or covering is utilized to increase the concentration of anesthetic vapor within the area more readily. This also restricts the ingress of atmospheric air and to some extent the elimination of carbon dioxide.

Insufflation method. The insufflation method (Fig. 6-4) is accomplished by vaporizing a volatile anesthetic agent by air or oxygen under pressure, and the resultant mixture is transported by a catheter into the upper respiratory passages.

The open, semiopen, and insufflation methods present the nearest approach to normal breathing since resistance is at a minimum and no dead space of any consequence, other than the anatomical dead space, is encountered. The prime disadvantage of these three methods is the inability to control the oxygen tension adequately or to augment the inspiratory effort.

Semiclosed method. The semiclosed method (Fig. 6-5) is accom-

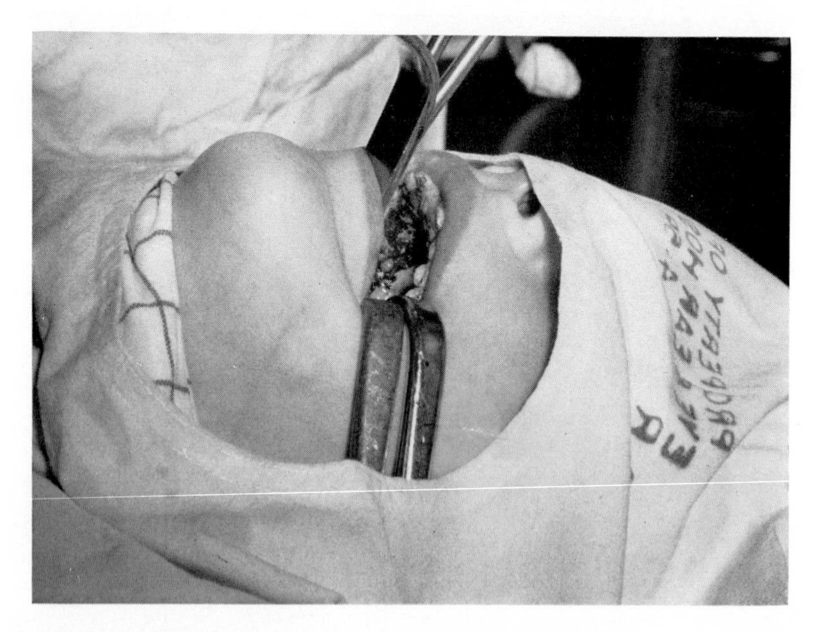

Fig. 6-4. Insufflation method.

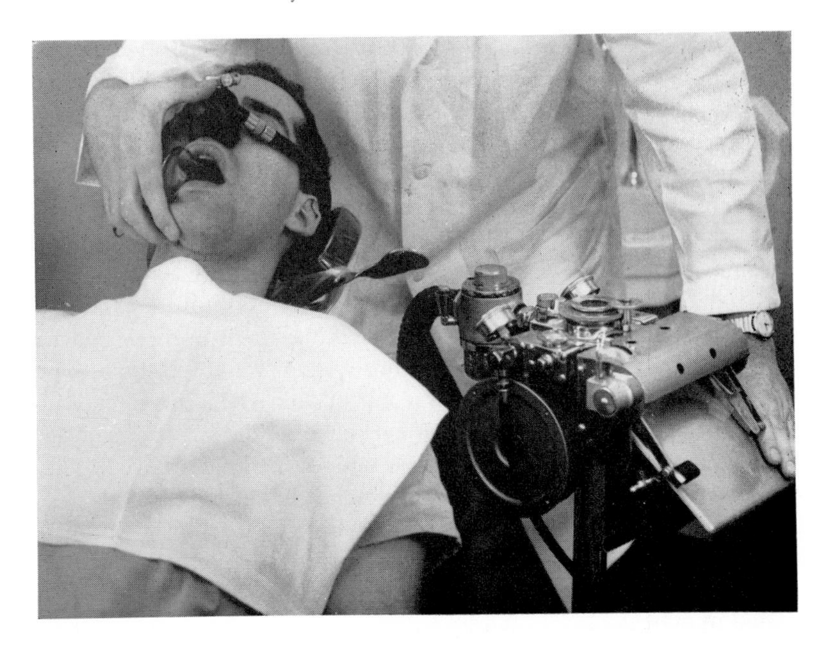

Fig. 6-5. Semiclosed method.

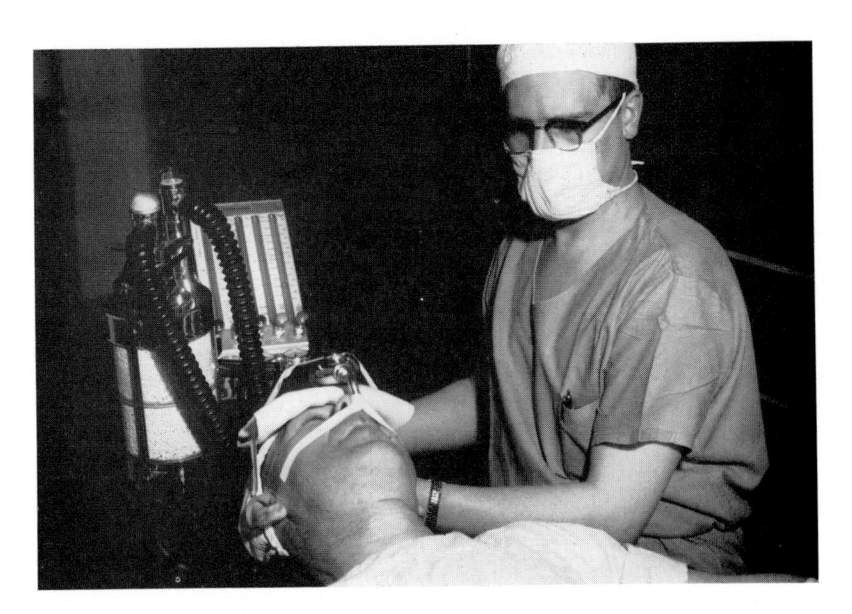

Fig. 6-6. Closed method. Nasotracheal intubation permits the operator unimpeded access to the oral cavity.

plished by using an anesthetic apparatus by which controlled amounts of anesthetic agent and oxygen are delivered by means of gauges, vaporizers, breathing tubes, and a mask. In this method the exhalations or portions thereof are blown into the atmosphere. This maintains an equilibrium of gases, reduces mechanical dead space, and affords an efficient elimination of carbon dioxide.

Closed method. The closed method (Fig. 6-6) is accomplished in the same manner as the semiclosed method, with the exception that the exhalations are not forced into the atmosphere but are confined to a closed system. This is achieved by making the anesthetic machine and the external part of the respiratory system (conducting and ventilating portions) one continuous circuit. When the closed method is used, a means to eliminate enough carbon dioxide to prevent a detrimental buildup of this gas within the body must be employed. This is done by routing either the exhalations or inhalations through a suitable chemical compound capable of absorbing the carbon dioxide from the anesthetic-oxygen mixture. This compound is contained within a canister strategically located in the mechanical system. The closed method may be accomplished by using either a circle filter or a to-and-fro system.

In the *circle filter* method, the canister is attached to the face mask by two breathing tubes, one for exhalations and the other for inhalations. The canister, which contains a chemical (soda lime) for absorbing carbon dioxide, is usually located on the exhalation side. The gases pass over the soda lime only during the exhalation phase. In the *to-and-fro* method, the canister containing the soda lime is located adjacent to the face mask. The gases therefore pass over the soda lime during both exhalation and inhalation.

The soda lime consists of a mixture of calcium hydroxide and sodium hydroxide. The sodium hydroxide imparts the initial chemical activity to the soda lime, and the calcium hydroxide increases the capacity for reaction. The moisture present combines with carbon dioxide to form carbonic acid, which in turn reacts with sodium hydroxide.

$$CO_2 \quad 2NaOH \longrightarrow Na_2CO_3 \quad H_2O \quad + \quad \text{Heat}$$
$$Na_2CO_3 \quad Ca(OH)_2 \longrightarrow 2NaOH \quad CaCO_3$$

The reaction of sodium hydroxide with carbon dioxide is a rapid one and removes the carbon dioxide from the exhalations primarily.

The reaction of sodium carbonate and calcium hydroxide is a slower one and regenerates the sodium hydroxide to increase markedly the carbon dioxide–absorbing capacity of the soda lime.

The semiclosed and closed methods have the advantage of being able to increase the oxygen tension and to augment or control the degree of pulmonary ventilation so as to increase the uptake of both oxygen and the anesthetic gases. Their principal disadvantage is the necessity for an expensive mechanical apparatus; also there is increased resistance to the expiratory effort. The closed method has the added disadvantage of a slight increase in the mechanical dead space; at times a harmful accumulation of carbon dioxide may be in evidence if the absorber fails to function properly, mainly because of spent soda lime.

Intravenous route. The intravenous route (Fig. 6-7) is the most direct one for inducing unconsciousness since the anesthetic agent is carried directly into the venous circulation. Two distinct techniques are widely used: the intermittent and the continuous drip.

Intermittent technique. With the intermittent technique, a suitable intravenous agent is injected slowly into the bloodstream until the desired plane of anesthesia is reached. Then the patient is watched carefully, the signs of anesthesia are observed, and additional intravenous agent is administered when necessary to maintain the proper level of anesthesia.

Continuous drip technique. The continuous drip technique employs the anesthetic agent in a much weaker concentration and allows it to drip constantly into the venous circulation. The rate of the drip is

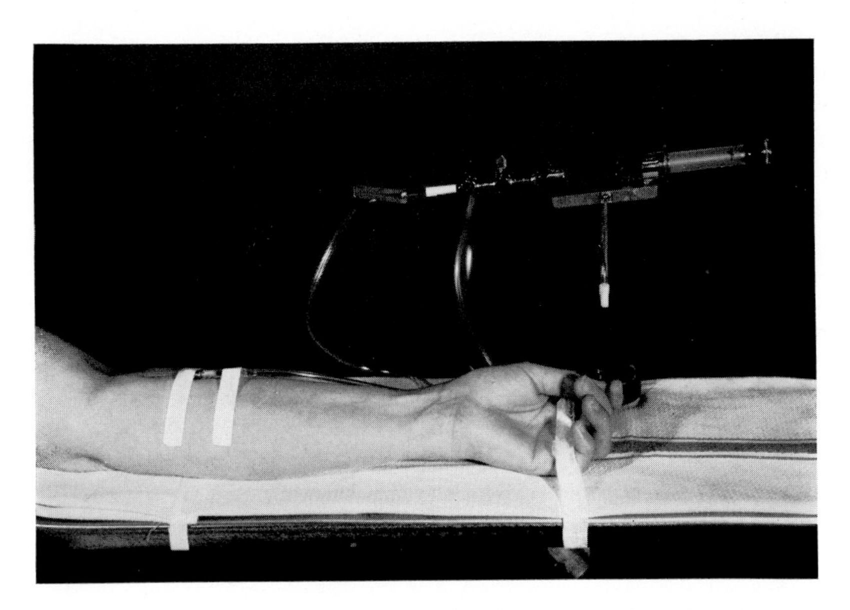

Fig. 6-7. Intravenous administration using Thomas arm board and syringe holder.

increased or decreased as desired to maintain the proper plane of anesthesia.

The methods previously discussed are those most frequently used to secure anesthesia for dental and oral surgery. They afford the anesthetist a fairly accurate control of the degree of depression of the central nervous system. Since the vast majority of dental procedures are elective, with no great degree of relaxation required, and are often employed for ambulatory patients and outpatients, it is essential that the anesthetist employ a method that will permit him minute-to-minute control over the degree of depression of the central nervous system.

Rectal route. The rectal route, although not too widely used in dental practice, does have its indicated place. In this method the anesthetist does not have minute-to-minute control over the depth of anesthesia since the anesthetic is administered rectally in a single dose. Therefore, this method is employed most often when basal narcosis is indicated and is supplemented by inhalation anesthesia. The rectal agent is absorbed through the rectal mucosa and, as with the other methods, must be absorbed eventually into the bloodstream in order to become effective.

Intramuscular route. In the intramuscular method the drug of choice is injected into the muscle tissues, whence it is absorbed into the bloodstream to produce the desired effect. This method affords the anesthetist little if any accurate control of the drug once it is administered, and therefore it is employed primarily for premedication since even basal narcosis would be difficult to obtain with any degree of consistency. In this method, as in the others, the drug must be absorbed eventually into the bloodstream to become effective.

Intraoral route. In the intraoral method, the patient is instructed to swallow a previously calculated dose. This, like the intramuscular method, permits the anesthetist no accurate control other than determination of the desired effect on the basis of previous experience. This procedure at best is inaccurate and unreliable for anything other than premedication. The drugs employed are eventually absorbed through the gastric mucosa into the bloodstream. The intraoral method has long been the method of choice among dentists to premedicate patients. Its shortcomings, while many, are overlooked for the sake of the convenience of administration.

An anesthetic may be administered by judiciously combining two or more of the various methods and the agents employed in each of them. This procedure was given impetus by Lundy in his introduction of balanced anesthesia.

MODES OF ACTION

Regardless of the method of administration, the anesthetic agent, be it volatile, nonvolatile, or gaseous, must eventually reach an effective concentration in the blood in order to depress the sensitive portions of the central nervous system. The first type of body tissue to be depressed is the brain. With a satisfactory anesthetic agent it should be possible to regulate the concentration so that the brain cells will be depressed in a selective manner while other tissue cells remain unaffected. This is possible primarily because the brain is more readily susceptible to the depressant action of anesthetic agents and secondarily because these particular tissues receive a proportionately higher percentage of the circulating blood volume. These agents not only are capable of depressing the brain tissues in advance of other body tissues but also will selectively depress specific cells of the brain so that vital functions are lost in a predetermined manner. It is this predetermination of depression that makes possible the classification of the stages and signs of anesthesia.

The concentration of a general or blood-borne anesthetic comes about by its solution in the bloodstream, regardless of the original method of administration. The anesthetic agents dissolved in the blood are then transported to all the tissues of the body in proportion to their blood supply. The anesthetic diffuses from the capillaries of the bloodstream into the extracellular fluid and then into the tissue cells.

Since the water content of tissue cells is high, water solubility plays an important part in the action of general anesthetics. The blood-borne anesthetics are transported from the site of their entrance into the bloodstream to the cells, which they eventually affect by circulating blood containing 70% water. The extracellular fluid through which they pass from the bloodstream to the cells is from 90 to 99% water. It is evident that the anesthetic agent, in order to reach the sensitive cells eventually, must possess a certain solubility in water.

Since water solubility plays a vital part in the action of the anesthetic agent, primarily by its transportation in the bloodstream and its diffusion through the extracellular fluid, the actual effect upon any particular body tissue depends on the liquid-water content of the cell and the oil-water partition coefficient of the anesthetic. According to Harris, there is no direct proof of the specific function of lipids, and it is probable that lipid solubility does nothing more than assist anesthetic agents to concentrate at the site of their fixation.

Control of the concentration of the anesthetic in the bloodstream depends on the rate of uptake of the anesthetic agent thereby and its excretion from the circulating blood. As we have seen, the anesthetic agents may be introduced into the body by the lungs, rectum, or stomach or may be administered by injection into the tissues or directly into the bloodstream. The three organs mainly responsible for the excretion of anesthetic agents from the circulating blood and eventually the body are the lungs, the kidneys, and the liver.

The so-called nonreactive anesthetic agents, having exerted their effect on the cells of the central nervous system, are excreted unchanged by the lungs or kidneys. Reactive agents are probably eliminated from the body in the urine as degradation products. They are usually detoxified in the liver by oxidation, reduction, hydrolysis, or conjugation before being eliminated through the kidneys. Some reactive agents may be eliminated unchanged through the lungs, as well as through the kidneys.

The eventual elimination of the reactive, as well as the nonreactive, agents may be greatly reduced by poor or inefficient function of the liver, kidneys, or lungs.

Whether they are volatile or nonvolatile, reactive or nonreactive, the anesthetic agents are dissolved in the circulating blood and transported by this means through the circulatory system. During each circuit of the blood a certain proportion of the dissolved agent is carried to the brain, while other parts are carried to other tissues. At the same time a certain proportion is being excreted, and still another part remains in the circulating blood to reinitiate the previous action. This action continues, the direction of diffusion being from the bloodstream to the tissues as long as the concentration in the bloodstream remains higher than that in the tissues. When the concentration in the bloodstream falls below that of the tissues because of detoxification, elimination, or reduced administration, the direction of diffusion is reversed. In this manner the anesthetic agent may reach a sufficient concentration in the cells to exert a depressant action, and it is also in this manner that the agent leaves the cells, which reverses the temporary paralysis and returns the cells to normal.

With the brain receiving a proportionately higher percentage of the circulating blood, it is evident that its tissues will consequently receive a higher proportion of the anesthetic agent during its initial round in the circulating blood. By the same token, since the brain receives a higher proportion of the anesthetic agent during the early circulation, it is reasonable to expect that the brain tissues will reach an equilibrium with the circulating blood earlier than other tissues and that the diffusion from brain tissues to bloodstream will be initiated prior to that from any other body tissues. It is, in fact, possible and indeed highly probable that the brain tissues will relinquish the anesthetic agent to the bloodstream while its concentration in other body tissues, both nervous and nonnervous, is still below that in the bloodstream; therefore these other tissues continue to absorb the agent.

The concentration of the anesthetic agent in the bloodstream will depend on the rapidity of its detoxification and elimination as compared to that of its uptake. It is desirable that during the induction phase the rate of uptake into the bloodstream surpass the rate of which it is being detoxified and eliminated. During the maintenance phase, the balance between the bloodstream and the intracellular tissues and between uptake and elimination should be kept as even as possible. During recovery it is essential that the concentration of the anesthetic agent in the bloodstream be below that in the tissue cells so that the diffusion of the agent will be from the tissues to the blood stream, which constantly reduces the affected concentration in the cells of the central nervous system and eventually allows them to return to normal.

Chapter 7

Phases, stages, and signs of anesthesia

Shortly after the introduction of nitrous oxide by Wells in 1844 and ether by Morton in 1846, anesthetists spoke about and recognized various depths of anesthesia. In 1847 Plomley described three stages of anesthesia, and later in the same year John Snow added a fourth stage, which he called the stage of overdose. From that time until 1920, when Guedel's classic work was published, very little had been written about this subject.

Guedel's stages and signs of anesthesia were the first to give a clear, descriptive terminology by which the depth of anesthesia could be recognized and taught. This work was conducted on unpremedicated patients, using the open drop method with ether as the anesthetic agent. While we shall be forever indebted to Dr. Guedel, time has brought changes and progress in the form of many new drugs and techniques. These advances have made necessary a reclassification of the phases, stages, and signs of anesthesia.

Most of the terminology in use today is arbitrary, and many texts are not in full agreement on the terms or their meanings. It is not unusual to speak glibly about these stages and signs, but, when pinned down to exact expressions, one often finds it difficult to express oneself without reservations.

Many texts refer to the first stage of anesthesia as the induction stage and the second stage as the stage of analgesia. Others refer to the first stage as analgesia and to the second stage as excitement. In Guedel's classic work, the stages of anesthesia are divided as follows.

First stage—analgesia
Second stage—delirium
Third stage—surgical
  First plane
  Second plane
  Third plane
Fourth stage—respiratory paralysis

Guedel's classification was fairly accurate and advantageous when ether was used on the unpremedicated patient, but this same terminology applied to the present-day drugs and techniques leaves the student at a loss, since the characteristics of the various stages may be ill defined and confusing.

The phases, stages, and signs of anesthesia should be all-inclusive so that the student, particularly, may have a clear-cut picture of the degree of depression of the central nervous system as exhibited by the characteristic signs. The stages and signs should be definable and possess physiological meaning.

First and foremost, general anesthesia and regional analgesia should be accepted as two distinct entities. Regional analgesia produces an absence of pain sensation without loss of consciousness by physiochemical interruption of the pathways of painful impulses. On the other hand, general anesthetics effect the loss of consciousness and unawareness of pain by the obliteration of perception and reaction to painful impulses. Any diminishing of pain perception or pain reaction during the first and second stages of anesthesia will not be complete, as the true definition of the word analgesia denotes. However, the pain threshold will be raised (hypalgesia) within the limits afforded by the particular drug in use.

PHASES

Regardless of the agents used or the time consumed, all general anesthesias should be divided into three phases. A phase may be defined as an integral part of a whole procedure characterized by certain definite limitations as to time and circumstances. These phases I would designate induction, maintenance, and recovery. Although these terms have been taken from Flagg, a slightly different concept has been applied to them.

Induction phase. The induction phase forms the first integral part of all anesthetic procedures, including any or all premedication, until the patient is sufficiently anesthetized so that the surgeon may begin his work. This phase will differ in duration according to the agents used and the depth of anesthesia required.

Maintenance phase. The maintenance phase begins when the anesthesia is deep enough to permit surgical intervention and continues until the operation has been completed. It is desirable that the anesthetist provide the optimum working conditions for the surgeon and at the same time maintain the patient in as satisfactory a physiological condition as possible. It may be advisable to vary the depth of anesthesia during the maintenance phase.

Recovery phase. The recovery phase runs from the completion of surgical maneuvers until the patient is again in harmony with his surroundings and in control of his faculties. Literally, it might be said that a patient who has not returned to his preanesthetic state has not recovered from the anesthetic.

These three phases are clearly delimited; therefore it can be stated at any time and under any circumstances which phase the patient is in.

STAGES

The stages of anesthesia, in contrast to the phases, should describe the depth of narcosis (degree of depression of the central nervous system) produced by the anesthetic agent or agents at any given time. A single classification of these stages based on physiological states should embrace all anesthetic agents, and while various stages may have narrower margins with some agents than with others, the descriptive terminology should be applicable to all.

With this in mind, I believe that the following classification of the stages of anesthesia are more descriptive and physiologically definable.

- First stage—preparation
- Second stage—chemanesia*
- Third stage—surgical
  - Light
  - Moderate
  - Depressed

Stage of preparation. The first stage of anesthesia is called the stage of preparation in preference to induction or analgesia. Induction logically applies to a phase and not a stage of anesthesia. Further, there may be little or no analgesic effect, depending on the agent used. The patient is in harmony with his surroundings and retains the ability to obey commands, even though sluggishly. This stage begins with the very earliest premedication, the night before surgery in many patients, and continues until the patient is no longer in harmony with

*Some years ago I coined the word chemanesia to denote a patient in a state of amnesia produced by a chemical or drug. It is my belief that this aptly describes the second stage of anesthesia.

his surroundings. At no time will analgesia in its true definition be present, although some cortical depression may be in evidence. It is true that the patient may be in a state of hypalgesia, or have a raised pain threshold, depending on the preoperative drugs administered. It should be stressed, however, that under no circumstances will the patient, while remaining in harmony with his surroundings, have complete absence of pain perception or pain reaction, as the word analgesia denotes. It should be mentioned that pain may be absent in patients in whom the pain stimuli are not severe.

Stage of chemanesia. In the chemanesia stage the patient retains no memory but may exhibit many reflexes. This stage should be divided into two planes—coordinated and uncoordinated (Table 7-1).

In the coordinated plane the patient reacts with coordinated muscular movements directed toward the site of injury. For example, if pressure is applied to a tooth with a forceps while the patient is in

Table 7-1. Chemanesia

Agents	*Respirations*	*Eye signs*	*Muscular relaxation*
Pentothal	Slightly depressed Inspiration and expiration equal	Lid reflex present Eyeballs oscillate Pupils react to light	None Swallowing reflex present Vomiting reflex present Laryngeal reflex present Cough reflex present Response to painful stimuli
Nitrous oxide	Volume increased Rate increased Inspirations and expirations equal or irregular	Lid reflex present Eyeballs oscillate Pupils react to light Pupils will be dilated or constricted, depending on premedication	None Patient may be tense Swallowing reflex present Laryngeal reflex present Cough reflex present Response to pain, but pain threshold raised
Ether	Volume increased Rate increased Inspirations and expirations equal or irregular	Lid reflex present Eyeballs oscillate Pupils react to light Pupils will be dilated or constricted, depending on premedication	None Patient may be tense Swallowing reflex present Laryngeal reflex present Cough reflex present Response to pain, but pain threshold raised

Table 7-2. Surgical planes of anesthesia

Agents	*Respirations*	*Eye signs*	*Muscular relaxation*
		Light plane	
Pentothal	Depressed Inspirations and expirations equal Augmentation necessary to maintain oxygenation	Lid reflex present Eyeballs centric and fixed Pupils react to light sluggishly	None or very little Swallowing reflex absent Laryngeal reflex present Cough reflex absent Vomiting reflex absent No reaction to painful stimuli
Nitrous oxide	Volume increased Rate increased Inspirations and expirations regular and equal	Lid reflex absent Eyeballs may oscillate slightly Pupils react to light Pupils dilated or constricted, depending on premedication	None Swallowing reflex absent Laryngeal reflex present, but obtunded Cough reflex present No reaction to painful stimuli
Ether	Volume increased Rate increased Inspiration and expiration equal and regular	Lid reflex absent Eyeballs centric and fixed Pupils react to light sluggishly Pupils dilated or constricted, depending on premedication	Moderate Swallowing reflex absent Laryngeal reflex absent Cough reflex absent No reaction to painful stimuli
		Moderate plane	
Pentothal	Depressed Inspirations and expirations equal Augmentation definitely needed to maintain oxygenation	Lid reflex absent Eyeballs centric and fixed Pupils constricted and will not react to light	Slight, depending on individual patient Swallowing reflex absent Laryngeal reflex absent Cough reflex absent No reaction to painful stimuli
Nitrous oxide	When adequate oxygenation is maintained, it is difficult and many times impossible to carry a patient into the moderate plane when nitrous oxide is used; if it is used with barbiturates or ether, the signs of these drugs usually predominate.		
Ether	Volume decreased Rate increased Respirations regular; expirations slightly longer	Lid reflex absent Eyeballs centric and fixed Pupils will not react to light Pupils just beginning to dilate, depending on premedication	Moderate to good Swallowing reflex absent Laryngeal reflex absent Vomiting reflex absent Cough reflex absent No reaction to painful stimuli

Table 7-2. Surgical planes of anesthesia—cont'd

Agents	*Respirations*	*Eye signs*	*Muscular relaxation*
		Depressed plane	
Pentothal	Markedly depressed Inspirations and expirations still equal Augmentation definitely needed to maintain oxygenation	Lid reflex absent Eyeballs centric and fixed Pupils constricted and will not react to light	Slight, depending on individual patient Swallowing reflex absent Laryngeal reflex absent Cough reflex absent No reaction to painful stimuli
Nitrous oxide	When adequate oxygenation is maintained, it is difficult and many times impossible to carry a patient into the depressed plane when nitrous oxide is used; if it is used with barbiturates or ether, the signs of these drugs usually predominate.		
Ether	Volume decreased Rate decreased Expirations longer than inspirations	Lid reflex absent Eyeballs centric and fixed Pupils will not react to light Pupils just beginning to dilate, depending on premedication	Usually adequate Swallowing reflex absent Laryngeal reflex absent Vomiting reflex absent Cough reflex absent No reaction to painful stimuli

the coordinated plane, he will make a deliberate, coordinated muscular effort to remove or free himself of the source of stimuli. Even in this plane, however, the patient will have no memory of his experience.

In the uncoordinated plane, the patient reacts when painful stimuli are applied, but the movements are uncoordinated and no direct movement is made toward the site of injury. During this stage patients may struggle, fight, cry out, cough, vomit, or lie perfectly still. However, they will respond definitely to painful impulses, the degree of response depending on the degree of stimulus and the analgesic potency of the drugs being used. With the present-day agents and techniques, the fighting, struggling patient is a rarity, and therefore the term excitement stage no longer seems applicable. Our own experience over a period of years has proved that lack of memory is typical of this stage of anesthesia. Patients in the chemanesia stage should be under constant surveillance. They will remain in this stage until sufficient anesthetic agent is introduced into the system to produce the neurological changes required to bring on the characteristics of the third stage. Contrary to popular belief, many operative procedures, particularly in the field of dentistry, can be performed with the patient in the stage of chemanesia.

When in this stage the patient has sufficient cerebral cortical depression so that he is no longer in harmony with his surroundings. When he is in the coordinated plane of chemanesia, the cerebellum is not sufficiently depressed to interfere with coordinated movements. When he is in the uncoordinated plane of chemanesia, the cerebellum is sufficiently depressed to abolish muscular coordination.

Surgical stage (Table 7-2). In the surgical stage, which continues to bear the name originally given by Guedel, the spinal cord is depressed, and the patient exhibits no response to painful stimuli. However, it is believed that a broader classification, rather than a division of this stage into four planes with much overlapping, would be more appropriate. On many occasions it is extremely difficult to determine whether a patient is in the upper border of the second plane or the lower border of the first plane. For this reason, I have adopted Clement's classification of light surgical, moderate surgical, and depressed surgical as the three planes of the third stage. This affords a quicker and easier evaluation.

Whereas the beginning of this stage is characterized by paralysis of the spinal cord and inability to convey motor and sensory impulses, the ensuing three planes are characterized primarily by the degree of depression of the medullary centers of respiration and circulation.

• • •

The fourth stage of anesthesia has been purposely omitted since it is believed that under the present-day concept of anesthesia, particularly in dentistry, it is no longer necessary or desirable to carry the patient into respiratory arrest by depressing the respiratory center along with other vital functions. This should be understood in order to differentiate between the apnea produced by the direct depression (paralysis) of the respiratory center due to anesthetic agents and the absence of respiratory movements due to the paralyzing effects of the muscle relaxants on the muscles of respiration.

It is not advisable for a dental anesthetist to deliberately give a patient a sufficient amount of an anesthetic agent to produce respiratory arrest. When this arrest does occur, it should not be considered an additional plane or stage of anesthesia but simply an overdose, which usually occurs inadvertently.

Summary. The stages and planes of anesthesia just described accurately depict the degree of depression of the central nervous system. For example, when it is stated that a patient is in the stage of preparation, it means that he has had some preliminary medication that has definitely altered his previous physical or mental status. We do know that the patient is still in harmony with his surroundings and will answer questions correctly, even though sluggishly at times. The patient may or may not have some degree of hypalgesia, depending on the type of premedication used. He will still retain the ability to recall experiences.

During the stage of chemanesia, the cerebral cortex is depressed to the extent that the patient is no longer in harmony with his surroundings. There will be no memory of any experiences in this stage. Coordinated or uncoordinated movements will be present, depending on whether or not the cerebellum is depressed.

When the patient is in the third stage, the higher centers of the central nervous system are depressed down to and including the spinal cord in the irregular pattern previously outlined. Regular respirations are in evidence, with their rate and volume dependent on the degree of depression of the medullary centers. There will, of course, be no muscular response to painful stimuli.

The three planes within this stage are characterized by the degree of depression of the respiratory center. It is my concept that the patient could be classified as being in the light surgical plane when the spinal cord is depressed; he does not react to painful stimuli, and the respirations are still sufficient to maintain adequate oxygenation and efficient elimination of carbon dioxide. The moderate surgical plane will be in evidence when the respiratory center, in addition to the spinal cord, is also depressed so that adequate oxygenation and efficient elimination of carbon dioxide are impaired, and therefore occasional augmentation of respirations is necessary. The depressed surgical plane is manifested by depression of respiration so that constant augmentation is necessary to maintain adequate oxygenation and efficient elimination of carbon dioxide.

It should be stressed again that when the muscle relaxants are being used, constant augmentation or control of respiration may be necessary even though the patient is in the light surgical plane.

SIGNS OF ANESTHESIA

The terminology for the phases of anesthesia is a completely arbitrary one for expressing the degree or state of depression of the central nervous system. It is absolutely essential that one be able to recognize and interpret the various signs of anesthesia and that these signs be transposed into the arbitrary classification. In this way it will be possible at any time to determine the exact stage or plane of anesthesia and thus the degree of depression of the central nervous system.

The signs of anesthesia are nervous in origin and are exhibited through the muscular system. Although the physical signs may vary with each agent and combination of agents and even tend to vary in different persons, sufficient conformity exists to permit a satisfactory interpretation. This conformity will come, in some patients, only when all the available signs are studied as a group and not as individual factors. The signs most frequently used to determine the stages and planes of anesthesia are respiratory, ocular, and muscular. They should not be confused with the signs indicating the physiological condition of the patient, such as pulse, blood pressure, and color. It is evident that a patient could have a rapid pulse without its being an indication of any degree of depression of the central nervous system. In other words, a patient may exhibit tachycardia and be in the stage of chemanesia or light surgical anesthesia. On the other hand, a patient with tachycardia may be in the depressed surgical stage. Also, a patient could be hypotensive or hypertensive and be in a less depressed stage, or he could be hypotensive or hypertensive and be in a more depressed stage. I am sure that on many occasions patients have been slightly cyanotic and still struggling while other patients under a 100% potent anesthetic agent are in the depressed stage of anesthesia and still exhibit good color. Therefore, it is my opinion that the pulse, blood pressure, and color, not the stage of anesthesia, should be used to determine the condition of the patient.

The anesthetist should be fully cognizant of the patient's preanesthetic condition and any previous medication before attempting to interpret the signs of anesthesia, since these factors will definitely affect the onset or absence of the physical signs. Any or all the signs of anesthesia may be affected by the presence of hypoxia or anoxia, or the retention of carbon dioxide. If these factors are present, they should be recognized by close observation of the signs of the physiological condition of the patient, such as pulse, blood pressure, and color, since these signs will be altered to a greater extent than the signs of anesthesia.

Respiratory signs. Respiratory signs may be subdivided into rate, volume, and character.

The rate of respiration will increase or decrease, depending on the stimulation or depression of the respiratory center. In the preparatory stage of anesthesia, the respiratory rate and volume are usually normal or depressed, depending on the type and amount of premedication used. The character of respirations (relation of inspiration to expiration) will be normal, with any variation occurring in the increased duration of the pause following expiration. For all practical purposes, the respiratory signs exhibited during the preparatory stage are not significant in that the patient is awake and able to vary the respiratory pattern as permitted by conscious control.

In the stage of chemanesia the respiratory pattern is characterized by irregularity or even uncertainty. The respirations may follow a variety of patterns, depending on the individual patient's preoperative emotional and physical state, as well as on the preanesthetic medication. The anesthetic agent or agents being used will have a marked effect on the respiratory pattern exhibited during this stage.

The surgical stage is characterized by the regular rhythmic onset of respirations. Their volume and rate, however, will depend on the anesthetic agent or agents being used. Usually when the inhalation agents are used, the volume is greater than normal, with a slightly increased rate caused by the shortening of the pause that follows the expiratory phase. With the administration of intravenous agents, the rate and volume are slightly decreased and depressed, with a prolongation of the pause that follows expiration.

As an increasing amount of anesthetic agent is administered, with further depression of the central nervous system thus manifesting the moderate and depressed surgical planes, a further decrease in the rate and volume of respirations occurs. This is evidence of the further depression of the medullary centers and is a very important sign of anesthesia, particularly when the anesthetic agents are employed without the muscle relaxants. The stage of anesthesia required should be established and the signs should be observed before the muscle relaxants are introduced.

As previously stated, the plane of the surgical stage can be determined best by the extent of the augmentation or controlled respiration needed to maintain adequate oxygenation and efficient elimination of carbon dioxide.

All the respiratory signs show the depressing effects of the anesthetic agent on the respiratory center and the corresponding decrease in rate and amplitude of impulses passing over the phrenic and intercostal nerves to the muscles of respiration (diaphragmatic and intercostal muscles).

Eye signs. The eye signs may be subdivided into lid reflex, eyeball movements, tearing, and pupillary reactions.

The lid reflex is the earliest of the eye signs to be eliminated, and with all anesthetic agents, with the exception of Vinethene, this reflex is absent by the time the patient enters the coordinated plane of the second stage.

The movements of the eyeballs vary with the anesthetic agent being used. When inhalation agents are used, movements of the eyeballs are much more active than when intravenous agents are administered. In the second stage of anesthesia, in both the coordinated and uncoordinated planes, the eyeballs oscillate because of an imbalance in the tone of the ocular muscles.

In lighter planes of anesthesia, the eyeball is moist, and tearing is sometimes in evidence, particularly in the second stage. The eyeball loses its luster in the depressed plane of the surgical stage, more so with the administration of the inhalation agents than with the intravenous agents. An apparently lusterless or dry eyeball is usually indicative of deep anesthesia.

Pupillary reactions may be of extreme interest during the various stages of anesthesia since the pupil's ability to dilate and contract is altered by various drugs and conditions. In order to interpret these reactions, one must understand the anatomy and physiology of the structures concerned.

The iris is a structure involved in contraction and dilation of the pupil. The muscles of the iris responsible for these phenomena are the circular fibers, or sphincter pupillae, and the radiating fibers, or dilator pupillae.

Both sympathetic and parasympathetic innervations serve the iris, the sympathetic controlling the dilator pupillae and the parasympathetic controlling the sphincter pupillae. Sympathetic innervation originates in the spinal cord at the level of Th-1 and Th-2 and passes to the sympathetic chain and the superior cervical ganglion, where excitor cells are located. The postganglionic fibers pass along the sheath of the internal carotid artery and into the skull, where they enter the cavernous plexus. From here they continue to the sympathetic root of the ciliary ganglion and along the short ciliary nerves to the radiating fibers that make up the dilator pupillae.

There is an alternate route for the sympathetic innervation from the cavernous plexus. It may be through the semilunar ganglion to the ophthalmic branch of the fifth cranial nerve and then by the nasociliary and long ciliary nerves to the eye.

The parasympathetic fibers originate from Edinger's nucleus, which is a group of cells located in the midbrain. Connector fibers that pass into the oculomotor, or third cranial, nerve are often referred to as the mibrain outflow. This outflow leaves the third cranial nerve to end in the ciliary ganglion, where a synapse occurs. The postganglionic, or excitor, fibers continue in the short ciliary nerves to the ciliary muscles and the sphincter pupillae.

A third center, probably of cortical origin, also exerts an effect on the parasympathetic constrictors. Thus a moderate dilation of the pupil is produced by inhibition of the oculomotor nerves, but when this nerve becomes paralyzed, miosis, or constriction, results because of the prevalence of parasympathetic fibers over the cervical sympathetic fibers when the inhibitors of the former have been removed.

This complex system is influenced by all factors producing stimulation or paralysis of one of the three described centers.

During the stage of preparation the pupil is normal except when premedication (morphine or atropine) has exerted its characteristic influence on the musculature of the pupil. (Morphine constricts, whereas atropine dilates.)

When the patient is in the stage of chemanesia, the pupil reacts to sympathetic stimulation and also to the excitation of the antagonistic cortical centers of the parasympathetic fibers.

In the surgical stage, the pupil may be greatly constricted, particularly when morphine has been used for premedication. This miosis is also characteristic of the more potent inhalation agents and is probably due to the paralysis of the antagonistic cortical centers of the parasympathetic fibers. As a result, the fibers accompanying the oculomotor nerve are no longer inhibited and have a decided predominance over the dilation fibers of the cervical sympathetic system.

With the onset of the moderate or depressed surgical planes of the third stage, the pupil begins to dilate, particularly when the inhalation agents are used, and may even produce paralysis of the oculomotor centers.

It must be remembered that dilation or constriction alone should not be the sole guide as to the depth of anesthesia since primary dilation may occur in the chemanesia stage. It is therefore important to utilize all the available signs, such as the reaction of the pupil to light, movements of the eyeballs, and moisture of the eyeball, so that confusion between the primary dilation in the second stage and secondary dilation in the depressed plane may be avoided.

Muscular signs. The manifestations of muscular signs during anesthesia depend primarily on the degree of relaxation of the skeletal muscles and the absence or presence of certain reflexes, namely the pharyngeal reflex, the laryngeal reflex, the swallowing reflex, and the vomiting reflex.

During anesthesia for the ambulatory dental patient, skeletal muscle relaxation is not required or desired. In most cases temporary relaxation of the masseter and buccinator muscles great enough to permit the insertion of an oral mouth prop will suffice. Even when an anesthetic for a hospitalized patient requiring intubation is being administered, it is no longer necessary to depend on the depth of anesthesia for adequate relaxation.

Although the muscle relaxants have to a great degree practically revolutionized general anesthesia, the dental anesthetist must be constantly cognizant of the laryngeal and pharyngeal reflexes. It would not be incorrect to state that in a fair percentage of ambulatory patients these reflexes are present and in some patients are active since they are not obtunded or completely depressed until the patient approaches or enters the moderate plane of the surgical stage.

The laryngeal and pharyngeal reflexes seem more capable of stimulation with the intravenous agents than with the inhalation agents. This is possibly due to the rapid cortical depressant effect of the intravenous agents before a corresponding depression of other centers.

Since the depth of anesthesia sufficient to depress or eliminate the laryngeal and pharyngeal reflexes is not required or desired for ambulatory dental patients, the anesthetist and dental surgeon should cooperate as a team to eliminate or prevent any unnecessary laryngeal or pharyngeal stimuli that might result in coughing spasms, laryngospasms, or regurgitation initiated by pharyngeal reflexes.

SUMMARY

The dentist or any other person administering an anesthetic should be constantly aware of the phase and stage of anesthesia at any given time. This is possible only by minute-to-minute or, better yet, second-to-second observation of the patient. The signs of anesthesia must be observed and interpreted so that at all times the anesthetist will be cognizant of the degree of depression of the central nervous system. This is possible only if he is completely familiar with the signs of anesthesia and constantly observes them for possible variation. This in itself eliminates the possibility of any one person acting as both anesthetist and operator.

Although close observation of the signs of anesthesia is of tremendous importance, this alone is not enough since it is the duty of the anesthetist not only to maintain the patient in a proper plane of anesthesia but also to monitor his physiological condition constantly. It is thus mandatory that the anesthetist, in addition to observing and interpreting the signs of anesthesia, observe and evaluate the physiological condition of the patient as manifested by the pulse, blood pressure, and color.

Chapter 8

The anesthetic agents

To induce and maintain general anesthesia for dental and oral surgery in the office or in the hospital, the dentist or anesthetist has at his command a variety of anesthetic agents. Each has its advantages and disadvantages, as well as indications and contraindications. The more familiar a person is with the chemistry and pharmacology of the various agents, as well as with their advantages, disadvantages, indications, and contraindications, the better able he will be to use the various agents or combination of agents to the best advantage for all concerned.

Not all the available anesthetic agents are adaptable for office use, nor are they all indicated for dental procedures in the hospital. The following discussions will include not only those agents commonly used for dental procedures in the office or the hospital but also some agents, such as cyclopropane and ethylene, that are mentioned occasionally as being used for dental anesthesia. The techniques of administration are discussed in Chapter 20. For purposes of discussion, anesthetic agents may be classified as volatile, gaseous, intravenous, and rectal.

VOLATILE AGENTS*

There are eight volatile agents that may be used for anesthesia in dental and oral surgery. They are diethyl ether, divinyl ether, tricholorethylene, ethyl chloride, ethyl-vinyl ether, fluothane, fluroxene, and methoxyflurane.

DIETHYL ETHER (ETHER)

History. Diethyl ether was first prepared by Valerius Cordus in 1543, and its first reported use for anesthesia was by William T. G. Morton

*See Table 8-1, p. 144.

in 1846. It has been authentically stated, however, that W. E. Clark and Crawford W. Long had used ether in 1842. Clark used it for the extraction of a tooth and Long for the removal of a growth from the neck. Neither of these men reported or publicized his experiences until after Morton's demonstration in 1846.

Physical properties. Ether is a colorless, volatile liquid that produces an irritating vapor with a characteristic odor. The molecular weight is 74.12; specific gravity, −0.718 at 15° C.; specific gravity of vapor, −2.6 (air = 1); and boiling point, −34.60° C. Ether is flammable and is explosive when mixed with air and oxygen.

Chemistry (Fig. 8-1). Ethyl ether— $(C_2H_5)_2O$ —is a saturated aliphatic ether usually prepared by the dehydration of ethyl alcohol with sulfuric acid at −140° C.

$$C_2H_5OH + H_2SO_4 \longrightarrow C_2H_5HSO_4 + H_2O$$
$$C_2H_5HSO_4 + C_2H_5OH \longrightarrow C_2H_5 - O - C_2H_5 + H_2SO_4$$

Ether is comparatively stable and does not react with alkalis, but it oxidizes when exposed to air, moisture, or light. Decomposition may yield peroxides. The peroxides, while not totally toxic, are unstable and may increase the explodability of ether when it is mixed with air and oxygen.

Ether is stored and shipped in metal containers that are usually copper lined. The copper lining is oxidized readily, thereby preventing the oxidation of the contents. When exposed to air, ether oxidizes rapidly and therefore it should be kept in closed containers.

Pharmacology. Ether is a 100% potent anesthetic agent, in that it will produce depressed levels of anesthesia and respiratory arrest without oxygen deprivation. It may be administered by inhalation or rectally. In dental or oral surgery the inhalation route is always indicated.

Ether has an irritating effect on the mucous membrane of the upper respiratory tract and tracheobronchial tree. This effect may be materially reduced if the administration is extremely gradual, which thus avoids sudden high concentrations. We have used low concentra-

```
  H H   H H
  | |   | |
H-C-C-O-C-C-H
  | |   | |
  H H   H H
```

Fig. 8-1. Diethyl ether.

tions to supplement nitrous oxide and oxygen for ambulatory dental patients with surprisingly little irritation.

According to Adriani, a concentration of 3.5 to 4.5% is required for anesthesia, whereas 6.7 to 8% may cause respiratory arrest. This agent possesses a wide margin of safety and is the safest of all general anesthetic agents in use today. When it is given with adequate oxygenation, respiratory arrest will precede circulatory failure.

Diethyl ether is eliminated unchanged through the lungs primarily, 85 to 90% being lost in this way. The remainder is eliminated through the skin and the urine or other body fluids.

Recovery is usually prolonged when deep anesthesia has been maintained for an hour or more. It has been our experience that low concentrations of ether to supplement nitrous oxide and oxygen for short periods prolong the recovery time but little.

During light anesthesia, respirations are stimulated. Deeper planes for dental and oral surgery are rarely indicated unless the patient is to be intubated under ether anesthesia. Salivation is increased in light anesthesia during both induction and recovery. It is markedly reduced, however, by low concentrations, which also tend to prevent coughing and laryngeal irritation. Vomiting is most likely to occur in the second stage of anesthesia.

Cardiac rate and output may be increased during induction, but these increases are probably caused by a reflex release of catecholamines, and not by a direct effect upon the heart. The blood pressure may increase slightly or remain unchanged.

On rare occasions convulsions occur with the administration of ether. They are not necessarily attributed to the ether but usually result from a combination of circumstances, primarily hypoxia and hyperthermia.

For dental or oral surgery, ether has the following indications, contraindications, advantages, and disadvantages.

Indications

1. As a supplement to nitrous oxide and oxygen.
2. As a complement to Avertin.
3. For very young patients (6 years of age or under) when preceded by divinyl ether.

Contraindications

1. When cautery or any open flame is to be used.
2. Acidosis from any cause.
3. Previous convulsions or other unpleasant experience with ether.

Advantages

1. 100% potent.
2. Possesses a wide margin of safety.
3. Comparatively stable.
4. Inexpensive.
5. Can be used with open drop, semiopen drop, semiclosed, closed, or insufflation method.

Disadvantages

1. Flammable and explosive.
2. Irritating to respiratory passages in strong concentrations.
3. Induction may be prolonged when nitrous oxide and oxygen administration is difficult.
4. Nausea and vomiting are frequent.
5. Recovery may be prolonged when higher concentrations are used.

It must be borne in mind that the vast majority of dental and oral surgical procedures are elective, and that most patients with respiratory infection, uncontrolled diabetes, or severe hepatic or renal disease should not be subjected to general anesthesia for dental surgery unless their physical condition, in the opinion of the internist, anesthesiologist, and dentist or oral surgeon, warrants the procedure. This in itself tends to eliminate some of the contraindications to and disadvantages of ether for dental and oral surgery.

DIVINYL ETHER (VINYL ETHER, VINETHENE, DIVINYL OXIDE)

History. Divinyl ether was first prepared by F. W. Semmler in Germany in 1887. Its anesthetic properties were first observed by Leake and Chen in 1930. The drug was first used clinically by Gelfan and Bell in 1933. Goldschmidt and Ravdin presented a comprehensive work on the pharmacology and clinical evaluation of divinyl ether in 1933.

Physical properties. Divinyl ether is a highely volatile clear fluid with a slightly purple fluorescence that produces a mildly irritating vapor with a characteristic strong odor. The molecular weight is 70.09; specific gravity, −0.767 at 20° C.; specific gravity of vapor, −2.2; and boiling point, −28.3° C. Divinyl ether is slightly soluble in water and completely miscible with alcohol, chloroform, and ethyl ether. It is flammable and highly explosive when mixed with air and oxygen.

Chemistry (Fig. 8-2). Divinyl ether—$(C_2H_3)_2O$—is an unsaturated aliphatic ether most often prepared by dehydrochlorination of dichlo-

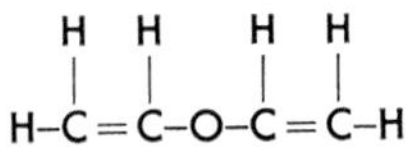

$$\begin{array}{c} H\ \ H\ \ \ \ H\ \ H \\ H{-}\overset{|}{C}{=}\overset{|}{C}{-}O{-}\overset{|}{C}{=}\overset{|}{C}{-}H \end{array}$$

Fig. 8-2. Divinyl ether.

roethyl ether with potassium hydroxide, with ammonia as a catalyst.

$$(C_2H_4Cl)_2O + NaOH \longrightarrow (C_2H_3)_2O$$

Divinyl ether is unstable and highly volatile and decomposes rapidly when exposed to light, heat, or air. It is not affected by contact with alkalis. Pure divinyl ether cannot be used alone because of undesirable qualities. Vinethene contains 4% absolute alcohol to prevent exhaled vapor from freezing on the mask and 0.01% N-phenyl-alpha-naphthylamine, an oxidation inhibitor, which acts as a stabilizer to prevent polymerization. The drug is stored and shipped in tightly sealed dark bottles and has an approximate shelf life of 2 years (the expiration date is marked on the label). Once a bottle is opened, the contents vaporize rapidly unless the container is kept tightly sealed.

Pharmacology. Divinyl ether, which is 100% potent, is administered by inhalation with the open drop, semiopen drop, semiclosed, or closed, or closed technique. The induction is extremely rapid and may be pleasant. The drug is mildly irritating to the upper respiratory passages and may produce copious salivation if administered rapidly in strong concentration. Slow, careful administration reduces salivary flow and irritation.

According to Adriani, a concentration of 4%, or 16 to 28 mg. per 100 ml., is required for surgical anesthesia; a concentration of 10 to 12%, or 68 mg. per 100 ml., usually produces respiratory failure.

The major part of divinyl ether is eliminated unchanged through the lungs, only a small part being eliminated through the urine and other body secretions. Recovery occurs in 2 to 3 minutes; the time required depends on the duration and depth of anesthesia. We have experienced some retarded recoveries when anesthesia was more prolonged (10 to 20 minutes for complete recovery).

During lighter anesthesia respirations are stimulated, with rapid, shallow respirations more or less typical. Higher concentrations and deeper planes depress respirations. Mild laryngeal spasm and phonation may occur during the early stages of administration with comparatively strong concentrations. This may be due to increased salivation rather than to a direct irritating effect of the agent. The drug also has a bronchodilating effect.

When this agent is administered with adequate oxygen, there is no apparent effect on the myocardium or the conductive system of the heart. The drug may have a deleterious effect on the liver with prolonged or repeated doses, particularly when there is hypoxia or anoxia.

Convulsions may occur when the semiopen drop method is used. In our experience they occurred more frequently in deeper planes of anesthesia. Lightening of the anesthesia, together with administration of oxygen under pressure, has been successful in controlling the convulsive seizures.

Divinyl ether has the following indications, contraindications, advantages, and disadvantages.

Indications

1. By the open drop method for short procedures on children (5 minutes or less).
2. As a supplement to nitrous oxide and oxygen.
3. For rapid induction preliminary to open drop or semiopen drop etherization.

Contraindications

1. Where cautery or any open flame is to be used.
2. For use on extremely apprehensive *unpremedicated* children.
3. Without the use of supplemental oxygen by hook or machine.
4. Prolonged procedures (15 minutes or longer).

Advantages

1. Rapid induction.
2. Rapid recovery.
3. No effect on vital centers in light anesthesia.
4. Sufficiently potent to produce adequate anesthesia.
5. Low incidence of nausea and vomiting when properly given, without struggling, hypoxia, or anoxia.

Disadvantages

1. Flammable and explosive.
2. Very volatile and expensive.
3. Signs of anesthesia sometimes unreliable.
4. Excessive salivation if improperly administered.
5. An extremely potent and toxic agent, which if not properly managed may produce convulsions and rapid overdosage.

In summary, divinyl ether is a potent, toxic, flammable, and explosive anesthetic agent which, in spite of its many advantages, possesses serious disadvantages. When given by the open drop method with oxygen for very short procedures on premedicated or cooperative children, it probably has no equal. The danger of explosions is practically eliminated, and if open flames and cautery are not used, the flammability of the agent should be of no concern. However, when it is used in a machine with nitrous oxide and oxygen, explosions caused by static electricity are a constant hazard.

TRICHLOROETHYLENE (TRILENE)

History. Trichloroethylene was first described in 1864 by Fisher. Its analgesic properties were noted by Plessner in 1915. It was first used clinically by Dennis Jackson of Cincinnati in 1934. Trichloroethylene experienced a period of disuse until Hewer of England, in his search for a potent nonflammable agent, revived interest in this drug in 1939.

Physical properties. Trichloroethylene is a colorless, heavy fluid possessing a characteristic pungent odor. The molecular weight is 131.4; specific gravity, −2.47 at 15° C.; specific gravity of vapor, −4.53 (air = 1); and boiling point, −86.7° C.

Trichloroethylene is nonflammable and nonexplosive when mixed with room air. Mixtures of 10% trichloroethylene and 90% oxygen are explosive, but this is an improbable mixture since 2.5% is the maximal concentration indicated for dental surgery.

Chemistry (Fig. 8-3). Trichloroethylene—C_2HCl_3—is an unsaturated chlorinated hydrocarbon prepared by the dehydrochlorination of tetrachloroethane with lime. It is the only reactive inhalation agent.

$$CH = CH + Cl_2 \longrightarrow CHCl_2 - CHCl_2$$

$$CHCl_2 - CHCl_2 \; Ca(OH)_2 \; CCl_2 = CHCl$$

This agent is stable under ordinary conditions but may be decomposed by light, heat, or air to dichloroacetyl chloride, hydrochloric acid, and phosgene. Trichloroethylene is stored in amber bottles for protection from light. A blue dye (0.61% 1/200,000 Waxoline blue) is routinely added for identification. Thymol (0.01%) is also added to prevent deterioration. When trichloroethylene comes in contact with an alkaline substance, dichloroacetlylene and phosgene gases are

```
   Cl  Cl
   |   |
H–C = C–Cl
```

Fig. 8-3. Trichloroethylene (Trilene).

formed. For this reason, trichloroethylene should never be used in a closed system with soda lime since both dichloroacetylene and phosgene are extremely toxic when inhaled.

Pharmacology. Trichloroethylene is a 100% potent, reactive anesthetic agent. It may be administered by the semiclosed system only, because its low volatility renders it unsuitable for use by the open drop method. Also, as previously noted, it cannot be used in a closed system. This agent should not be given simultaneously with epinephrine, levarterenol (Levophed), or nordefrin (Cobefrin). It may, however, be used with phenylephrine (Neo-Synephrine).

When administered cautiously in low concentrations, trichloroethylene is not irritating to the mucous membrane of the upper respiratory passages. Sudden strong concentrations may be slightly irritating—enough to produce coughing and salivation.

Trichloroethylene possesses high analgesic potency; a concentration of 0.5 to 1.5% will produce marked hypalgesia, and 1.5 to 2.5% anesthesia. This agent affords comparatively rapid, pleasant induction, particularly when combined with nitrous oxide and oxygen. The drug is eliminated mostly unchanged through the lungs; recovery is usually rapid after short dental procedures but may be prolonged following longer procedures, particularly if deeper planes of anesthesia are utilized. Nausea and vomiting may occur in 15 to 20% of the patients.

Caridac arrhythmias, which are infrequent when trichloroethylene is used in low concentrations (0.5 to 1.5%), may occur frequently with higher concentrations. Respirations are stimulated during light anesthesia, with a pronounced increase in the respiratory rate.

Liver function is unaffected by low concentrations, particularly when the agent is administered with adequate oxygen. Prolonged or repeated usage, however, may impair liver function. As a rule the kidneys are unaffected.

Trichloroethylene is most often used in dentistry to produce hypalgesia or analgesia or to supplement nitrous oxide and oxygen mixtures to potentiate the action of nitrous oxide and permit the administration of metabolic oxygen. The agent has the following indications, contraindications, advantages, and disadvantages.

Indications

1. To produce hypalgesia or analgesia with oxygen or air mixtures.
2. To potentiate nitrous oxide and oxygen mixtures for light surgical anesthesia of short duration (30 minutes, preferably less).

Contraindications

1. Should not be used simultaneously with epinephrine, levarterenol, or nordefrin.
2. Should never be used in a closed system with soda lime.
3. Should not be used in the proximity of an open flame since traces of phosgene may be formed.

Advantages

1. Nonflammable and nonexplosive in anesthetic mixtures with air or oxygen.
2. Produces rapid induction and rapid recovery when mixed with nitrous oxide and oxygen.
3. Possesses analgesic properties.
4. Stable.
5. Inexpensive.

Disadvantages

1. Cannot be used in a closed system.
2. May produce cardiac arrhythmias.
3. May be hepatotoxic when used repeatedly in strong concentrations.
4. Signs of anesthesia may be confusing.
5. Nausea and vomiting may occur in a comparatively high percentage of patients unless concentrations are kept at a minimum.

Trichloroethylene is a valuable agent for anesthesia in dental surgery. Its true worth will be best appreciated by those who have learned to employ nitrous oxide and oxygen mixtures to their fullest advantage and add trichloroethylene to supplement and potentiate the nitrous oxide—not to replace it. The judicious use of trichloroethylene with nitrous oxide and oxygen should permit the administration of metabolic oxygen at all times without unduly retarding the patient's recovery. The failure to utilize nitrous oxide to its fullest degree, with the resultant sharp increase in trichoroethylene concentrations to maintain adequate anesthesia, can be hazardous.

ETHYL CHLORIDE

History. Ethyl chloride as a specific compound was discovered by Glauber in 1648, and its narcotic properties were first observed by Heyfelder in 1848. Carlson, a Swedish dentist, in 1894 accidentally produced general anesthesia while spraying the gingival tissues for local anesthesia.

Physical properties. Ethyl chloride is a gas at ordinary temperatures but is easily compressed to a fluid. It posseses a characteristically sweet odor and is slightly irritating to the mucous membrane of the upper respiratory passages. The molecular weight is 64.52; specific gravity, −0.921 at 20° C.; specific gravity of vapor, −2.28 (air = 1); and boiling point, −12.57° C. This agent is flammable and explosive but has a high ignition temperature.

Chemistry (Fig. 8-4). Ethyl chloride—C_2H_5Cl—is a halogenated hydrocarbon prepared commercially by (1) adding hydrogen chloride gas to ethylene or (2) treating ethanol with hydrogen chloride.

$$(1)\ C_2H_4 + HCl \longrightarrow C_2H_5Cl$$

$$(2)\ C_2H_5OH + HCl\ C_2H_5Cl + H_2O$$

Ethyl chloride is stable at room temperatures but is decomposed by light or air. It is hydrolyzed by acids and alkalis to alcohol and chlorides. The fluid is usually stored in glass containers from which it can be sprayed. Caution is to be exercised to keep the container free of excessive heat since even body heat from the hand has been known to cause it to explode. Vaporization reduces temperatures to below freezing, thus enabling the spray to produce refrigerated anesthesia over a small gingival area.

Pharmacology. Ethyl chloride is a 100% potent anesthetic agent and for dental and oral surgery is administered solely by the open drop technique. It offers rapid, pleasant induction but should be used only as an induction agent preliminary to the administration of ether or for short procedures for children. Anesthesia requires a concentration of 3.5 to 4.5%; respiratory failure occurs with only 6% concentration. Not only is there a narrow margin of safety, but also cardiac arrest may closely follow or precede the cessation of respiration. For this reason, the popularity of ethyl chloride has diminished since the introduction of more favorable agents. However, this drug has been and still is being used as the anesthetic of choice for short procedures at the Forsyth Dental Clinic for Children in Boston, where it has been administered to over 300,000 patients without a fatality. The duration of anesthesia is limited to 2 minutes or less.

```
  H H
  | |
H-C-C-Cl
  | |
  H H
```

Fig. 8-4. Ethyl chloride.

Ethyl chloride is eliminated unchanged by exhalation. However, small amounts are eliminated through the urine and through perspiration. Recovery from ethyl chloride anesthesia is extremely rapid.

Ethyl chloride depresses the myocardium and decreases cardiac output. Cardiac arrhythmias and ventricular fibrillation may occur on account of increased irritability of autonomic tissues. Respirations are not stimulated during induction but may become rapidly depressed in deeper planes with a toxic overdose. Respirations are the only accurate signs of anesthesia since eye signs are unreliable. Liver function may be reduced with larger doses in the presence of hypoxia.

For dental and oral surgery, ethyl chloride has the following indications, contraindications, advantages, and disadvantages:

Indications

1. As a preliminary agent to ether induction.
2. For very short procedures in children (2 or 3 minutes by open drop technique only).
3. As a refrigerated spray on small areas of gingival tissues (not very satisfactory).

Contraindications

1. In the presence of cautery or open flame.
2. For procedures over 2 or 3 minutes in duration.
3. For children who are anything but A risks.

Advantages

1. Rapid induction and rapid recovery.
2. Minimum of nausea and vomiting.
3. Stable and inexpensive.

Disadvantages

1. Has a narrow margin of safety.
2. Circulatory failure may occur before cessation of respirations.
3. Buccinator and masseter spasms may occur.
4. Rapidity of induction sometimes makes signs of anesthesia difficult to follow.

ETHYL-VINYL ETHER (VINAMAR)

History. Ethyl-vinyl ether was discovered by Frankel in 1930, and its anesthetic properties were investigated by Leake in the same year.

$$C_2H_5—O—C_2H_3$$

Fig. 8-5. Ethyl-vinyl ether.

Physical properties. Ethyl-vinyl ether is a clear, colorless, volatile liquid with a characteristic pungent odor. The molecular weight is 72.10; specific gravity, –0.7590 at 20° C.; specific gravity of vapor, –2.49 (air = 1); and boiling point, –35.8° C. Ethyl-vinyl ether is flammable and explosive when mixed with air and oxygen.

Chemistry (Fig. 8-5). Ethyl-vinyl ether–$C_2H_5OC_2H_3$–is an unsaturated ether compound having a chemical structure intermediate between diethyl ether and divinyl ether. The drug is prepared by the reaction of acetylene and ethyl alcohol under pressure in the presence of a catalyst.

$$C_2H_2 + C_2H_5OH \xrightarrow{\text{Catalyst}} C_2H_5OC_2H_3$$

Ethyl-vinyl ether is comparatively stable when treated with 0.01% N-pheny-alpha-naphthylamine and 3% absolute ethanol. In the absence of stabilizers, however, it tends to undergo oxidation and other reactions. Acids and moisture catalyze the polymerization and hydrolysis of ethyl-vinyl ether to form aldehydes and other derivatives. The drug is stored in dark, tightly stoppered bottles, and any contacts with acids must be avoided.

Pharmacology. Ethyl-vinyl ether is a 100% potent anesthetic agent that may be administered by the open drop, semiopen drop, semiclosed, or closed technique. When administered by the open drop or semiopen drop method, it is mildly irritating, especially when the concentration is high.

For anesthesia a concentration in the blood of approximately 25 mg. per 100 ml. is required. A concentration of approximately 65 to 75 mg. per 100 ml. is required for respiratory arrest. The margin of safety lies between that for ethyl ether and divinyl ether. This agent is eliminated primarily through the lungs, as are ether and divinyl ether.

The induction time for ethyl-vinyl ether is more rapid than that for ethyl ether but slower than that for divinyl ether. Recovery times for ethyl-vinyl ether and divinyl ether are within the same range for short procedures. For longer ones, recovery time for ethyl-vinyl ether is slightly prolonged, but not enough to constitute a serious disadvantage.

In the dog, ethyl-vinyl ether anesthesia produces no functional liver damage. In experimental work on dogs and monkeys the drug produced no histopathological changes in the liver and kidneys.

Ethyl-vinyl ether has the following indications, contraindications, advantages, and disadvantages.

Indications

1. By open drop method for short procedures on children.
2. As a supplement to nitrous oxide and oxygen.
3. For rapid induction preliminary to open drop or semiopen drop etherization.

Contraindications

1. When cautery or any open flame is to be used.
2. Without the use of supplemental oxygen by hook or machine.
3. Prolonged procedures (10 minutes or longer) with the open drop or semiopen drop method.

Advantages

1. Rapid induction.
2. Rapid recovery.
3. No effect on vital centers in light anesthesia.
4. Sufficiently potent to produce adequate anesthesia.
5. Low incidence of nausea and vomiting when properly given, without struggling, hypoxia, or anoxia.

Disadvantages

1. Flammable and explosive.
2. Comparatively expensive.
3. Signs of anesthesia unreliable.
4. Excessive salivation if improperly administered.

FLUOTHANE (HALOTHANE)

History. Fluothane was synthesized by Raventos and Suckling in 1956 while they were investigating a series of fluorinated hydrocarbons in search of a potent nonexplosive anesthetic agent. The first clinical trial was reported by Johnstone in 1956.

Physical properties. Fluothane is a clear, colorless liquid with a characteristic pleasant odor. The molecular weight is 197.418; specific gravity, –1.86 at 20° C.; specific gravity of vapor, –6.8; and boiling point, –50.2° C. at 760 mm. Hg. This drug decomposes slowly when exposed to light, forming volatile acids. This decomposition is prevented by storing it in amber-colored bottles and adding 0.01% thymol.

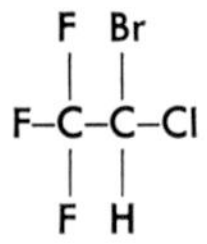

```
    F  Br
    |  |
F—C—C—Cl
    |  |
    F  H
```

Fig. 8-6. Fluothane (Halothane).

Fluothane is nonflammable, nonexplosive, and stable in the presence of soda lime.

Chemistry (Fig. 8-6). Fluothane—$CF_3CH\,Cl\,Br$—is a halogenated ethane, 2 bromo, 2 chloro-1-1-1-trifluoroethane, and should not be confused with fluomar (trifluoroethyl-vinyl ether), which is a flammable fluorinated ether. Liquid fluothane may affect certain metals, such as tin and aluminum, and has a softening effect on rubber.

Pharmacology. Fluothane is a 100% potent anesthetic agent and may be administered by the open drop, semiopen drop, closed, or semiclosed method. It is nonirritating to the buccal, laryngeal, and tracheal mucosa and is considered to be four times as potent as ether. Therefore, only a controlled and known amount of fluothane should be administered. Induction should be slow and gradual because of the agent's high potency. A decrease in depth or rate of respirations should be avoided, and if necessary, respirations should be assisted. However, during assisted respirations care should be exercised so that an excessive concentration of fluothane is not delivered. With this agent the myocardium and the conductive system of the heart are susceptible to increased concentrations, and hypotensive episodes may be brought about by them. It is believed that this hypotension is related to the degree of sympatheticotonia or the depth of anesthesia. Some investigators think that fluothane intensifies the vagal action on the heart, which enhances the movement of the pacemaker, with resultant nodal rhythms. Cardiac arrhythmias occur most often during rapid induction and in the deeper stages of anesthesia. Investigators have demonstrated that with slow induction, lightened anesthesia (due to decreased concentrations) and adequate oxygenation reduce or eliminate these irregularities.

It was believed previously that *d*-tubocurarine or its chemically related compounds, as well as epinephrine or norepinephrine, should not be used when fluothane is the anesthetic agent. If a muscle, relaxant is required, succinylcholine is the drug of choice. However, it is now known that *d*-tubocurarine or its related compounds can be used when fluothane is the anesthetic agent, but the relaxant should be used sparingly and with caution, as there is an additive or synergistic effect between fluothane and *d*-tubocurarine that produces a prolonged effect of the relaxant. However, it is still our belief that epinephrine or nonepinephrine should not be used when fluothane is the anesthetic agent. If a vasopressor drug is needed, methamphetamine (*d*-desoxyephedrine), methoxamine (Vasoxyl), or phenylephrine (Neo-Synephrine) should be used.

Most clinicians who have had extensive experience with this drug agree that a nonrebreathing technique is the safest for administering fluothane. The open drop method is also practical and reasonably safe if the patient is observed closely; however, this method is not advocated. Curare is not recommended, but succinylcholine may be used for rapid intubation or occasional relaxation if the concentration of fluothane is observed closely during augmentation of controlled breathing.

Rapid, pleasant induction with a quiet awakening is possible. Nausea and vomiting are uncommon if no hypoxia exists, and hypotensive episodes are avoided. One to 3 vol.% of fluothane are required for inductions, whereas 0.5 to 1 vol.% is required for maintenance. The greatest advantage of fluothane appears to be as an adjunct to nitrous oxide and oxygen. The induction can be hastened by using just enough intravenous barbiturate to produce amnesia and unconsciousness before giving the nitrous oxide–oxygen mixture and fluothane when and if indicated.

Fluothane possesses no analgesic properties, and patients often react to painful stimuli in the very early period of anesthesia and immediately after the return to consciousness. For this reason it has been advantageous to use narcotics preoperatively or intravenously during the procedure to raise the pain threshold.

Approximately 5 years after the introduction of halothane, isolated reports that tended to incriminate the drug as a contributor to hepatic damage and necrosis appeared in the literature. It was suggested that the agent be investigated more thoroughly. In December, 1961, the Committee on Anesthesia of the National Academy of Sciences–National Research Council (NAS–NRC) designated a knowledgeable, prestigious committee to gather as much data as possible on the relationship of halothane anesthesia to hepatic necrosis. Following a 4-year study (1958-1962), the Committee concluded the following:

1. Fatal postoperative massive hepatic necrosis was a rare occurrence. It could usually be explained on the basis of circulatory shock, sepsis, or previous hepatic disease. The possible rare occurrence of halothane-induced hepatic necrosis following single or multiple administrations could not be ruled out.

2. Halothane, rather than being a dangerous anesthetic, had a record of safety as reflected in an overall mortality of 1.87%, compared to an average for all anesthetic practices of 1.93%. This overall parity of halothane holds up when imbalances in patient populations are taken into account by detailed statistical adjustments. No evidence was found to support the imputed risk of halothane in operations performed on the gallbladder or bile ducts, or in craniotomies.*

At the present time our experience with fluothane has been extensive, and it is felt that the agent has a definite place in anesthesia for dental and oral surgery. When used with nitrous oxide and oxygen, its rapidity of induction, ease of maintenance, and rapidity of recovery offer definite indications for the use of fluothane for ambulatory patients. To date, halothane has proved to be an effective, safe general anesthetic for both hospitalized and ambulatory dental patients.

FLUROXENE (FLUOROMAR)

History. Fluroxene was synthesized by Shukys in 1951. Its anesthetic properties were discovered in 1953 by Krantz, and it was first used clinically in the same year by Sadove.

Physical properties. Fluroxene is a clear, colorless, volatile liquid with a mild, sweet, etheral odor. It has a molecular weight of 126, specific gravity of 1.13, a vapor density of 4.4 (air = 1), and a boiling point of 43.2° C. at 760 mm. Hg. The drug is very stable and can be used with soda lime. Fluroxene is flammable, but the lower limits of flammability make is very difficult to ignite; as a result, the explosion and fire hazards are definitely reduced and are almost nonexistent.

Chemistry (Fig. 8-7). Fluroxene–$CF_3–CH_2–O–CH=CH_2$–is trifluoroethyl vinyl ether. It is a very stable compound but may polymerize under favorable conditions; therefore, 0.01% *n*-phenyl-a-napthylamine is added to prevent this occurrence. The appearance of a yellowish tint to the drug is due to the *n*-phenyl-a-napthylamine and does not affect the anesthetic properties of the agent.

Pharmacology. Fluroxene is a 100% potent anesthetic agent with a volatility about midway between diethyl ether and fluothane. It can be administered by the closed, semiclosed, open, or semiopen technique. When the semiclosed or closed method is used, no special vaporizer is needed. It has been our experience that the drug is far more advantageous when used by the closed and semiclosed methods as a supplement to nitrous oxide and oxygen. In many cases the induction time may be reduced by using an intravenous agent followed with nitrous oxide–oxygen–fluroxene mixtures.

*From Summary and conclusions of the National Halothene Study, J.A.M.A. **197**:786, 1966.

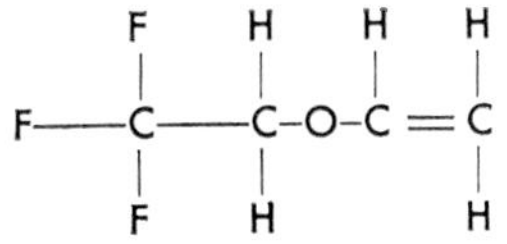

```
      F     H     H     H
      |     |     |     |
F-----C-----C-O-C ═ C
      |     |           |
      F     H           H
```

Fig. 8-7. Fluroxene (Fluoromar).

Although the induction time with fluroxene is a little longer than with halothane, excitement is usually minimal, and due to its non-objectionable odor, secretions are not increased. During this period, however, sudden stimulation should be avoided.

During the first stage of anesthesia, when the central nervous system is depressed slightly, a marked degree of hypalgesia (analgesia) is in effect. This elevation of the pain threshold is evident throughout the anesthetic and lasts for 10 to 30 minutes after the termination of the anesthetic. For this reason, the use of narcotics is not necessary to raise the pain threshold during fluroxene anesthesia, and procedures may be performed in lighter planes of anesthesia.

Signs of anesthesia closely resemble those for cyclopropane; thus there is no effect upon the respiratory pattern in the lighter planes of anesthesia. There is, however, a sufficient reduction in tidal volumes during deeper planes to require augmentation of the ventilation. During fluroxene anesthesia for oral surgery there is no reason to carry the patient beyond the light plane of the surgical stage. The pulse and blood pressure seem to remain unaltered during the lighter planes of anesthesia.

Fluroxene is compatable with practically all drugs associated with anesthesia, particularly the catecholamines and the muscle relaxants. Atropine is especially indicated preceding the use of this agent. Dornette states, "Patients who have developed a tolerance to the narcotic agents, the barbiturates, or alcohol will in all likelihood possess a cross-tolerance to fluroxene."*

This agent seems to be worthy of additional study and consideration as a supplement to nitrous oxide–oxygen mixtures for ambulatory patients.

METHOXYFLURANE (PENTHRANE)

History. Methoxyflurane was synthesized by Larsen in 1958, and its anesthetic properties were discovered in the same year by Lar-

---

*From Dornette, W. H. L.: Clinical anesthesia with fluroxene. In Artusio, J. F., editor: Halogenated anesthetics, Philadelphia, 1963, F. A. Davis Co.

Table 8-1. Physical and chemical properties and pharmacology of volatile anesthetic agents

Agent	*Diethyl ether* $(C_2H_5)_2O$	*Divinyl ether* $(C_2H_3)_2O$	*Trichloro-ethylene* C_2HCl_3	*Ethyl chloride* C_2H_5Cl	*Ethyl-vinyl ether* $C_2H_5OC_2H_3$	*Fluothane* $CF_3CHClBr$	*Fluroxene* $CF_3\text{-}CH_2\text{-}O\text{-}CH=CH_2$	*Methoxyflurane* $CHCl_2\text{-}CF_2\text{-}OH_3$
Physical and chemical properties								
First used clinically	1842 by Long; 1846 by Morton	1933 by Gelfan and Bell	1934 by Jackson	1894 by Carlson	1947 by Krantz	1956 by Johnstone	1953 by Sadove	1959 by Artusio and Van Poznak
Type of compound	Saturated ether	Unsaturated ether	Unsaturated chlorinated hydrocarbon	Halogenated hydrocarbon	Unsaturated ether	Halogenated ether	Halogenated ether	Halogenated hydrocarbon
Molecular weight	74.12	70.09	131.4	64.52	72.10	197.39	126	155
Specific gravity Air = 1 at 25° C.	2.56	2.42	4.53	2.22	2.49	1.95 (1.86 at 20° C.)	1.13	1.42
Boiling point in degrees C.	34.6	28.4	86.7	12.57	35.8	50.2 at 760 mm. Hg	43.2	104.8
Oil-water distribution ratio at 37° C.	3.2	41.3	34.4	15.3	45.5	330	94	400
Flammability	Explosive in anesthetic range	Explosive in anesthetic range	Nonflammable in ordinary percentage concentration	Explosive in anesthetic range	Explosive in anesthetic range	Nonflammable	Flammable but difficult to ignite; fire hazard almost nonexistent	Nonflammable
Stability	Moderately stable	Unstable; stabilized with aromatic amine and alcohol	Stable	Moderately stable	Moderately stable	Stable	Stable	Stable

Reaction with soda lime	Traces of aldehydes may be formed	Stable	Dehydrochlorination to dichloroacetylene	Alcoholic solution of KOH may be hydrolized to HCl and C_2H_5OH	Stable	Stable	Stable	Stable
Commercial preparation	Dehydration of ethanol with sulfuric acid	Dehydrochlorination of (chloroethyl) ether with potassium hydroxide	Dehydrochlorination of tetrachloroethane with lime	Addition of hydrogen chloride to ethylene; treatment of ethanol with hydrogen chloride	Reaction of acetylene and ethyl alcohol under pressure			
Pharmacology								
Administered	Open drop; semiopen drop; semiclosed; closed; insufflation	Open drop; semiopen drop; semiclosed; closed	Semiclosed	Open drop	Open drop; semiclosed	Open drop; semiclosed; closed; semiopen	Open; semiopen; closed; semiclosed	Open; semiopen; closed; semiclosed
Eliminated	Unchanged through lungs; nonreactive	Unchanged through lungs; nonreactive	Mostly unchanged through lungs; only reactive; volatile agent	Mostly unchanged through lungs	Unchanged through lungs; nonreactive	Unchanged through lungs; nonreactive	Unchanged through lungs; nonreactive	Unchanged through lungs; nonreactive
Effect on central nervous system	Depressed in proportion to depth of anesthesia	Depressed in proportion to depth of anesthesia	Depressed in proportion to depth of anesthesia	Depressed in proportion to depth of anesthesia	Depressed in proportion to depth of anesthesia	Depressed in proportion to depth of anesthesia	Depressed in proportion to depth of anesthesia	Depressed in proportion to depth of anesthesia

Table 8-1. Physical and chemical properties of volatile anesthetic agents—cont'd

Agent	*Diethyl ether* $(C_2H_5)_2O$	*Divinyl ether* $(C_2H_3)_2O$	*Trichloro-ethylene* C_2HCl_3	*Ethyl chloride* C_2H_5Cl	*Ethyl-vinyl ether* $C_2H_5OC_2H_3$	*Fluothane* $CF_3CHClBr$	*Fluroxene* $CF_3\text{-}CH_2\text{-}O\text{-}CH = CH_2$	*Methoxyflurane* $CHCl_2\text{-}CF_2\text{-}OH_3$
				Pharmacology—cont'd				
Effect on respiratory center	Stimulated light planes; depressed deep planes	Stimulated light planes; depressed deep planes	Stimulated light planes; depressed deep planes	Stimulated light planes; depressed deep planes	Stimulated light planes; depressed deep planes	Depressed	Depressed in deeper planes	Depressed in deeper planes
Effect on circulation	Vasomotor center not affected; heart rate normal; cardiac output increased; blood pressure slightly increased or unchanged	Vasomotor center not affected; heart rate little changed; blood pressure little changed	Vasomotor center not affected; heart rate decreased; blood pressure little changed	Vasomotor center depressed; heart rate increased; output decreased; blood pressure decreased	Vasomotor center not affected; heart rate little changed; blood pressure little changed	Vasomotor center depressed; vasodilation; bradycardia	Depressed in deeper planes	Depressed in deeper planes
Effect on kidneys	Renal function depressed; urine volume diminished	Function unimpaired in short anesthesia without hypoxia	Function unimpaired in short anesthesia without hypoxia	Function unimpaired in short anesthesia without hypoxia	Function unimpaired in short anesthesia without hypoxia	No marked effect	No marked effect	No marked effect
Potency	100%	100%	100%	100%	100%	100%	100%	100%
Toxic effects	Moderate on diseased kidneys	Toxic effects on liver	Large doses may produce arrhythmias	Overdose may be toxic to liver and heart	May have toxic effect on liver with hypoxia	May produce hypotension	Hypotension in deeper planes	Depresses vital centers in deeper planes

sen, Chenoweth, and Shea. The drug was first used clinically by Artusio and Van Poznak in 1959. It is a fluorinated hydrocarbon and one of the large series that has been closely investigated in recent years.

Physical properties. Methoxyflurane is a clear, colorless liquid with a sweet, pungent odor. The molecular weight is 155, specific gravity is 1.42 at 25° C., the boiling point is 104.8° C., and the oil-water distribution coefficient is 400, as compared to 330 for fluothane and 3.8 for diethyl ether. The saturated vapor pressure at 20° C. is 25 mm. Hg. Dibenxylamine 0.01% is added to methoxyflurane to stabilize the drug, and it is marketed in amber bottles. It is nonflammable, and its explosive limits are approximately 4% at 60° C., which puts it beyond the limits of explosibility for the concentration used clinically.

Chemistry (Fig. 8-8). Methoxyflurane is 2,2-dicholor-1, 1 difluro-ethyl methyl ether, with a structural formula as indicated in Fig. 8-7.

Pharmacology. Methoxyflurane is a 100% potent anesthetic agent and may be administered by the open, semiopen, closed, or semiclosed technique. No special vaporizers are essential when this drug is used by the closed or semiclosed method. Induction with this agent when the open method is used may take from 5 to 15 minutes. This period may be reduced when the closed or semiclosed system is used. An intravenous barbiturate will markedly shorten the induction time.

The drug is pharmacologically compatible with other drugs ordinarily used during the conduct of anesthesia. Therefore, a variety of drugs may be used as premedication or to supplement methoxyflurane.

The signs of anesthesia with methoxyflurane differ from those of other inhalation agents. The eye signs, particularly, are of no value in the use of this agent, as the pupils change very little and the eyes are fixed early in anesthesia. During anesthesia for oral surgery, when only light planes of anesthesia are required, it is very difficult to determine accurately when this state has been reached. In our experiences, methoxyflurane has been used only with nitrous oxide and oxygen; the onset of regular respirations plus a lack of response to painful stimuli have been our most reliable signs. In the light

```
    Cl F       H
    |  |       |
H—C—C—O—C—H
    |  |       |
    Cl F       H
```

Fig. 8-8. Methoxyflurane (Penthrane).

planes of anesthesia, which are needed for dental and oral surgery, the vital signs—pulse, blood pressure, respirations—are not sufficiently depressed to be consistently indicative for this stage of anesthesia.

Although it is often stated that there are no contraindications to methoxyflurane as a general anesthetic, it is my opinion that at present all halogenated agents should be used with caution in patients with a history of liver disease. Also, when methoxyflurane is being used as the anesthetic agent, epinephrine or similar catecholamines should be avoided or used in minimal amounts.

At present, judging from our experiences with methoxyflurane, Halothane, and fluroxene, it is my opinion that the slower action of methoxflurane is the greatest disadvantage of its use as an anesthetic for outpatients. For the outpatient, for whom time of induction and recovery are so important, Halothane and fluroxene seem superior to methoxyflurane.

GASEOUS AGENTS*

There are three gaseous agents that may be used for anesthesia in dental and oral surgery. They are nitrous oxide, ethylene, and cyclopropane.

NITROUS OXIDE

History. Nitrous oxide was discovered by Joseph Priestley in 1772, but it was not until 1795 that its anesthetic properties were suspected by Sir Humphry Davy. The true value of the gas as an anesthetic agent was not proved until 1844, when Horace Wells demonstrated its ability to alleviate pain in the extraction of a tooth. Andrews, in 1868, first suggested and used oxygen with nitrous oxide.

Physical properties. Nitrous oxide is a colorless, tasteless gas with a faint sweetish odor. The molecular weight is 44.02; specific gravity, −1.53 (air = 1 at 25° C.); and boiling point, −89.5° C.

Nitrous oxide is stored and shipped in cylinders at 70° C. as a liquid under pressure. On the release of pressure the liquid immediately vaporizes. Nitrous oxide is nonflammable but will support combustion approximately one seventh as well as oxygen. Commercial preparations are packaged in blue cylinders.

Chemistry (Fig. 8-9). Nitrous oxide—N_2O—is the only inorganic gas

N_2O

Fig. 8-9. Nitrous oxide.

*See Table 8-2, p. 156.

commonly used to produce anesthesia. It is prepared for commercial use by heating ammonium nitrate to 240° C.

$$NH_4NO_3 \xrightarrow{\text{Heat}} N_2O + 2H_2O$$

Nitrous oxide is stable under pressure at ordinary temperatures but will form nitric oxide when heated above 450° C. Nitric oxide is the principal impurity present in nitrous oxide, but it is not present at room temperatures. The gas is nonreactive with soda lime.

Pharmacology. Nitrous oxide is a 15% potent anesthetic agent that may be administered by the semiclosed or closed technique. It is nonirritating to the mucous membranes of the tracheobronchial tree. Its action within the bloodstream is purely physical, and it combines chemically with no tissues. Nitrous oxide is the weakest of all the anesthetic agents and is effective primarily through the replacement of nitrogen. In most instances light surgical anesthesia is the greatest depth that can be obtained with the gas, and in some patients even this is achieved with difficulty, if at all.

A concentration of 30 to 50% with air or oxygen is required to produce a satisfactory degree of hypalgesia or analgesia. A concentration of 50 to 75% will produce amnesia, whereas 75 to 90% may be required to produce light surgical anesthesia.

In practically all patients, it would be difficult to administer a lethal dose of nitrous oxide if it is administered with metabolic oxygen. The prime danger in the administration of nitrous oxide is from hypoxia or anoxia, which are produced when the percentage of nitrous oxide is increased to secure anesthesia at the expense of the oxygen flow.

Nitrous oxide acts rapidly, and light surgical anesthesia may be obtained in 3 to 4 minutes. The gas is also rapidly eliminated unchanged through the lungs, and complete recovery may be effected in 2 to 3 minutes. The gas diffuses rapidly through the alveolar membrane, and even this rate may be increased when the gas is administered with increased pressure by augmenting the inspiratory phase.

Nitrous oxide has no detrimental effects on the heart, liver, or kidneys when administered with metabolic oxygen or when no hypoxia is present. The agent does have a depressing effect on the cerebral cortex, even when administered with metabolic oxygen. Nitrous oxide does have analgesic properties, and when it is administered with 50% oxygen, it will raise the pain threshold to approximately 15 mg. of morphine.

Muscle relaxation is poor with the administration of nitrous oxide and oxygen, and rigidity and spasm may occur because of hypoxia if the gas is administered in higher percentages with decreased oxygen in an attempt to obtain deeper anesthesia and more relaxation.

Indications

1. As a supplement to the administration of barbiturates intravenously or Avertin rectally.
2. As a complement to ether, trichloroethylene, divinyl ether, or ethyl-vinyl ether.
3. For very short procedures when no relaxation or depth beyond the light surgical plane is required.
4. For hypalgesia or analgesia in general dentistry.

Contraindications

1. As the sole anesthetic agents when it is necessary to increase the nitrous oxide percentage by decreasing the oxygen percentage to hypoxic levels.
2. For very small infants who are breathing against the pressure of the machine and when the increased dead space is hazardous.

Advantages

1. Rapid induction.
2. Rapid recovery.
3. Nonirritating.
4. No deleterious effect on any body tissues when given with metabolic oxygen.
5. Produces a minimum of nausea and vomiting.
6. Produces hypalgesia.
7. Nonflammable and nonexplosive.

Disadvantages

1. Is the weakest of all anesthetic agents, with the result that hypoxia must be constantly guarded against.
2. Relaxation is inadequate.
3. Maintenance is difficult unless this agent is combined with other agents.

Nitrous oxide, after approximately 113 years of use in dentistry, is still the anesthetic of choice for the office and is still widely used in operating rooms. With the introduction of more potent agents, such as divinyl ether, trichloroethylene, ethyl-vinyl ether, and the intravenous drugs, the value of nitrous oxide as an anesthetic for dental and oral surgery has increased. The more potent agents have served to potentiate the weak nitrous oxide, with the result that anesthetists are now able to utilize the advantages that nitrous oxide offers and to eliminate most of its disadvantages.

It is suggested that any person administering anesthesia for dental or oral surgery should be thoroughly familiar with this agent and the technique for its administration. Unfortunately, with the introduction of the more potent agents, many dentists have discarded nitrous oxide until its administration has almost become a lost art. It is my conviction that nitrous oxide, when supplemented by more potent intravenous or volatile agents to permit the constant administration of metabolic oxygen and to potentiate the action of nitrous oxide, offers the greatest degree of safety while maintaining rapid induction and recovery and satisfactory ease of maintenance.

ETHYLENE (OLEFIANT GAS)

History. Ethylene was first discovered by Ingenhousz in 1779. Its anesthetic properties were first described by L. Hermann, a physiologist, in 1864. In 1908, Crocher and Knight of the Hull Botanical Laboratories noted the toxicity of ethylene to plants. In 1923, Luckhardt and Carter introduced ethylene as an anesthetic agent and discussed its properties. The first series of cases (106) was reported by Dr. Isabella Herb in 1924. In a Pittsburgh hospital in 1926, two consecutive fatalities during induction with ethylene caused its use to be restricted. The fatalities were proved to have been caused by carbon monoxide since ethylene contains 0.003% carbon monoxide. The Explosives Division of the United States Bureau of Mines, in consultation with Dr. John McCurdy and Dr. George J. Thomas of the Department of Anesthesiology of St. Francis Hospital and the University of Pittsburgh, began a cooperative research program for purifying ethylene. In 1927, this same group presented a process for the manufacture of carbon monoxide-free ethylene.

Physical properties. Ethylene is a colorless, tasteless, nonirritating gas with a characteristic odor. The molecular weight is 28.05, and the specific gravity is −0.97. Ethylene liquefies at 10° C. and has a boiling point of 103.9° C. This substance is highly flammable and explosive. It is available commercially as a compressed gas in a red cylinder.

Chemistry (Fig. 8-10). Ethylene—C_2H_4—is an unsaturated hydrocarbon, prepared for commercial use by the catalytic dehydration of ethyl alcohol.

$$C_2H_5OH \xrightarrow[\text{Catalyst}]{\text{Heat}} H_2C = CH_2 + H_2O$$

Ethylene is stable under ordinary circumstances. The most danger-

$H_2C{=}CH_2$

Fig. 8-10. Ethylene.

ous impurity was carbon monoxide, but improvement of standards of purity has eliminated this hazard. This agent may be used in a closed system since it is nonreactive with soda lime.

Pharmacology. Ethylene is a 25% potent anesthetic agent that may be administered by the closed or semiclosed technique. It is nonirritating to the mucous membranes of the tracheobronchial tree. This agent is 10% more potent than nitrous oxide. Muscular relaxation is poor, and the inherent weakness of the gas prevents the attainment of deeper anesthesia (beyond the light surgical plane) without supplementation by more potent agents.

According to Adriani, a concentration of 20 to 25% is required for hypalgesia or analgesia, and 80 to 90% for anesthesia. It is difficult to administer a lethal dose when adequate oxygen is maintained. As with nitrous oxide, the prime danger in the administration of ethylene is hypoxia, with the added hazard of explosibility.

Ethylene affords rapid induction (2 to 3 minutes) and rapid recovery. The gas is rapidly eliminated by exhalations and has high lipophilic qualities.

Ethylene has no detrimental effects on the heart, liver, or kidneys when administered with metabolic oxygen. It does have a depressant effect on the cerebral cortex, even when administered with metabolic oxygen. Its analgesic properties are equal to those of nitrous oxide.

Muscle relaxation, as with nitrous oxide, is poor, and any attempt to obtain more relaxation by deepening the anesthesia at the expense of the oxygen concentration will lead to muscular spasm and rigidity.

For dental or oral surgery, ethylene has the following indications, contraindications, advantages, and disadvantage.

Indications

1. As a supplement to the administration of barbiturates intravenously or Avertin rectally.
2. As a complement to ether, trichloroethylene, divinyl ether, or ethyl-vinyl ether.
3. For short procedures when no relaxation or depth beyond the light surgical plane is required.
4. For hypalgesia or analgesia.

Contraindications

1. As a sole anesthetic agent when it is necessary to increase the ethylene percentage by decreasing the oxygen percentage to hypoxic levels.
2. For very small infants who are breathing against the pressure of the machine and when the increased dead space is hazardous.

Advantages

1. Rapid induction.
2. Rapid recovery.
3. Nonirritating.
4. No deleterious effect on any body tissues when given with metabolic oxygen.
5. Produces a minimum of nausea and vomiting.
6. Produces a high degree of hypalgesia.

Disadvantage

1. Flammable and explosive.

Ethylene, as an anesthetic agent, more closely approaches the ideal for dental and oral surgery than any other agent. It possesses just enough more potency than nitrous oxide to permit the light surgical anesthesia necessary for dental surgery, without hypoxia. When it is combined with other, more potent agents, a correspondingly smaller concentration of these agents is needed. It is nonirritating and possesses satisfactory analgesic properties. However, its flammability and explosibility are constant hazards, particularly for dental and oral surgery. Despite this, some oral surgeons advocate ethylene as the anesthetic of choice for treatment of patients in the office. It is my opinion that ethylene, besides having the other advantages of nitrous oxide, possesses enough increased potency to make it the ideal agent for office use. However, since the explosibility of ethylene is an ever-present hazard, nitrous oxide will continue to be the anesthetic of choice when it is used with nonexplosive agents.

CYCLOPROPANE (TRIMETHYLENE)

History. Cyclopropane was first prepared by Freund in 1882, but he did not mention its anesthetic properties. Henderson and Lucas first reported its anesthetic properties in 1929 after experimentation on animals. Ralph M. Waters first administered cyclopropane to a human patient in December, 1930. The first extensive clinical report was prepared by Stiles, Neff, Rovenstine, and Waters in 1933.

Physical properties. Cyclopropane is a colorless, nonirritating gas

```
   H     H
   |     |
H—C——C—H
    \  /
     C
    /  \
   H    H
```

Fig. 8-11. Cyclopropane (Trimethylene).

having a sweetish taste and odor. The molecular weight is 42.1; specific gravity, −1.46; boiling point, 32.89° C.; and freezing point (approximate), 126° C.

Cyclopropane is highly flammable and explosive when mixed with air and oxygen. It is shipped commercially as a liquid in an orange-colored container.

Chemistry (Fig. 8-11). Cyclopropane—C_3H_6—is a saturated cyclic hydrocarbon and an isomer of propane. It is stable and relatively inert chemically. The gas is prepared by the treatment of 1,3 dichlor propane in the presence of zinc or by progressive thermol chlorination of propane.

$$C_3H_6Cl_2 \xrightarrow{Zn} C_3H_6 + ZnCl_2$$

Pharmacology. Cyclopropane is a 100% potent and expensive anesthetic agent and is usually administered by the closed method only. It gives rapid induction and fairly rapid recovery. According to Adriani, a concentration of 6 to 8% will produce unconsciousness, and a concentration of 7 to 23% is required for the three planes of the third stage of anesthesia. A concentration above 23% may produce respiratory arrest. The agent is not altered in the body, the main portion being eliminated by exhalations in 5 to 10 minutes.

Cyclopropane will produce all planes of anesthesia with adequate oxygenation. The cerebral cortex is depressed by cyclopropane. The respiratory center is not affected early but is depressed in later stages of anesthesia. There are no significant effects on the myocardium during light surgical anesthesia. Arrhythmias may occur frequently in deeper stages of anesthesia. Cyclopropane should not be used with epinephrine or related amines. The liver is not affected by repeated uses of this agent. The formation of urine is suppressed, as it is by most other anesthetic agents, but the kidneys themselves are not affected.

The indications, contraindications, advantages, and disadvantages of cyclopropane will not be discussed since this agent is rarely used for dental patients. Recent articles, particularly from England and Scotland, discuss and advocate the use of cyclopropane for dental anesthesia. However, it is my opinion that the extreme potency, explosibility, flammability, and cost of this agent render it impractical for dental use. This is particularly so because other more satisfactory agents and techniques are now available.

INTRAVENOUS AGENTS*

There are three intravenous agents that may be used for anesthesia in dental or oral surgery. They are thiopental sodium (Pentothal), thiamylal sodium (Surital sodium), and methohexital sodium (Brevital). Other intravenous agents—hexobarbital sodium (Evipal sodium), methitural sodium (Neraval), hydroxydione sodium (Viadril), and glutethimide (Doriden)—are now of historic interest only.

The introduction of barbital in 1903 may be considered the beginning of modern intravenous anesthesia. However, many years lapsed before a suitable intravenous agent became available. The long-acting compounds (barbital and phenobarbital) required excessive doses and produced prolonged residual effects. As shorter-acting barbiturates were introduced, each was tried and evaluated. The acceptance of intravenous anesthesia was established with introduction of newer short-acting barbiturates—Evipal (1933), Nembutal (1930), Pentothal (1933), Surital (1948), Neraval (1954), Viadril (1956), and Doriden (1958).

With the exception of Viadril and Doriden, all the intravenous anesthetic agents are barbiturate derivatives. Anesthesia produced by the intravenous agents differs in many respects from that produced by the inhalation drugs. The level of anesthesia is more readily controlled when the inhalation agents are used since the concentration of the drug can be altered by hyperventilation of the patient.

The intravenous agents must be metabolized and then eliminated, whereas the inhalation agents, with the exception of trichloroethylene, are eliminated completely unchanged through the lungs. The intravenous barbiturates are almost completely metabolized in the body; only a minute percentage is excreted unchanged in the urine. Although the primary site of detoxification is the liver, the degradation of barbiturates is largely determined by their chemical structure. The mechanisms of metabolism are mainly three: side chain oxidation, nitrogen dealkylation, and desulfuration of thiobarbiturates. A single compound may be affected by one or more of these mechanisms.

The intravenous barbiturates are lost from the blood plasma at a

*See Table 8-3, p. 166.

Table 8-2. Physical and chemical properties and pharmacology of gaseous anesthetic agents

Agent	*Nitrous oxide* N_2O	*Ethylene* C_2H_4	*Cyclopropane* C_3H_6
Physical and chemical properties			
First used clinically	1846 by Wells	1923 by Luckhardt	1933 by Waters
Type of compound	Oxide of nitrogen	Unsaturated hydrocarbon	Cyclic hydrocarbon
Physical state in cylinder	Liquid and gas	Gas	Liquid
Approximate pressure at 70° F.	755	1,250	75
Molecular weight	44.02	28.05	42.08
Specific gravity, air = 1 at 25° C.	1.53	0.97	1.48
Boiling point at degrees C.	−89.5	−103.9	−32.8
Oil-water distribution ratio at 37° C.	3.2	14.4	34.43
Flammability	Nonflammable; supports combustion	Explosive in anesthetic range	Explosive in anesthetic range
Stability	Stable; decomposes above 450° C.	Stable but adds halogens and acids	Moderately stable
Reaction with soda lime	Stable	Stable	Stable
Commercial preparation	Decomposition of ammonium nitrate by heat	Dehydration of ethanol; cracking of fuel gases	Treatment of 1 chloro 3 bromo propane with zinc for ring closure

Pharmacology

Administered	Closed or semiclosed	Closed or semiclosed	Closed or semiclosed
Eliminated	Through lungs; unchanged	Through lungs; unchanged	Through lungs; unchanged
Effect on central nervous system	Cortex depressed; other areas unaffected; without hypoxia	Cortex depressed; other areas unaffected; without hypoxia	Cortex deeply depressed; subcortical centers depressed; vagus centers stimulated
Effect on respiratory center	Not affected; without hypoxia	Not affected; without hypoxia	Depressed; bronchial muscles not relaxed
Effect on circulation	Unaffected; without hypoxia	Heart rate moderate; increased without hypoxia	Arrhythmias common; heart rate decreased; cardiac output increased; blood pressure elevated during anesthesia
Effect on liver	Unaffected; without hypoxia	Unaffected; without hypoxia	Unaffected; without hypoxia
Effect on kidneys	Unaffected; without hypoxia	Unaffected; without hypoxia	Urine secretion depressed during anesthesia and increased after anesthesia
Potency	Weakest of anesthetic agents; Guedel rating 15%	25% potent	100% potent
Toxic effects	No toxic effects; without hypoxia	No toxic effects; without hypoxia	Cardiac pacemaker affected; conduction system occasionally

rapid rate since they readily diffuse into all tissues. This rate of diffusion is dependent on the concentration in the fat and other nonsensitive tissues, as compared to that in the bloodstream.

THIOPENTAL SODIUM (PENTOTHAL)

History. Thiopental sodium was synthesized by Volwiler and Taburn and introduced clinically by Lundy in 1933.

Physical properties. Thiopental sodium is a bitter-tasting, yellow hygroscopic powder with a characteristic odor. It is soluble in water or alcohol and forms a solution that is comparatively unstable, decomposing in 24 to 72 hours. The solution has a pH between 10 and 11.

Chemistry (Fig. 8-12). Thiopental sodium—$C_{11}H_{17}O_2N_2SNa$—is sodium methy-l-butyl-thiobarbiturate, which is the sodium salt of thiopentobarbituric acid. The thiobarbiturates are made by condensing malonic acid with thiourea.

Pharmacology. Thiopental sodium is a rapid-acting thiobarbiturate. It may be administered by the intermittent technique (2% solution), by continuous drip (0.5% solution), or rectally for children. This drug primarily depresses the cerebral cortex to produce hypnosis and anesthesia, the degree of which depends on the dose. Respirations are depressed in direct proportion to the dose used. Smaller hypnotic doses may have no depressant effect on the respiratory center. However, hypnotic or light anesthetic doses that do not ordinarily depress respirations may, if given rapidly, produce moderately severe or severe respiratory depression. The medullary centers are depressed in proportion to the dose and the speed of administration. The blood pressure, which is usually not affected by ordinary doses, may be significantly lowered by larger or smaller doses when the drug is given rapidly. Ordinary anesthetic doses with slow administration produce no myocardial changes, but the heart rate may be increased. Arrhythmias are uncommon with adequate oxygenation. The heart is not sensitized to epinephrine or other sympathomimetic amines.

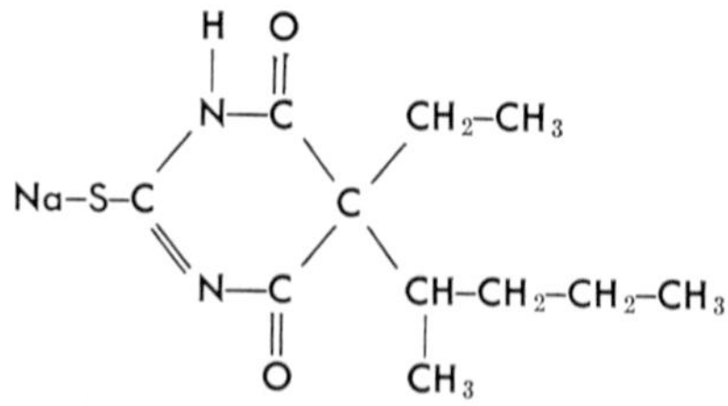

```
          H  O
          |  ||
          N—C      CH2–CH3
         /    \   /
Na–S–C         C
        \\    /  \
          N—C      CH–CH2–CH2–CH3
            ||     |
            O      CH3
```

Fig. 8-12. Thiopental sodium (Pentothal).

Laryngeal reflexes are not abolished except in the deeper planes of anesthesia. They may even be hyperreactive in the lighter planes. The salivary glands are not stimulated and there is no excessive production of mucus. The vomiting center is depressed, and postanesthetic nausea or vomiting is uncommon. The vagal reflexes may be hyperactive. Muscle relaxation is inadequate during light anesthesia, but the masseter and buccinator muscles may be relaxed early.

Thiopental sodium is mainly detoxified in the liver. Larger doses may be shunted into adipose and other nonsensitive tissues, from which the drug is diffused back into the circulation. Smaller doses are rapidly removed from the bloodstream. Patients who have had larger doses may show retarded recovery time because of the release of the drug from nonsensitive tissues.

For dental or oral surgery, thiopental sodium has the following indications, contraindications, advantages, and disadvantages.

Indications

1. As a controlled premedication preceding and with nitrous oxide and oxygen.
2. As the sole anesthetic for short procedures (5 minutes or less).

Contraindications

1. As the sole anesthetic for longer procedures (5 to 10 minutes or more).
2. In young patients (12 years of age or under).
3. For difficult procedures without the use of an intratracheal tube.
4. For patients who are allergic to barbiturates.

Advantages

1. Rapid, pleasant induction.
2. Rapid recovery with smaller doses.
3. Nausea and vomiting uncommon.
4. Nonflammable and nonexplosive.
5. Ideal as controlled premedication for nitrous oxide and oxygen.

Disadvantages

1. Laryngeal reflexes remain active.
2. Low analgesic potency.
3. Venipuncture may be difficult.
4. Action is cumulative.

Thiopental sodium has been a valuable addition to the armamentarium of the oral surgeon and the dental anesthetist. In my opinion many of the shortcomings of the drug have been due to its misuse rather than to the drug itself.

In the office, thiopental sodium should be employed as a controlled premedication with nitrous oxide and oxygen. If used alone, it should be confined to very short procedures requiring no extensive manipulation. The use of thiopental sodium alone for long office procedures should be condemned. When the drug is to be used to produce longer periods of anesthesia for the hospitalized patient, the intratracheal method should always be employed and nitrous oxide and oxygen should be administered. Unless the patient is intubated and the respirations are augmented with nitrous oxide and oxygen or oxygen alone, the use of thiopental sodium as the only anesthetic for long dental procedures is hazardous.

Thiopental sodium should never be used under any circumstances unless trained personnel are employed and resuscitation equipment is readily available.

THIAMYLAL SODIUM (SURITAL)

History. Thiamylal sodium is an ultrashort-acting thiobarbiturate. It was introduced by Seevers in 1948.

Physical properties. Thiamylal sodium is a whitish-yellow hygroscopic powder that may be mixed with water or saline solutions to form a comparatively unstable solution (24 to 72 hours). It has a pH between 10 and 11. It has a molecular weight of 276.33.

Chemistry (Fig. 8-13). Thiamylal sodium—$C_{12}H_{17}O_2N_2SNa$—is the sodium salt of 5-allyl-5 (methylbutyl)-2-thiobarbituric acid. Chemically it is quite similar to thiopental sodium, which is apparent if one compares their chemical structures.

Pharmacology. Thiamylal sodium is similar to thiopental sodium in every respect. When blind tests to discriminate between the two drugs are conducted, it is extremely difficult if not impossible to determine any outstanding variations between the two drugs. The indications,

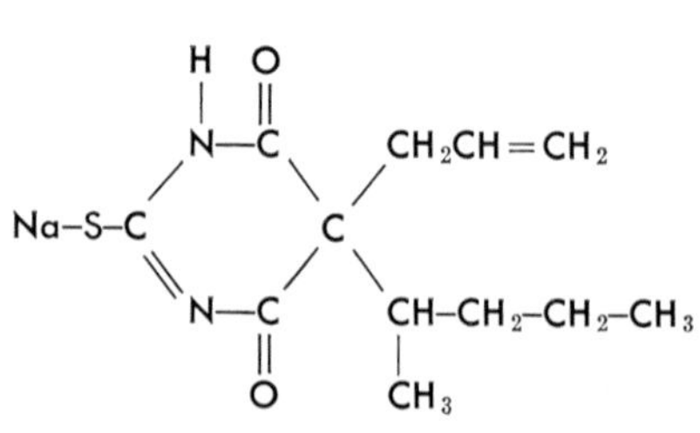

```
            H  O
            |  ||
            N—C     CH2CH=CH2
          /     \  /
  Na–S–C         C
          \\    /  \
            N—C     CH–CH2–CH2–CH3
               ||    |
               O     CH3
```

Fig. 8-13. Thiamylal sodium (Surital).

contraindications, advantages, and disadvantages of both these agents are identical.

METHOHEXITAL SODIUM (BREVITAL)

History. Methohexital sodium was synthesized in 1954 and was first used clinically in the latter months of 1955.

Physical properties. Methohexital sodium is a white hygroscopic powder. It is soluble in aqueous solution, and at room temperature (25° C.) it is stable for 4 to 6 weeks. It has a pH of approximately 11 and, as the other barbiturates, is not compatible with acid solutions.

Chemistry (Fig. 8-14). Methohexital sodium—$C_{13}H_{18}O_3N_2Na$—is sodium a-dl-1-methyl-5-allyl-5-(1-methyl-2-pentynyl) barbiturate. This compound differs from the other intravenous barbiturates in that it contains no sulfur in the molecule.

Pharmacology. Methohexital sodium is a rapid-acting sodium barbiturate. It has a greater potency than the other intravenous anesthetic agents used at the present time.

We have used this drug quite extensively and continue to administer it in a 1% solution by the intermittent technique. The actual recovery time for comparatively short procedures does not seem to be any shorter than for the other intravenous barbiturates. However, the patients do seem to be more mentally alert. The occurrence of hiccups is still a frequent complication (10 to 12%), but they do not persist and do not seem significant.

The same precautions and techniques of administration were observed as with the other intravenous agents. Also similar are the indications, contraindications, advantages, and disadvantages.

METHITURAL SODIUM (NERAVAL)

History. Methitural sodium is an ultrashort-acting thiobarbiturate introduced in 1954 after its development by Zima, von Werder, and

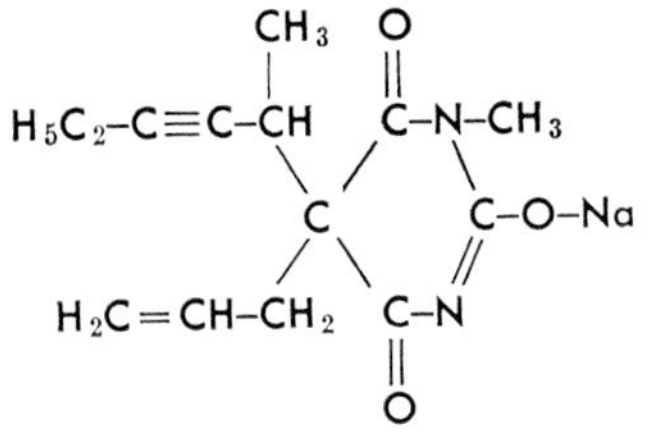

```
                 CH3   O
                  |    ||
H5C2-C≡C-CH    C-N-CH3
            \  /      \
              C         C-O-Na
            /  \      //
H2C=CH-CH2     C-N
                 ||
                 O
```

Fig. 8-14. Sodium methohexital (Brevital).

Hotovy. To the best of my knowledge, it is no longer commercially available.

Physical properties. Methitural sodium is a pale-yellow hygroscopic crystalline powder that dissolves readily in water, 5% dextrose, or saline to form a clear solution with a characteristic sulfurous odor. These solutions contain 50 mg. of anhydrous sodium carbonate per gram of methitural sodium to act as a buffer for stabilization. Even then the solution is comparatively unstable. The pH varies from 10.5 to 10.6.

Chemistry (Fig. 8-15). Methitural sodium—$C_{12}H_{19}O_2N_2SNa$—is the sodium salt of methyl-thio-ethyl-2 pentyl-thiobarbituric acid.

Pharmacology. In percentage strength, methitural sodium is the weakest of the intravenous anesthetics. Otherwise, its actions affect techniques of administration. Precautions to be taken are very similar to those for thiopental sodium and thiamyal sodium, with the exception that the percentage strength can be increased to 3, 4, or 5%.

The indications, contraindications, advantages, and disadvantages are identical with those of thiopental sodium and thiamylal sodium.

HEXOBARBITAL SODIUM (EVIPAL SODIUM)

History. Hexobarbital sodium was introduced as an anesthetic agent in Germany in 1932. It was the first of the intravenous agents to be widely used as a general anesthetic.

Physical properties. Hexobarbital sodium is a white, readily soluble hygroscopic powder which, when dissolved in saline solution or water, produces a solution with a pH of 10.

Chemistry (Fig. 8-16). Hexobarbital sodium—$C_{12}H_{15}O_3N_2Na$—has the chemical formula of sodium 5 (1-cyclohexenyl 1, 5 dimethyl barbiturate).

Pharmacology. When hexobarbital sodium was first introduced, it was generally used in 5% solution. This caused adverse side effects that tended to hold back the widespread acceptance of the drug. We

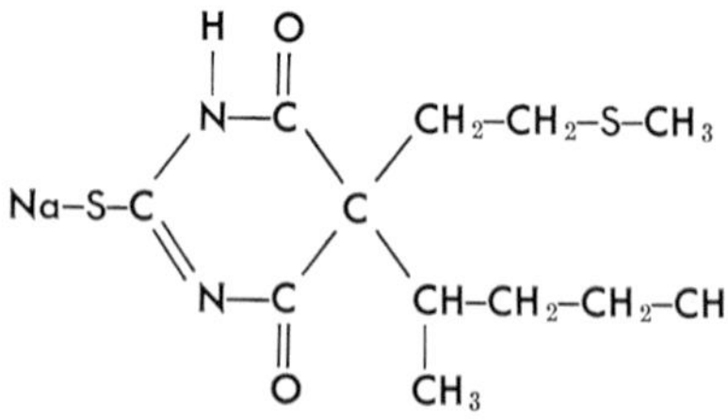

H O
N—C CH_2–CH_2–S–CH_3
Na–S–C   C
N—C   CH–CH_2–CH_2–CH_3
O CH_3

Fig. 8-15. Methitural sodium (Neraval).

have used the agent in 2% concentration and find it quite similar to the other intravenous agents.

The indications, contraindications, advantages, and disadvantages of hexobarbital sodium are identical with those of the other intravenous agents. It does, however, have a longer reaction time than the other commonly used intravenous agents.

HYDROXYDIONE SODIUM (VIADRIL)

History. Selye in 1941 reported the anesthetic activity of a large series of steroids. Hoeffer and Glaser in 1950 reported electroencephalographic changes suggesting cortical suppression following steroid therapy. While investigating various steroids for their anesthetic potency and other properties, Laubach and associates found that hydroxydione was the most satisfactory.

Physical properties. Hydroxydione sodium is a nonvolatile, readily soluble, crystalline solid with a pH of 7.8 to 10.2. It is supplied commercially in dry powder from 100 ml. vials containing 0.5 Gm. of the drug.

Chemistry (Fig. 8-17). Hydroxydione sodium—$C_{25}H_{36}O_6$—is a sodium salt of 2-1-hydroxy pregnane-3, 2-0 dione hemiscuccinate. A vial of Viadril contains 0.476 Gm. of hydroxydione, 0.123 Gm. of sodium carbonate, and 0.085 Gm. of sodium chloride.

Pharmacology. Hydroxydione sodium (Viadril) is the first steroid that has so far been used to any extent to produce anesthesia in man with no hormonal effects. Most of the pharmacological data to date have been derived from laboratory studies. These studies have shown that the drug causes pronounced depression of the central nervous system and that surgical anesthesia can be produced. The onset of anesthesia is slow but smooth, with a fairly rapid recovery. The duration of anesthesia is said to vary with the dose. Experimentation on laboratory animals has shown the following results: (1) The degree of respiratory depression was slight. (2) In dogs, no cardiac arrhythmias

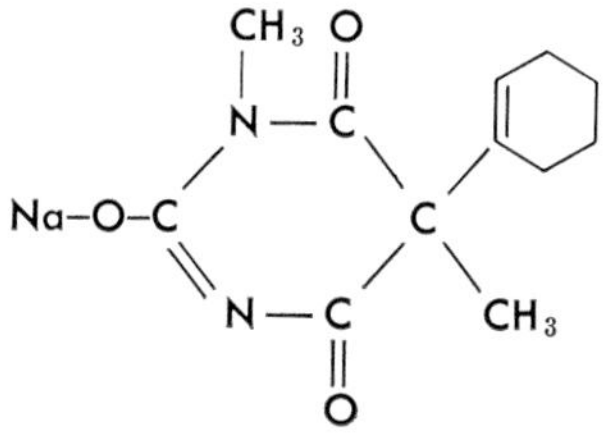

Fig. 8-16. Hexobarbital sodium (Evipal).

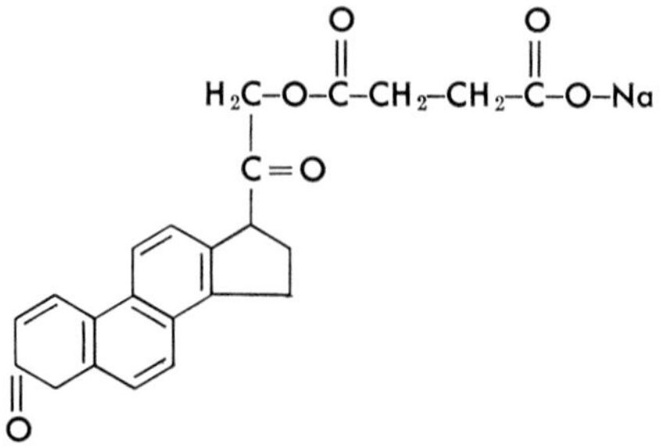

Fig. 8-17. Hydroxydione sodium (Viadril).

were observed. (3) Renal activity was decreased, which was a reaction similar to that induced by other anesthetics.

Hydroxydione sodium is the only intravenous anesthetic that is not stored in fat since the drug undergoes metabolic inactivation in the liver, as do the physiological steroids. Experimental evidence with rats suggests that hydroxydione sodium is detoxified in the liver by enxymatic reduction to urinary end products.

When it is administered intravenously to human subjects, hydroxydione sodium is capable of producing anesthesia and cerebral metabolic changes similar to those produced by the barbiturates. Induction is comparatively slow but smooth. The pharyngeal and laryngeal reflexes are usually obtunded more thoroughly than with other intravenous agents.

Hydroxydione sodium did not prove sufficiently effective or advantageous for anesthesia in dental or oral surgery. Its comparatively slow induction plus other disadvantages made it unsuitable as a general anesthetic for dentistry or oral surgery. These same disadvantages have excluded it from the armamentarium of the anesthesiologist.

GLUTETHIMIDE (DORIDEN)

History. Glutethimide was used only experimentally as an intravenous anesthetic. While it has been used widely as a soporific, it has never achieved any value as an anesthetic.

Physical properties. Glutethimide is a white crystalline compound with a melting point of 85° to 87° C. and a molecular weight of 217.3. The compound is insoluble in water but readily soluble in organic solvents.

Chemistry (Fig. 8-18). Glutethimide–$C_{13}H_{20}NO_2$–is an ethyl-a-phenyl-glutarimide and is a short-acting nonbarbiturate, nonnarcotic an-

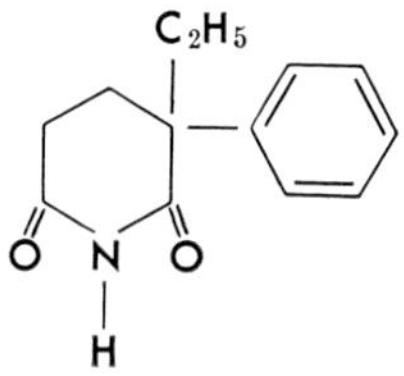

Fig. 8-18. Glutethimide (Doriden).

esthetic. It is the first of its type to be used as an intravenous anesthetic. Since glutethimide is poorly soluble in water, an organic solvent, polyethylene glycol, is used to prepare the solution.

Pharmacology. Our experience with this drug was limited to experimental use only. While no ill effects were demonstrated, its disadvantages far outnumbered the advantages and prevented its acceptance as a general anesthetic agent.

Animal experimentation showed no deleterious effects when the drug was used in anesthetic doses. When administered to dogs in larger doses, it occasionally produces a certain amount of hemolysis. This has not been observed in human beings.

Because our series of cases was so small, no definite opinion has been expressed. Whereas the current literature should be observed for any future developments or opinions concerning this agent, it is very doubtful whether any will appear.

RECTAL AGENTS

There are two rectal agents that may be used for anesthesia in dental and oral surgery. They are tribromoethanol (Avertin) and thiopental sodium (Pentothal).

TRIBROMOETHANOL (AVERTIN)

History. Tribromoethanol was first produced by Willstätter and Duisberg in Germany in 1923. It was first used clinically as an anesthetic by F. Eicholtz in 1926.

Physical properties. Tribromoethanol is a white crystalline compound soluble in water at 40° C. and has a characteristic ethereal odor. The drug is commonly used in fluid form, which is made by dissolving tribromoethanol in amylene hydrate. Tribromoethanol is a clear, heavy fluid that must be kept sealed in a dark bottle. Air will cause the amylene hydrate to vaporize, which allows tribromoethal crystals to precipitate. The fluid has a specific gravity of 1.4 at 20° C. The amylene hydrate is flammable but not explosive.

Table 8-3. Physical and chemical properties and pharmacology of intravenous agents

Agent	*Thiopental sodium (Pentothal)*	*Thiamylal sodium (Surital)*	*Methitural sodium (Neraval)*	*Hexobarbital sodium (Evipal)*	*Methohexital sodium (Brevital)*	*Hydroxydione sodium (Viadril)*	*Glutethimide (Doriden)*
Physical and chemical properties							
First used clinically	1934 by Lundy	1948 by Seevers	1954 by Zima	1932	1955 by Stoelting	1956 by Laubach	1958
Type of compound	Barbiturate	Barbiturate	Barbiturate	Barbiturate	Oxybarbiturate	Steroid	Nonbarbiturate
pH	10-11	10-11	10.5-10.6	10	10-11	7.8-10.2	
Solubility in water	Soluble	Soluble	Soluble	Soluble	Soluble	Soluble	Nonsoluble
Solubility in sodium chloride	Soluble	Soluble	Soluble	Soluble	Soluble	Soluble	Nonsoluble
Solubility in glucose	Soluble	Soluble	Soluble	Soluble	Soluble	Soluble	Nonsoluble
Stability	48-72 hours	24-72 hours	24-48 hours	24-48 hours	24-72 hours	24 hours	Stable
How supplied	Hygroscopic powder, 1 and 5 Gm. ampules	Hygroscopic powder, 1 and 5 Gm. ampules	Hygroscopic powder, 1 and 5 Gm. ampules	Hygroscopic powder, 1 Gm. ampules	Hygroscopic powder, 0.5, 2.5, 5 Gm. ampules	Dry powder, 0.5 Gm. ampules	Experimental

Percent of concentration commonly used	1-2½	1-2½	2-4	2-2½	1	1-2 Experimental	Experimental
Chemical formula	$C_{11}H_{17}O_2N_2SNa$	$C_{12}H_{17}O_2N_2SNa$	$C_{12}H_{19}O_2N_2SNa$	$C_{12}H_{15}O_3N_2Na$	$C_{12}H_{17}O_3N_2Na$	$C_{25}H_{36}O_6$	$C_{13}H_{20}NO_2$
Pharmacology							
Effect on central nervous system	Depressed in proportion to depth of anesthesia	Depressed in proportion to depth of anesthesia	Depressed in proportion to depth of anesthesia	Depressed in proportion to depth of anesthesia	Depressed in proportion to depth of anesthesia	Depressed in proportion to depth of anesthesia	Depressed in proportion to depth of anesthesia
Effect on respiration	Depressed in light planes; apnea in deep planes	Depressed in light planes; apnea in deep planes	Depressed in light planes; apnea in deep planes	Depressed in light planes; apnea in deep planes	Depressed in light planes; apnea in deep planes	Slight depression in all planes	In anesthetic doses no marked respiration depression
Effect on circulation	Slight vasomotor depression; pulse rate increased; blood pressure normal after initial lowering	Slight vasomotor depression; pulse rate increased; blood pressure normal after initial lowering	Slight vasomotor depression; pulse rate increased; blood pressure normal after initial lowering	Slight vasomotor depression; pulse rate increased; blood pressure normal after initial lowering	Slight vasomotor depression; pulse rate increased; blood pressure normal after initial lowering	Slight vasomotor depression; pulse unchanged; moderate hypotension	None noted yet

Continued on next page.

Table 8-3. Physical and chemical properties and pharmacology of intravenous agents—cont'd

Agent	***Thiopental sodium (Pentothal)***	***Thiamylal sodium (Surital)***	***Methitural sodium (Neraval)***	***Hexobarbital sodium (Evipal)***	***Methohexital sodium (Brevital)***	***Hydroxydione sodium (Viadril)***	***Glutethimide (Doriden)***
			Pharmacology—cont'd				
Effect on liver	Glycogen content decreased; no toxic effects	Glycogen content decreased; no toxic effects	Glycogen content decreased; no toxic effects	Glycogen content decreased; no toxic effects	Glycogen content decreased; no toxic effects	No toxic effects	Experimental
Effect on kidneys	No reduction in function; oliguria in renal disease	No reduction in function; oliguria in renal disease	No reduction in function; oliguria in renal disease	No reduction in function; oliguria in renal disease	No reduction in function; oliguria in renal disease	Function unimpaired in short anesthesia; without hypoxia	Experimental
Metabolized	Stored in adipose tissue; degradated in liver	Stored in adipose tissue: oxidized and degradated in liver more slowly than Pentothal	Stored in adipose tissue; oxidized and degradated in liver more quickly than Pentothal	Stored in adipose tissue; oxidized and degradated in liver	Stored in adipose tissue; degradated in liver	No fat storage; detoxified in liver by enzymatic reduction	Experimental
Toxic effects	Nontoxic, except on diseased liver and kidneys	Nontoxic, except on diseased liver and kidneys	Nontoxic, except on diseased liver and kidneys	Nontoxic, except on diseased liver and kidneys	Nontoxic, except on diseased liver and kidneys	Relatively nontoxic	Experimental

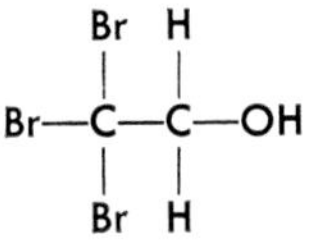

```
    Br  H
    |   |
Br—C—C—OH
    |   |
    Br  H
```

Fig. 8-19. Tribromoethanol (Avertin).

Chemistry (Fig. 8-19). Tribromoethanol–CBr_3CH_2OH–is produced by first treating ethyl alcohol with bromine to form tribromacetaldehyde (bromal). This compound is then reduced with aluminum ethoxide is an atmosphere of nitrogen. The resulting tribromoethanol crystals are then dissolved in amylene hydrate at a ratio of 1 Gm. of tribromoethanol to 0.5 Gm. of amylene hydrate to form 1 ml. of tribromoethanol.

Pharmacology. Tribromoethanol with an amylene hydrate is used rectally solely as a basal anesthetic. The solution is absorbed from the colon, about 95% being absorbed within half an hour. The solution is nonirritating to the rectal mucosa but may become irritating if the solution is decomposed or used repeatedly within a short period.

The drug is broken down in the liver by conjugation with glycuronic acid and is excreted almost completely through the kidneys. The amylene hydrate portion of the solution is eliminated unchanged in the urine and a small portion through the lungs. Tribromoethanol depresses the cerebral cortex but does not possess analgesic properties. The respiratory center is also depressed, whereas the threshold of stimulation from carbon dioxide is raised. An overdose may produce severe respiratory depression or apnea. Basal anesthetic doses usually cause no damage to the liver in a patient who has received adequate oxygen. Larger doses may depress liver function and produce a cloudy swelling of this organ. Severely reduced kidney function is common during tribromoethanol narcosis, with polyuria manifested after recovery.

The myocardium is unaffected by smaller doses, although the cardiac output may be mildly decreased. Larger doses may markedly depress the myocardium. The systolic pressure is usually lowered, whereas the diastolic pressure remains unchanged, showing reduced pulse pressure. The pharyngeal and laryngeal reflexes may be slightly obtunded but not abolished. The patient should be aided in the maintenance of a patient airway while under the influence of tribromoethanol.

The effects of the drug usually last for 2 to 4 hours. depending on the dose. Six to 10 mg. per 100 ml. of blood will produce unconsciousness. Emergence is usually gradual, but the patient may experience pain since tribromoethanol possesses no analgesic properties. For dental or oral surgery tribromoethanol has the following indication, contraindications, advantages, and disadvantages.

Indication

1. As a basal anesthetic for apprehensive children, to be followed with ether or nitrous oxide.

Contraindications

1. Presence of colitis or any disease of the colon.
2. Presence of hepatic or renal disease.

There are many medical contraindications to the use of tribromoethanol. However, these same contraindications would also delay most dental or oral surgical procedures, and therefore they are not listed as specific contraindications. For these patients before any procedures are attempted, medical consultation with both the internist and anesthesiologist should be sought.

Advantages

1. Can be given in the patient's room; thus an apprehensive patient can come to the operating room asleep.
2. Reduces markedly the amount of inhalation agent needed.

Disadvantages

1. Is administered in a single dose, which may be inaccurate.
2. May depress respirations.
3. Possesses no analgesic properties.
4. Definitely retards recovery time.

Rectal tribromoethanol, while not very widely used for dental and oral surgery, may prove highly advantageous for extremely apprehensive patients. It is particularly indicated when oral barbiturates are inadvisable and a trip to the operating room may be a terrifying and traumatic experience. Because of the prolonged recovery time, its use should be restricted to the hospital.

THIOPENTAL SODIUM (PENTOTHAL)

Thiopental sodium is discussed in detail under the intravenous agents; therefore it will suffice to state here that its principal rectal use should be as a basal anesthetic for children. The dose should be underestimated when one is in doubt. The technique of administration is discussed in Chapter 20.

Chapter 9

Drugs associated with anesthesia

Many drugs, although they are not anesthetic agents, are so closely associated with anesthesia that no discussion of the subject would be complete without them. Some of these drugs are absolutely essential to the administration of the anesthetic, whereas others, although not essential, greatly enhance the procedure.

OXYGEN (O_2)

History. Oxygen was discovered by Priestley in 1771. Although other experimenters may have observed this element, they did not recognize it at the time.

Physical Properties. Oxygen is a clear, colorless, odorless gas, with a molecular weight of 32 and a specific gravity of 1.015. It will liquefy at −119° C. at 50 atmospheres of pressure. The gas will boil at −183° C. and will solidify at −218° C.

Oxygen itself is neither flammable nor explosive, but it readily supports combustion and will thus enhance the flammability of other materials. In proper concentrations, it is a necessity in forming explosive mixtures with other gases.

Oxygen is marketed as a compressed gas and distributed in green cylinders. It constitutes 20.94% by volume of ordinary air.

Chemistry. Oxygen is usually prepared by the fractional distillation of liquid air. In this method, the nitrogen boils off first, leaving the oxygen as a liquid. It is also prepared by the electrolysis of water or by the reaction of water and sodium peroxide.

Pharmacology. Oxygen is essential for the maintenance of life and is a necessary constituent of all anesthetic mixtures. Its concentration should be at least sufficient to maintain normal body metabolism or any increased demands required at any particular time. Oxygen is transported within the bloodstream in chemical combination with the hemoglobin in the red cells as oxyhemoglobin and in physical solution in the plasma.

Oxygen diffuses rapidly across the alveolar membranes, the rate of diffusion depending on the gradient ratio of pressures. Under ordinary circumstances and for a reasonable length of time, oxygen is nonirritating to the tissues. However, prolonged inhalation of pure oxygen under pressure can act as an irritant to the mucous membranes. If 100% oxygen is inhaled under moderate pressure, the dissolved oxygen in the plasma may be increased fourfold. This increase has little or no effect on the oxygen-carrying qualities of the red cells.

Oxygen deficiency can result from the following conditions: (1) asphyxia, in which an inadequate supply of oxygen reaches the lungs; (2) hypoxia, in which oxygen unsaturation of the hemoglobin occurs; (3) anemia, in which there is a deficiency of hemoglobin in the blood; (4) ischemia, in which there is an inadequate circulation of the blood through the body; and (5) histotoxic anoxia, which is the incapacity of tissue cells to utilize oxygen.

Under normal circumstances, oxygen exerts a pressure of 152 mm. Hg in the atmosphere, a pressure of 105 mm. Hg in the lungs, and a pressure of approximately 100 mm. Hg in arterial blood. In a normal person, ordinary air may be diluted until it contains only 15% oxygen without producing any immediate ill effect. At a concentration of 10%, symptoms of anoxia such as dizziness, shortness of breath, deeper and more frequent respirations, quickened pulse, and cyanosis are noticeable. With a concentration of 7%, the symptoms become more serious and stupor sets in, and with a slightly lower percentage, unconsciousness occurs. Five percent is the minimal concentration compatible with life, and death may occur in this situation within a short time. Different persons vary in sensitivity to oxygen deficiency. Patients with cardiac and pulmonary diseases are more susceptible because their compensation is impaired. Thyrotoxic patients develop anoxia more easily because of their greater consumption of oxygen. Conversely, hypothyroid subjects are more tolerant of oxygen lack.

CARBON DIOXIDE (CO_2)

History. Carbon dioxide was first isolated by Black in 1757. Its chemical nature was explained later by Lavoisier, who showed it to be an oxide of carbon. In 1774, T. Bergman in working with carbon dioxide called it "acid of air."

Physical properties. Carbon dioxide is a colorless gas with a pungent odor and taste. It gives a tingling sensation to the nostrils when inspired. The gas has a molecular weight of 44 and a specific gravity of 1.54. Carbon dioxide liquefies at 30.9° C. and 77 atmospheres of pressure. The liquid is a colorless, mobile fluid that floats on water. It boils at −59° C. and solidifies at approximately −78° C. Faraday first liquefied carbon dioxide in 1823, and it is now a commercial preparation dispensed in steel containers. Solid carbon dioxide evaporates into air without melting and gives off carbon dioxide gas. Carbon dioxide is marketed as a compressed gas and distributed in gray cylinders. It is also distributed as a 90 to 10 mixture (90% oxygen and 10% carbon dioxide) in gray-green cylinders. Carbon dioxide constitutes about 0.03% of atmospheric air by volume.

Chemistry. Carbon dioxide is an inorganic, highly stable gas. It is nonflammable and is often used as a diluent for oxygen to smother flammable mixtures. It is readily absorbed by alkalis and combines with water to form carbonic acid, with 105 ml. dissolving in 100 ml. of water at 20° C.

Carbon dioxide is prepared by the oxidation of coke and by the heating of alkaline earth carbonates–$CaCO_3 \longrightarrow CaO + CO_2$. It is also formed from the fermentation of sugar, which decomposes into ethyl alcohol and carbon dioxide.

Pharmacology. Carbon dioxide is a primary stimulant of the respiratory center and as such triggers the inspiratory effort. It is a by-product of all cellular metabolism. An increase of alveolar carbon dioxide of 0.1% doubles ventilation, whereas a decrease of 0.1% may produce apnea for a short period. An excess of carbon dioxide increases the volume first and then the rate. This early stimulation may be followed by depression when carbon dioxide in excess of 10% is utilized. Increased carbon dioxide tension above that required to stimulate the respiratory center may stimulate respirations by way of the carotid body. The cardiac output is initially increased by small increases. Excessive retention may produce cardiac arrhythmias. Carbon dioxide favors dissociation of oxyhemoglobin but does not increase the oxygen-carrying capacity of the blood. The clotting time is shortened by an increase in carbon dioxide tension of the blood.

Carbon dioxide is capable of producing anesthesia and is used for this purpose in experimental animals. A concentration of 30% or more with oxygen is required to produce anesthesia. Excess carbon dioxide in man may produce convulsions. In general anesthesia, efficient elimination of carbon dioxide is essential for successful administration of the anesthetic. Although small increases in carbon dioxide may be an early stimulant, the stimulation is followed by depression when the carbon dioxide is further increased. With still greater increases the gas continues to act as a depressant and not as a stimulant.

NITROGEN (N)

History. Nitrogen was first discovered and isolated by Rutherford in 1772. Cavendish confirmed it in 1785. Chaptal suggested calling the gas nitrogen, from the Greek words *nitron,* meaning niter, and *genesis,* meaning to generate.

Physical properties. Nitrogen is an inert gas that comprises approximately 80% of the total volume of atmospheric air. It is colorless and tasteless and does not combine with water or other substances. It has a molecular weight of 28 and a specific gravity of 0.967. It liquefies at −149° C. at 75 atmospheres of pressure, solidifies at −214° C., and boils at −186° C. Nitrogen is nonflammable and will not support combustion. It is dispensed as a compressed gas in steel cylinders with an orange top and gray bottom.

Chemistry. Nitrogen is a diatomic element prepared on a large scale by the liquid air process as a by-product during the manufacture of oxygen. While nitrogen is commonly known as an inert gas under ordinary circumstances, it will combine with other elements. It is highly active chemically when in a combined form. This is illustrated by nitrogen chloride, which is a violent explosive. The inertness of nitrogen is overcome by high temperatures at which the gas will combine with some metals to form nitrides.

Pharmacology. All living matter and the waste products of animals contain considerable amounts of nitrogen in a combined state. While plants depend on nitrogen for food, they cannot obtain it directly from the atmosphere. Nitrogen has no known effect on tissues but can produce anoxia if inhaled in excessive quantities. It is present in simple solution (as an inert gas) in plasma, interstitial tissues, and cells. It is present in all body fluids and exists in identical concentrations in arterial and venous blood. The gas will diffuse from tissues as do other inert gases. Alveolar and expired air has a nitrogen tension of 576 mm. Hg when the inspired air is at a tension of 590 mm. Hg. The primary use of nitrogen is as a diluent to reduce high oxygen tension during inhalation anesthesia. It may also be utilized to reduce the flammability of other anesthetic agents when helium is not available.

HELIUM (He)

History. The presence of helium was first detected on the sun in 1608, but the element was not recognized as such. With the invention and subsequent use of the telescope and spectroscope, more careful observation of the sun was achieved. In 1866, J. Norman Lockyer of England originated a method for solar investigation that used the spectroscope. In 1868 Lockyer and Janssen, a Frenchman, made observations of the sun's spectrum. Since these were the first observations of this kind, both men were given equal credit by the French Academy of Science, but Janssen had not noted a new, unclassified line that Lockyer had noted and referred to as D3, or the new element, helium. In 1895 Professor William Ramsay and Lord Rayleigh discovered helium in the earth.

Physical properties. Helium is a rare, monatomic, inert gas found in the air in proportions of 1 volume of helium in 185,000 volumes of air. The gas has an atomic weight of 4 and a molecular weight of 4. It is colorless, odorless, tasteless, nonpoisonous, nonflammable, and nonexplosive. The gas is not only inert but also chemically nonreactive. The specific gravity of helium is 0.1381; it is next to the lightest element known. It is seven and a quarter times as light as air. Helium has high thermal conductivity and diffuses at a very fast rate. When liquefied at–207° C. and 2.26 atmospheres of pressure it forms a colorless, mobile, transparent fluid.

Chemistry. Helium exists in the atmosphere in proportions too small to be recovered economically. The readiest source of helium is natural gas, particularly that occuring in Texas, which provides the most practical source. Helium is marketed as a compressed gas in brown steel cylinders. When helium is mixed with oxygen, the tank is colored green and brown.

Pharmacology. Helium has no physiological effect on the tissues because of its inertness and low solubility in water and body fluids. It is used in combination with oxygen to facilitate breathing. The gas was first used in anesthesia as a diluent by Dr. G. J. Thomas of Pittsburgh.

Except for its possible use as a diluent, helium has no practical value in anesthesia for dental surgical procedures.

ATROPINE AND SCOPOLAMINE

Atropine and scopolamine are both alkaloid derivatives of belladonna. As alkaloids, they are basic in reaction when in aqueous solution, and they form salts with mineral acids. The clinical history of these drugs is obscure, although it is known that they were used in the Middle Ages.

ATROPINE

History. Atropine was first recognized by Vaequelin is 1809 and described as an alkaloid by Brandes in 1819.

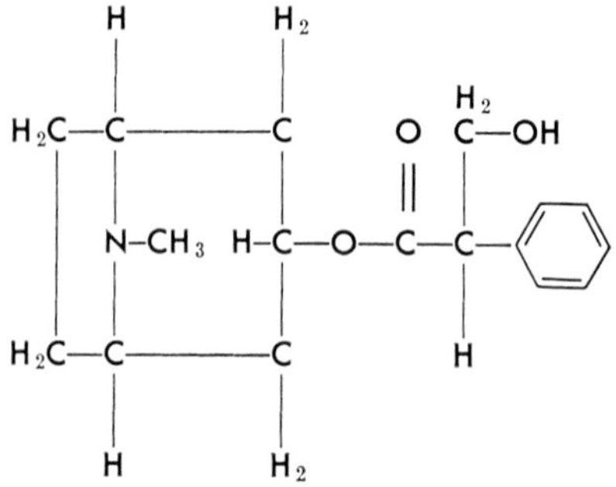

Fig. 9-1. Atropine.

Physical properties (Fig. 9-1). Atropine, as an organic base, is a white crystalline powder with a characteristic bitter taste. The base is poorly soluble in water but will combine with acids to form salts. The most commonly used salt is the sulfate, which is a white powder soluble in water.

Pharmacology. Atropine is primarily used in anesthesia for premedication, usually combined with a narcotic or a barbiturate. Atropine stimulates autonomic nerve endings centrally and depresses them peripherally. In small doses it stimulates the medulla, particularly the vagus center, which produces bradycardia. Small doses also stimulate the respiratory center but have so particular effect on the cortex. Atropine is used mainly for its peripheral effect in inhibiting the normal reactions produced by parasympathetic stimulation, which it annuls by acting directly on the effector cells at the terminal ends of the parasympathetic postganglionic fibers. Atropine inhibits the secretary glands in the oral and nasal passages as well as in the tracheobronchial tree. As previously stated, while small doses may stimulate the respiratory center, this stimulation is insignificant as compared to the depressant effect of larger doses on respirations. Adequate doses of atropine produce relaxation of the smooth muscles of the trachea and bronchi.

The first effect of atropine on the heart rate is a slowing one, due to stimulation of the vagus center. This is followed, however, by an increase in heart rate due to paralysis of the vagal endings. Larger doses of atropine produce tachycardia and flushing of the skin. For many patients, atropine may be administered to overcome persistent bradycardia.

Atropine paralyzes the sphincter oculi muscle of the iris, causing dilation of the pupil. In addition, it produces paralysis of the ciliary

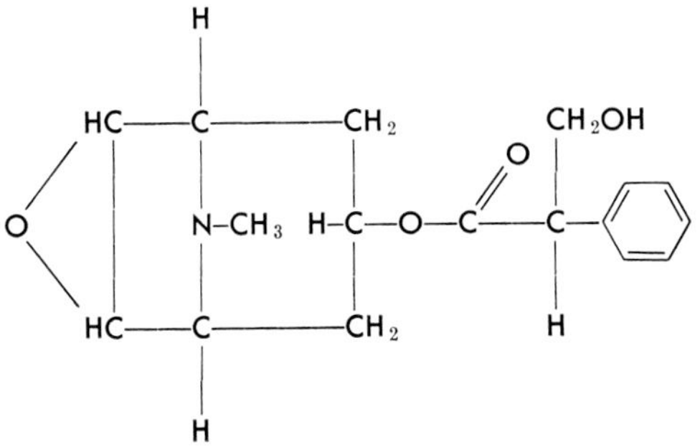

Fig. 9-2. Scopolamine.

muscle of the crystalline lens, causing failure of accommodation for near objects.

The degree of action of atropine on the laryngeal nerve is a questionable one, and the drug should not be relied upon to depress this nerve action sufficiently to prevent laryngospasm. The effect of atropine in preventing or treating laryngospasm is doubtful, and I have had very little success with this drug. The incidence of laryngospasm is almost directly proportional to the effectiveness of atropine in reducing secretions within the air passages, rather than to any direct action it may have on the laryngeal or vagus nerves. The use of atropine for routine premedication preceding intravenous anesthesia for short dental procedures in ambulatory patients is no longer required.

SCOPOLAMINE

History. Scopolamine was first discovered by E. Schmidt in 1888.

Physical properties. Scopolamine, as an organic base, is a colorless, heavy liquid. It may crystallize into a white powder with a melting point of approximately 59° C. The base is only slightly soluble in water but is readily soluble in alcohol, chloroform, or ether. The organic base will combine with acids to form salts, the most common of which is the hydrobromide. The salt is a white crystalline powder soluble in water and has a bitter taste.

Pharmacology (Fig. 9-2). Scopolamine, like atropine, is primarily used in anesthesia for premedication, in which it is generally combined with a narcotic or barbiturate. Again, like atropine, it is both a stimulant and a depressant. However, atropine stimulates centrally, whereas scopolamine is a cortical depressant. Scopolamine in preanesthetic doses (0.4 to 0.6 mg.) has a depressing effect on the central nervous system that results in drowsiness and even sleep. On the other hand, it has no analgesic properties; when it is given alone to patients who are in pain, restlessness, excitement, or hallucinations may be manifested. The heart rate is slowed with scopolamine, probably because of stimulation of the vagus center. Its direct effect on the vagus nerve is much less distinct than that of atropine.

In all respects, the peripheral effects of scopolamine are similar to those of atropine but less pronounced. The drying effect of scopolamine is greater than that of atropine but is shorter.

Scopolamine, because of its amnesic effects and fewer side reactions, offers some advantages over atropine, but it is contraindicated for elderly patients since it may cause excitement or hallucinations. The dosages of both drugs are similar.

NARCOTICS

The narcotics are an important group of drugs. Any person administering general anesthetics should have an understanding of them since they may be of inestimable value. Any dentist prescribing narcotics should be fully aware of the provisions of the Harrison Narcotic Act.

The narcotics may be divided into three groups: (1) opiates, or alkaloids of opium, which include morphine, pantopon, and codeine; (2) the synthetic opiates, which include dihydromorphinone (Dilaudid), diacetylmorphine (Heroin), hydroxydihydromorphinone (Numorphan), and methyldihydromorphinone (Metopon); and (3) opioids, or synthetic compounds, which include meperidine (Demerol), alphaprodine (Nisentil), methadone (Dolophine), levo-dromoran tartrate (Levorphan), and anileridine (Leritine).

NARCOTICS—OPIATES OR ALKALOIDS OF OPIUM

The naturally occurring narcotics are obtained from opium, which is in turn obtained from the milky exudate of the Oriental poppy seed. This exudate contains many alkaloids, of which 75% are resins and oils pharmacologically unfit for use. About 10% of opium is morphine; whereas codeine represents about 0.5%.

Since not all the narcotics are frequently used in conjunction with general anesthesia, only those drugs more commonly employed for premedication or in conjunction with the anesthetic shall be discussed.

MORPHINE

History. Morphine is the principal compound of the opium alkaloids and was isolated from opium by Serturner in 1805.

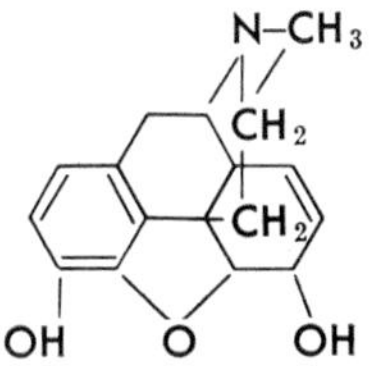

Fig. 9-3. Morphine.

Physical properties. Morphine is a white crystalline powder slightly soluble in water (1 Gm. dissolves in 5,000 ml.). It combines with acids to form salts, the most important of which is the sulfate. The sulfate salt is a white powder that is readily soluble in water and has a bitter taste.

Chemistry (Fig. 9-3). Morphine is the principal alkaloid of opium and has the following structural formula: $C_{17}H_{19}NO_3+H_2O$.

Pharmacology. Morphine is a potent analgesic agent that is believed to have a selective action on the pain centers in the optic thalami. Although it has a decided analgesic effect, it produces only a mild cerebral cortical depression, with the result that as average dose seldom produces amnesia but more often produces euphoria. Increased doses may cause a degree of hypnosis, anesthesia, and extreme respiratory depression. Death from an overdose is usually the result of respiratory depression. Morphine may produce an increased intracranial pressure that is enhanced by hypoxia.

The pupils usually constrict in patients who have received a single dose of morphine, whereas the respirations may be depressed in proportion to the dose and the susceptibility of the individual patient. Morphine may stimulate the vomiting center, with the result that nausea and vomiting are not uncommon, occurring in 15 to 25% of the patients. In addition, the drug may produce gastrointestinal immobility.

Morphine has little or no effect on the heart, but when it does affect the heart, it usually causes bradycardia due to stimulation of the vagus nerve. The blood pressure is not generally affected by ordinary dosages. The drug is detoxified in the liver, and the larger part is excreted by the kidneys as monoglucuronide.

Morphine may be administered intravenously, intramuscularly, or subcutaneously. The intravenous and intramuscular doses for the average adult are 8, 10, or 16 mg. (1/8, 1/6, or 1/4 grain). These doses should be scaled down correspondingly for children, infants, and geriatric patients.

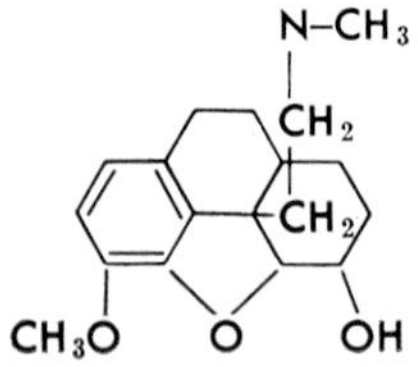

Fig. 9-4. Codeine.

PANTOPON

Pantopon is a mixture of purified opium alkaloids and contains 50% morphine by weight. The drug is given in doses ranging from 10 to 12 mg.; it closely resembles morphine in all respects. It can be administered orally as well as parenterally, and this is its only advantage over morphine.

CODEINE

Codeine (Fig. 9-4), or methylmorphine, constitutes about 0.5% of opium. It is available as a free base and is most often used as the phosphate or sulfate salt, which is soluble in water to about 3%.

Codeine is less potent than morphine, and maximum doses, which range from 15 to 60 mg. (¼ to 1 grain), raise the pain threshold by about 50%. The drug is one of the most effective analgesics available to the dentist since it is tolerated well when given orally and can be given intramuscularly. It can be combined with other drugs if desired.

Not only is codeine less potent than morphine, but its side effects are also less pronounced. This is a distinct advantage in many instances for an outpatient or when the oral route for premedication is desired.

Synthetic opiates

DIHYDROMORPHINONE (DILAUDID)

Dihydromorphinone (Fig. 9-5) follows the same pattern as morphine, with the exception that it is more potent and shorter acting. Dihydromorphinone does not cause constriction of the pupil, nor does it as readily induce nausea and vomiting. The dose used is one fourth to one fifth that of morphine.

NARCOTICS—OPIOIDS OR SYNTHETIC COMPOUNDS

Only the opioids, or synthetic compounds, commonly employed as premedication or in conjunction with general anesthetics will be discussed.

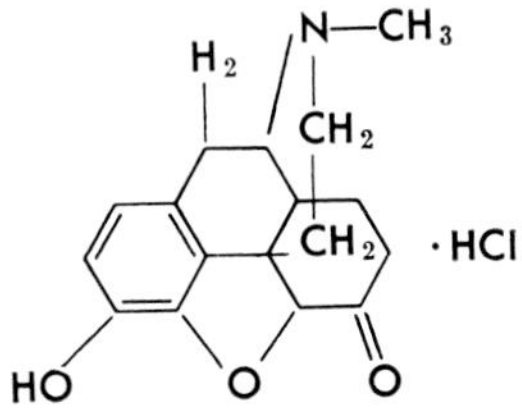

Fig. 9-5. Dihydromorphinone (Dilaudid).

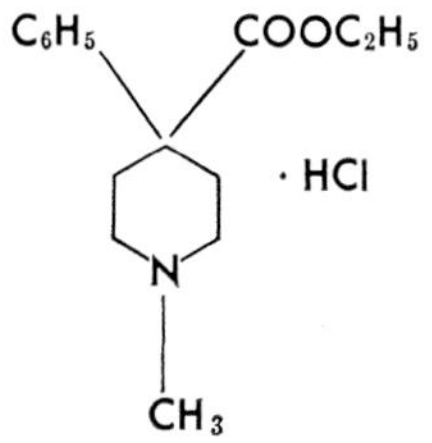

Fig. 9-6. Meperidine (Demerol).

MEPERIDINE (DEMEROL)

Meperidine is ethyl 1-methyl-4-phenylpiperidine-4-carboxylate hydrochloride (Fig. 9-6) and is the first synthetic narcotic and opioid. It is a white odorless crystal, soluble in water, and has a slightly bitter taste. It can be administered orally or intramuscularly in 50 to 100 mg. doses, but it is not recommended for subcutaneous use.

Meperidine possesses the properties of morphine, codeine, and atropine and has an analgesic potency between that of morphine and codeine. In average doses it is capable of raising the pain threshold by 60 to 65%.

This drug, although synthetic, is capable of producing addiction. It does not cause significant respiratory depression but will occasionally induce nausea or vomiting. Dizziness is the most common complication in ambulatory patients. The drug is detoxified by the liver, and a small percentage is excreted in the urine.

ALPHAPRODINE (NISENTIL)

Chemically, alphaprodine (Fig. 9-7) is dl-alpha-1, 3-dimethyl-4-phenyl-4-propionoxy-piperidine hydrochloride. It is a potent, short-acting analgesic capable of raising the pain threshold by 75 to 100%. The drug can be used both orally and parenterally and has a much more

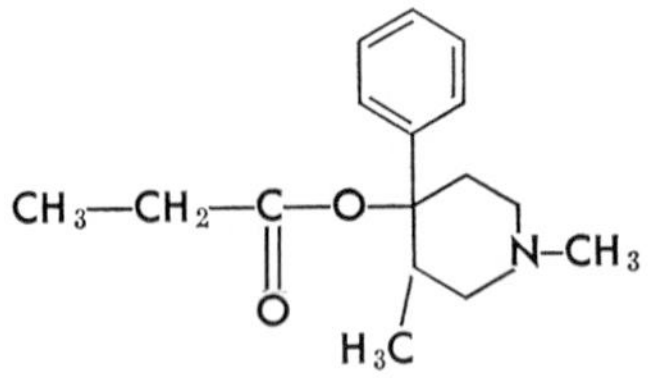

Fig. 9-7. Alphaprodine (Nisentil).

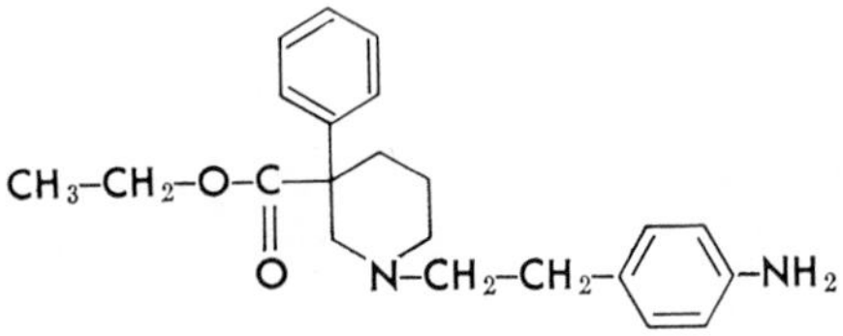

Fig. 9-8. Anileridine (Leritine).

rapid onset than morphine, codeine, or meperidine. The average dose is 20 to 40 mg.

The advantages of alphaprodine are its rapid onset, its short duration, its potency, and that fact that it is effective by any route of administration. Alphaprodine in usual doses should not be used with phenobarbital.

ANILERIDINE (LERITINE)

Anileridine is 1-(4-aminophenethyl)-4-phenylisonipecotic acid ethyl ester (Fig. 9-8). It is one of the newest of the potent opioids and is approximately two and one-half times as potent as meperidine. The drug can be used orally as well as parenterally. For maintenance during anesthesia we have used a solution containing 0.2 mg. per ml. (225 mg. of anileridine in 1,000 ml. of 5% dextrose). When given intramuscularly or intravenously in single doses, anileridine is used in doses approximately three eighths the amount used for meperidine and three times that for morphine.

Anileridine causes addiction and is also capable of depressing both respiration and circulation when larger doses are used. When necessary, the respiratory depression produced by anileridine can be reversed by the use of a narcotic antagonist. Larger doses of anileridine may cause stimulation of the central nervous system, excitement, and convulsions.

BARBITURATES

History. Barbital was first prepared by Fischer and von Mering in 1903. Phenobarbital was prepared by Horlein in 1911. These compounds are referred to as barbiturates, and according to Goodman and Gilman, over 2,500 such preparations have been synthesized since their inception.

Physical properties. The barbiturates are white powders, weakly acid and poorly soluble in water. They have a melting point ranging from 100° to 200° C. The weak acids dissolved in bases produce a salt that is readily soluble in water. The sodium salts are the most common preparation and have a pH of 9 to 10.

Chemistry (Fig. 9-9). The barbiturates are derivatives of barbituric acid (malonylurea), which is a combination of malonic acid and urea. Barbituric acid has no hypnotic properties, but replacement of hydrogen by various radicals produces many different drugs possessing hypnotic characteristics. The new compounds are varied in their actions, the potency and duration of action being markedly affected by the different substitutions.

Pharmacology. The barbiturates are primarily central nervous system depressants, and by varying the dose and method of administration, one may use them as sedatives, hypnotics, or general anesthetics. These drugs may be administered intraorally, intramuscularly, intravenously, or rectally, but they are usually administered intraorally or intramuscularly when used for premedication preceding general anesthesia. The intravenous route is more commonly employed when the barbiturates are used for controlled premedication or basal narcosis or as anticonvulsants.

The primary site of action of the barbiturates is not completely un-

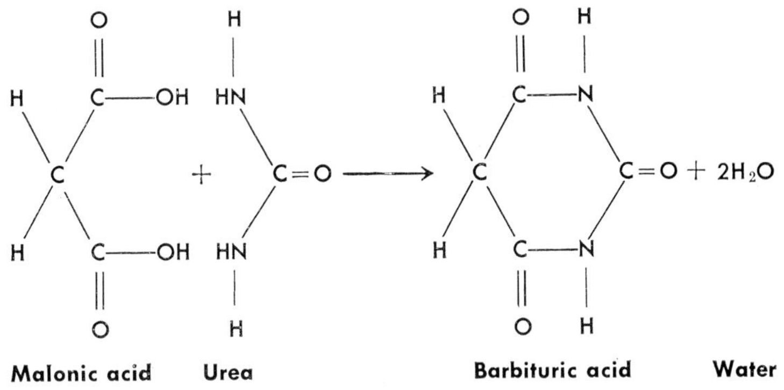

Malonic acid + Urea → Barbituric acid + $2H_2O$

Malonic acid **Urea** **Barbituric acid** **Water**

Fig. 9-9. Barbituric acid (malonic acid—urea).

derstood, but the hypothalamus is thought to be one of the first areas affected. It would seem logical to assume that the cerebral cortex is among the structures most sensitive to these drugs since they do depress cortical function and produce drowsiness and amnesia.

In doses that would ordinarily be used for premedication, the bar biturates have an extremely low incidence of untoward reactions, with so significant depressant effect on respiration or circulation. Larger doses usually depress the respirations and in many patients cause a sharp fall in blood pressure. The barbiturates in smaller therapeutic doses do not affect the heart muscle nor the cardiac output, but the myocardium may be depressed by larger doses. The barbiturates have no analgesic properties, and when they are given alone in hypnotic doses, they may lower the pain threshold rather than elevate it. They may, however, potentiate the action of other analgesic drugs.

There is a wide margin of safety between the hypnotic dose and the toxic dose when the drug is given orally. From five to ten times the hypnotic dose would be required to produce toxic symptoms. About the only valid contraindication to the use of barbiturates would be a history of allergy.

Toxic symptoms may be encountered in a particularly sensitive person who becomes unduly affected by a small dose of the drug. These symptoms will be manifested by drowsiness and, in some patients, sleep. Respiration is depressed in direct proportion to the depth of coma. Death, when it does occur, is usually the result of respiratory depression and hypoxia. This should never occur from the conservative hypnotic dose such as would be prescribed by the dentist for premedication.

Patients with an impaired cardiovascular, renal, or hepatic system should be given proportionately smaller doses of the barbiturates. It is extremely doubtful that any ambulatory patient able to present himself in the dental office would have a sufficiently impaired cardiovascular, renal, or hepatic system to be unable to detoxify and eliminate a smaller dose.

The barbituric acid derivates do not differ significantly in their pharmacological actions. Their main difference lies in the time of onset, duration of action, and manner of detoxification and elimination. They are divided, therefore, into four groups: ultrashort-acting, short-acting, intermediate-acting, and long-acting.

Since the ultrashort-acting and short-acting barbiturates are the only ones commonly employed for premedication preceding or is conjunction with general anesthesia, they will be the only groups discussed.

Ultrashort-acting barbiturates. The ultrashort-acting barbiturates most commonly used are Pentothal sodium, Surital sodium, Evipal sodium, and Brevital sodium. These drugs are thoroughly discussed in Chapter 8.

Short-acting barbiturates. The short-acting barbiturates most commonly used are pentobarbital (Nembutal) and secobarbital (Seconal).

These barbiturates are detoxified primarily by the liver and excreted in the urine. They may be administered orally, intramuscularly, intravenously, or rectally. The intraoral and intramuscular doses vary from 50 mg. (3/4 grain) to 200 mg. (3 grains), and the intravenous dose varies from 50 mg. to 100 mg. All doses will vary, depending on the age, body build, and physical condition of the patient, as well as on the effect to be obtained.

These drugs require 1 to 3 minutes for their maximum effect when given intravenously, and 20 to 45 minutes when given intraorally or intramuscularly. The duration of action ranges from 2 to 4 hours, with a residual effect lasting up to 6 hours.

Rectal administration of barbiturates is discussed in Chapter 20.

MUSCLE RELAXANTS

History. The history of muscle relaxants had its beginning in the sixteenth century. Sir Walter Raleigh mentioned the arrow poison of the Indians in his book *Discovery of Guiana,* which was published in 1595. The earliest scientifically planned investigation of the neuromuscular activity of curare was made by Claude Bernard in 1850. Renewed interest in the drug began in 1935 when King isolated *d*-tubocurarine from tubocurare. Curare was first used in anesthesia in 1942 by Griffith in the form of an aqueous solution of curare extract called Intocostrin. The synthetic compound succinylcholine was prepared by Hunt in 1906 but was not recognized as an almost ideal muscle relaxant until Bovet and Phillips, working independently, discovered its neuromuscular activity. The drug was first introduced into clinical practice in Austria by Brucke, Mayrhofer, and Hassfurther. Succinylcholine was introduced into the United States by Foldes.

The introduction of the muscle relaxants into anesthesia was a milestone and one of the greatest advancements in its development. The use of these drugs practically revolutionized the field of anesthesia, and for all intents and purposes has removed the need for deep narcosis. Intubation, particularly in anesthesia for oral surgery, became much more applicable and safe, and no longer was the insertion of an intratracheal tube a prolonged procedure and at times a hazardous one because of the deep anesthesia required. The availability of the rapid-acting and short-acting muscle relaxants practically reduced laryngospasm to a minor complication when intravenous agents were used.

Chemistry. Most of the naturally occurring muscle relaxants have been isolated from crude curare preparations. From these have been isolated quaternary ammonium bases called curarines. The three curare preparations are calabash curare, pot curare, and tubocurare. The relaxants from each are called curarines, protocurarines, and tubocurarines.

Pharmacology. The primary action of the muscle relaxants is to produce relaxation by paralyzing the skeletal muscles. They have no hypnotic or analgesic properties.

Before the pharmacology of the muscle relaxants is discussed, it is important to review briefly the mechanism of normal transmission of nerve impulses and the myoneural junction to facilitate a better understanding of these drugs. The myoneural junction is the terminal arborization between the nerve axon and the muscle fiber. It is in this area that the acetylcholine receptor substance and the acetylcholine esterase of the end-plate are found.

The resting nerve axon is in a polarized state, which indicates a difference in electrical potential between the two sides of its surface membrane. When a nerve impulse is propelled along the nerve axon, the surface membrane is depolarized. This wave spreading along the nerve fiber not only removes the polarity of the membrane, but also creates changes in its permeability. This increased permeability of the surface membrane allows for the rapid migration of sodium, chloride, and potassium ions in opposite directions until the membrane potential is restored and excitation ceases. Immediately following the passage of an impulse, acetylcholine is liberated.

The presence of acetylcholine at the myoneural junction prevents repolarization and permits the muscle to continue in a relaxed state. Ordinarily the acetylcholine is rapidly broken down into acetic acid and choline by an enzyme, cholinesterase. Any interference with the

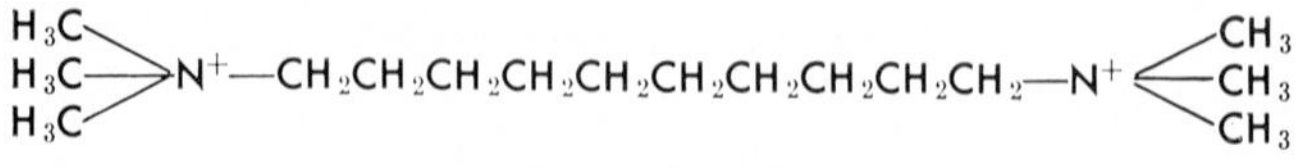

$$(H_3C)_3N^+{-}CH_2CH_2CH_2CH_2CH_2CH_2CH_2CH_2CH_2CH_2{-}N^+(CH_3)_3$$

Fig. 9-10. Decamethonium chloride (Syncurine).

breakdown and elimination of acetylcholine or the presence of an excess will produce paralysis and relaxation of the muscle fibers.

The commonly used muscle relaxants can be divided into two groups: (1) depolarizing agents, which are decamethonium chloride (Fig. 9-10), whose proprietary preparation is Syncurine, and succinylcholine (Fig. 9-11), whose proprietary preparations include Anectine and Quelicin; and (2) nondepolarizing agents, which include curare (Fig. 9-12) and its analogues.

The depolarizing agents, probably due to their slender molecular configuration, produce a biphasic block. The phase I, or depolarization, block is in effect when neuromuscular transmission is inhibited due to a sustained depolarization of the past junctional membrane. When this type of relaxant is administered over a prolonged period, the permeability of the past junctional membrane changes. The end-plate becomes repolarized and is accompanied by changes in the characteristics of the block or a phase II block. During this period a tachyphylactic effect of the drug is evident first, and later the block resembles that produced by the nondepolarizing agents.

The phase I block is usually preceded by muscular twitching, which can be eliminated if small amounts (3 to 6 mg.) of a nondepolarizing agent are given sufficient time preceding the administration of the depolarizing drug. The prolonged administration of the depolarizing drugs increases the patient's sensitivity to the nondepolarizing ones.

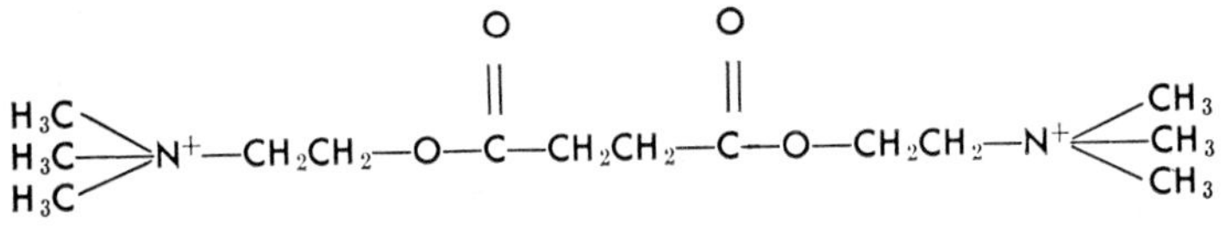

$$(H_3C)_3N^+{-}CH_2CH_2{-}O{-}\overset{O}{\overset{\|}{C}}{-}CH_2CH_2{-}\overset{O}{\overset{\|}{C}}{-}O{-}CH_2CH_2{-}N^+(CH_3)_3$$

Fig. 9-11. Succinylcholine (Anectine; Quelicin).

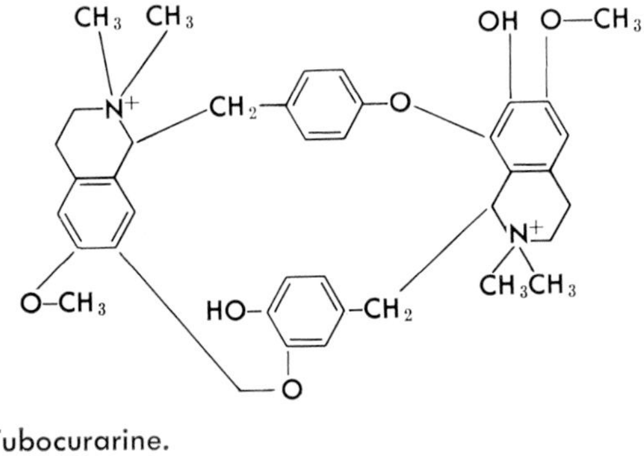

Fig. 9-12. *d*-Tubocurarine.

A sufficient amount of a muscle relaxant concentrated at the end-plate will produce a neuromuscular block that will be maintained as long as the plasma level is adequate to continue the end-plate concentration. When the administration of the drug is decreased or discontinued, the plasma level drops, permitting the drug to diffuse from the end-plate back into the plasma and thus restore neuromuscular transmission.

Small doses of a muscle relaxant are shunted from the end-plate back into the plasma and then into inactive tissue depots, bringing a termination of the block. Larger doses eventually saturate the tissue depots and are then metabolized or excreted in the urine. Succinylcholine is almost completely hydrolyzed by plasma cholinesterase, whereas *d*-tubocurarine is partly excreted unchange and partly metabolized.

The depolarizing agents, which are synthetic compounds, produce an acetylcholine-like action, and as long as a sufficient amount of the drug remains at the myoneural junction, the nerve will be in a depolarized state. At present, succinylcholine chloride is the most widely used depolarizing agent. The most frequent method of administration is the continuous drip. The drug has a rapid onset, and its action is of comparatively short duration. Within approximately 3 minutes the succinylcholine is hydrolyzed and its effect reversed. The hydrolysis is completed by the action of cholinesterase.

When the drug is administered rapidly, muscle twitching is produced because of rapid depolarization of the end-plate. Slow administration does not seem to duplicate this condition.

The nondepolarizing agents produce their effect by preventing access of the acetylcholine to the cholinergic receptors of the end-plate, and thus the acetylcholine is prevented from depolarizing the membrane. The administration of this type of muscle relaxant produces no twitching effect.

Although the muscle relaxants are of tremendous value in anesthesia, they are not without their inherent dangers. Primary among these dangers is the interference with pulmonary ventilation due to paralysis of the respiratory muscles. It is therefore essential that any person using these drugs in conjunction with anesthetic agents be well versed in their use and be capable of either augmenting or controlling the respirations.

At times any of the muscle relaxants may have a prolonged effect. In one instance, an apparently healthy 26-year-old woman was given succinylcholine to facilitate intratracheal intubation. None of the drug was given subsequently. Spontaneous respirations did not occur for a period of 3 hours, during which time controlled ventilation was continued. After this the patient made an uneventful recovery and was able to give a detailed report of what took place, stating that she was aware of her surroundings but was unable to breathe or move.

Some anesthetic agents have a potentiating effect when given with the muscle relaxants. Ether and halothane potentiate the effects of *d*-tubocurarine, whereas nitrous oxide and the intravenous agents have no effect on the action of the muscle relaxants.

Although we have used muscle relaxants (succinylcholine administered by the continuous drip technique) with nitrous oxide and intravenous agents for ambulatory patients, we do not recommend their routine use. Muscle relaxants in anesthesia for dental and oral surgery can best be utilized to facilitate intratracheal intubation or to combat laryngeal spasm. Since muscle relaxation is not usually required for this type of surgery, these drugs should be employed only when specifically indicated.

ATARAXIC DRUGS (TRANQUILIZERS)

History. Recently a tremendous amount of interest has centered on a new group of drugs called tranquilizers, or ataraxic agents. The term ataraxic was coined by Fabing in 1955 from a Greek word meaning without disturbance. Although many agents are classified in this group, not all of them are alike in chemical structure or pharmacological action.

The introduction of the phenothiazine derivatives into clinical usage could be considered a milestone in the field of sedation of the autonomic nervous system. The history of phenothiazine derivaties goes back to the synthesis of phenothiazine by Bernstein in 1883. French investigators in 1945 began screening the amine derivative of phenothiazine in the search for compounds possessing antiparkinsonian and antihistamine activity. Drowsy sedation was noted to be a frequent side effect associated with the clinical use of these drugs. The degree of sedation was often unrelated to the main clinical potency of the agent. In 1948 Winter noted a marked potentiating action of this drug on barbiturates.

Chemistry. The French scientists concerned themselves primarily with tertiary amine derivatives, whereas German investigators were engaged in the synthesis of a number of aromatic (ring) derivatives of phenothiazine.

Derivatives of phenothiazine include the following: (1) chlorpromazine (Fig. 9-13, *A*), (2) promethazine (Fig. 9-13, *B*), and (3) mepazine (Fig. 9-13, *C*).

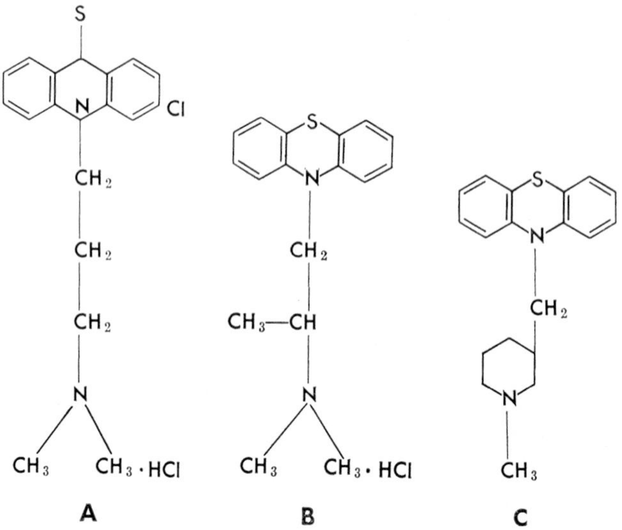

Fig. 9-13. A, Chlorpromazine hydrochloride (Thorazine), **B,** promethazine (Phenergan), **C,** and mepazine (Pacatal).

Pharmacology. The mode of action of the tranquilizing drugs is not clear. Many hypotheses have been outlined to explain their site of action, but as yet none have been substantiated.

At present the effect of the ataraxic drugs is thought to be due to their action on the midbrain and the reticular substance. The inversion of the stress responses may be related to suppression of the reflexes of the spinal cord caused by slowing or abolishing neuronal discharges.

The greatest usefulness of an ataraxic drug for dental anesthesia is as a potentiator for the barbiturates and the narcotics when used for premedication. Most of my experience has been with promethazine and hydroxyzine (Vistaril), which have proved to be valuable assets to the dental anesthetist. The combination of promethazine and meperidine has proved ideal for elevating the pain threshold while suppressing fear and apprehension. It has been possible to reduce greatly the amount of intravenous barbiturates required and at the same time to render mixtures of nitrous oxide and oxygen more effective. When employed alone, promethazine or hydroxyzine seems to produce no effects other than drowsiness. It has been by experience that patients receiving promethazine or hydroxyzine alone seem more susceptible to painful stimuli. Also, larger doses are required to produce drowsiness, and they may produce severe hypotension in some patients. This hypotensive state has not been observed frequently when smaller doses are combined with barbiturates or narcotics. The overall effect when smaller combined doses have been used has been more desirable.

Promethazine and hydroxyzine, when combined with meperidine, have also proved most effective for relieving painful experiences when patients emerge from a general anesthetic. This combination of drugs in 25 mg, doses of each has markedly elevated the pain threshold, with a minimum of cortical depression or associated nausea.

As research and clinical observation continue, undoubtedly the scope of usefulness of the ataraxic drugs will increase. They should be used with caution; however, and their potentiating effect on barbiturates and narcotics should be kept in mind.

NEUROLEPT AGENT

INNOVAR

Innovar is a combination of a potent narcotic analgesic, fentanyl (Sublimaze), and a powerful psychosedative drug, droperidol (Inapsine), in a 50:1 mixture (fentanyl, 0.05 mg., and droperidol, 2.5 mg.). In combination each exerts its own pharmacological action, with the droperidol potentiating the analgesic effect of the fentanyl and producing a high level of analgesia. Innovar should be a most advantageous adjunct to local anesthesia for the poor-risk patient.

Respiratory effects. The fentanyl component tends to produce a severe respiratory depression, particularly when given intravenously. In some cases verbal commands instructing the patient to breathe deeply will overcome the depression. In other cases the patient may have to have a muscle relaxant and intratracheal intubation to ensure adequate ventilation.

Cardiovascular effects. As a general rule, significant alterations in pulse rate and blood pressure are uncommon. There may be a slight decrease in the heart rate and blood pressure following injection. The heart rhythm is, as a rule, unaffected.

Chapter 10

Maintenance of the airway

The maintenance of a patent airway is, without a doubt, the most important factor in the administration of a general anesthetic. Nothing should be allowed to interfere in any manner with the free and unobstructed uptake of oxygen and the unimpeded elimination of carbon dioxide. This is so essential that it is impossible to overstress the importance of this exchange.

Whenever anyone undertakes the administration of a general anesthetic, he should be cognizant of the patient's respiratory ventilation and remain keenly aware of this situation throughout the anesthesia. At no time should the anesthetist allow himself to be in doubt as to the patient's respiratory efficiency. If at any time he has any doubt whatsoever as to the adequacy of the pulmonary ventilation, he should assume that it is inadequate and take measures to improve it. If an error is to be made, it is better to err on the side of safety.

One of the most insidious complications that occurs during the administration of a general anesthetic is gradually increasing hypoxia in a mildly obstructed or mildly depressed patient. The oxygen deficiency or carbon dioxide retention may be so slight that the inexperienced anesthetist may accept it as being of no consequence. It is therefore the slow but unrecognized onset of this serious complication that makes it so dangerous. A seemingly mild obstruction due to a poor position of the head and neck, a relaxed tongue, or blood and mucus in the postpharyngeal region may actually reduce the respiratory exchange by as much as 25 or even 50%. It is therefore self-evident why these conditions should not be tolerated.

The mechanical obstructions previously mentioned are the most frequent causes of inadequate pulmonary ventilation. They can best be recognized by watching and listening closely to every respiratory excursion of the patient. Normal unobstructed breathing is practically inaudible, and the patient's thoracic cage expands and relaxes with a synchronous rhythm. Whenever the normal exchange of respiratory gases is clearly audible and there are sounds of obstruction, steps should be taken to correct the deficiency.

The maintenance of a free and patent airway during the administration of a general anesthetic for any type of dental surgery is at times difficult and may even be hazardous. This situation is due to the fact that the operation is being performed within the air passages, and from time to time blood or mucus produced by the manipulations within the oral cavity may gravitate toward the oropharynx and laryngopharynx. Furthermore, the operator may sometimes find it necessary to apply varying degrees of pressure against the mandible, which creates a partial obstruction.

The anesthetist should be constantly on the alert for such happenings and immediately call to the attention of the operator or his assistant the presence of the obstructing factors. It is the fundamental duty of the anesthetist to see that these conditions are corrected so that insidious hypoxia of sufficient consequence to create a serious emergency does not occur. The anesthetist who tolerates a respiratory obstruction, hoping that in due time the operator will correct the situation on his own initiative, may misjudge the amount of hypoxia created or the elapsed time and thus permit the creation of a serious emergency while he is watchfully waiting.

It is always advisable to attempt to maintain a free and patent airway, first by adhering to a few basic rules and second by carrying out the more simple maneuvers. The chin should be held up, with the head and trunk in normal position and the tongue drawn forward. This position tends to maintain a free passage of air into and out of the tracheobronchial tree.

Obstructions are most likely to occur at the oropharyngeal, laryngopharyngeal, or glottal area of the conducting portion of the external respiratory system. In the oropharyngeal area, a relaxed tongue, blood, mucus, or a misplaced oropharyngeal partition may seriously interfere with the ingress or egress of respiratory gases. The laryngopharyngeal area is subject to these same interferences. The glottal opening into the trachea, protected by the true and false cords, could be considered the most hazardous area for the occurrence of mechanical, physiological, or pathological obstruction. In this area a relaxed tongue may permit the epiglottis to partially obstruct the free passage of gases into and out of the glottal opening. Also, it is in this area that foreign bodies may become impacted, completely obstructing the airway. Furthermore, the true cords may become spastic during adduction and thus prevent respiratory gases from entering the tracheobronchial tree. Respiratory complications are discussed in more detail in Chapter 15.

If the oropharynx and laryngopharynx are free of mucus, blood, or debris, practically all methods of maintaining a free and patent airway should be directed toward preventing any interference with the free passage of respiratory gases into and out of the tracheobronchial tree caused by muscular relaxation or muscle spasm, which interferes with normal pulmonary ventilation.

With the head and neck of the patient in the proper position, the most commonly used means of maintaining a patent airway are oropharyngeal airway, nasopharyngeal airway, and intratracheal intubation (orotracheal and nasotracheal).

OROPHARYNGEAL AIRWAY

The oropharyngeal airway is a suitably curved apparatus made of metal, plastic, or hard rubber (Fig. 10-1) which, when placed in the

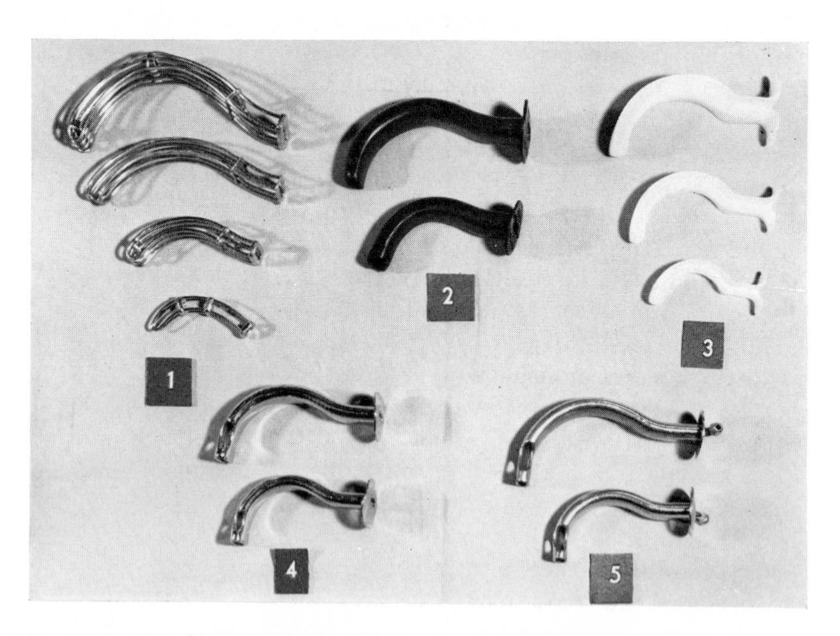

Fig. 10-1. Oropharyngeal airways. **1,** Wire; **2,** rubber; **3,** plastic; **4,** solid metal; **5,** metal, with oxygen attachment.

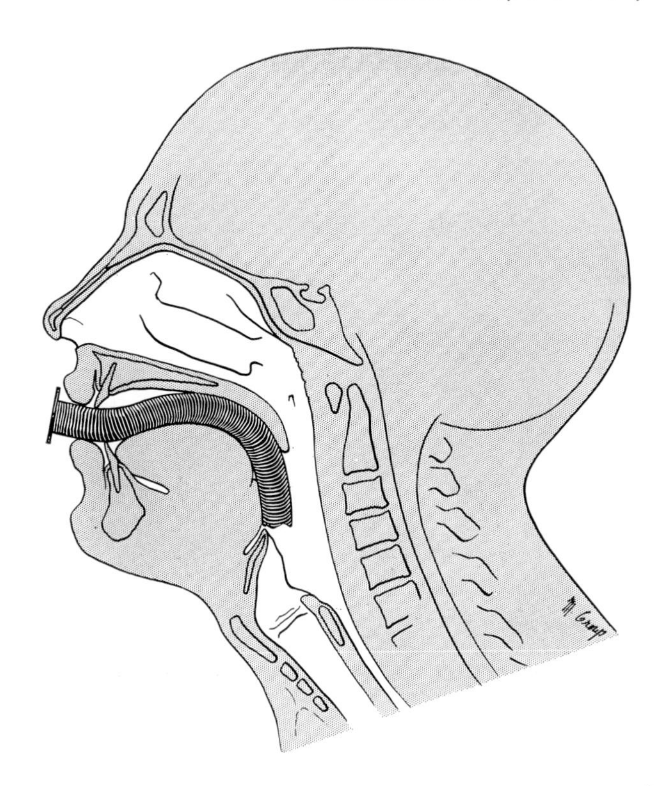

Fig. 10-2. Oropharyngeal airway in place; note that the airway holds the tongue forward.

oral cavity, extends posteriorly into the oropharynx. The curvature and stability of this apparatus are instrumental in maintaining the tongue in a forward position (Fig. 10-2) so that its musculature cannot relax posteriorly (Fig. 10-3), which would permit the epiglottis to obstruct the glottal opening. Anatomically and physiologically, the relationship of the musculature of the tongue to the epiglottis is such that pulling the tongue forward enhances the ingress of respiratory gases into the glottal opening. This is also shown by the fact that when the tongue is drawn forward, swallowing can be accomplished only with difficulty. In some situations it may be possible to accomplish the same end by placing a suture through the anterior portion of the tongue and drawing it slightly forward.

NASOPHARYNGEAL AIRWAY

The nasopharyngeal airway is composed of a rubber catheter of sufficient gauge, e.g., No. 29 or 30 French, No. 6 or 7 Magill (Fig.

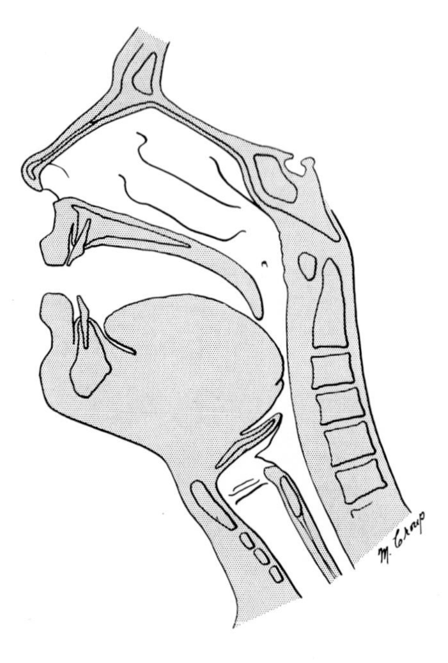

Fig. 10-3. Tongue is relaxed posteriorly, obstructing the airway.

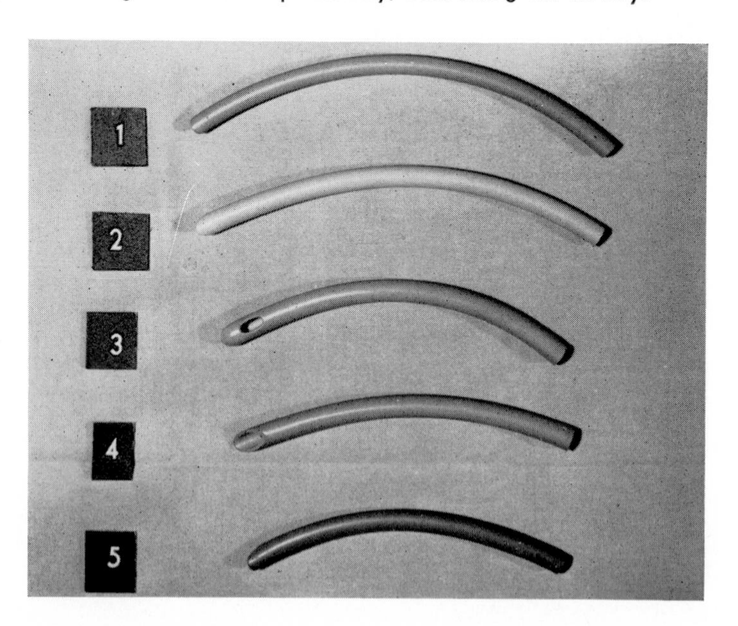

Fig. 10-4. Nasopharyngeal airways. Note various lengths and diameters. In **3** the airway has an additional opening opposite the bevel.

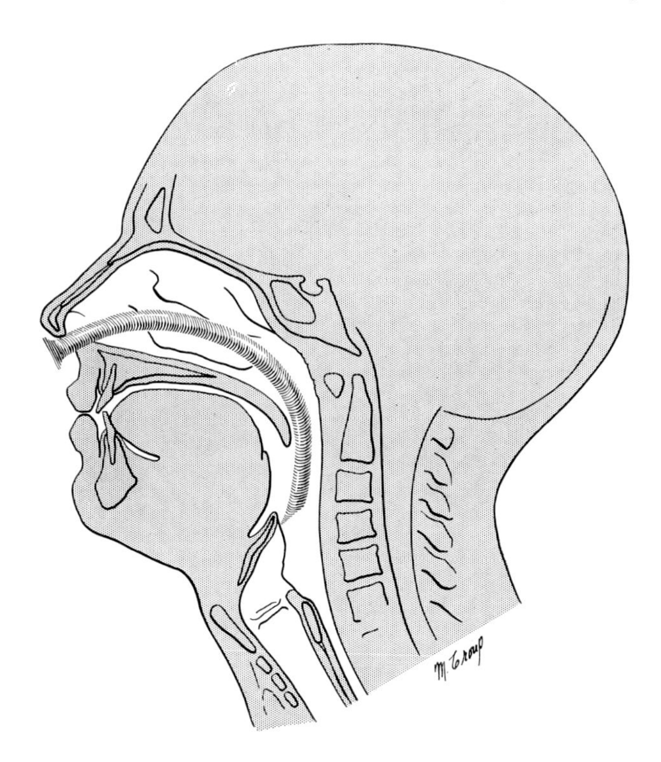

Fig. 10-5. Nasopharyngeal airway in place, maintaining patent airway.

10-4), to permit its insertion in the nasal passages and its extension into the nasopharynx and laryngopharynx (Fig. 10-5). The length of this airway should approximate the distance from the tip of the nose to the meatus of the ear (Fig. 10-6). The required length of the tube can thus be determined before its insertion. A suitable attachment (Fig. 10-7) should be affixed to the tube to prevent it from entering the anterior nares and slipping into the laryngopharynx, trachea, or esophagus.

INTRATRACHEAL INTUBATION

The ideal method of maintaining a patent airway is by the use of an intratracheal catheter. It can be inserted through the oral cavity and into the trachea (orotracheal, Fig. 10-8) or into the trachea via the nasal passages (nasotracheal, Fig. 10-9).

Since the introduction of the muscle relaxants, the use of intratracheal intubation for ambulatory patients has increased markedly. Whereas depressed planes of anesthesia were necessary for intubation,

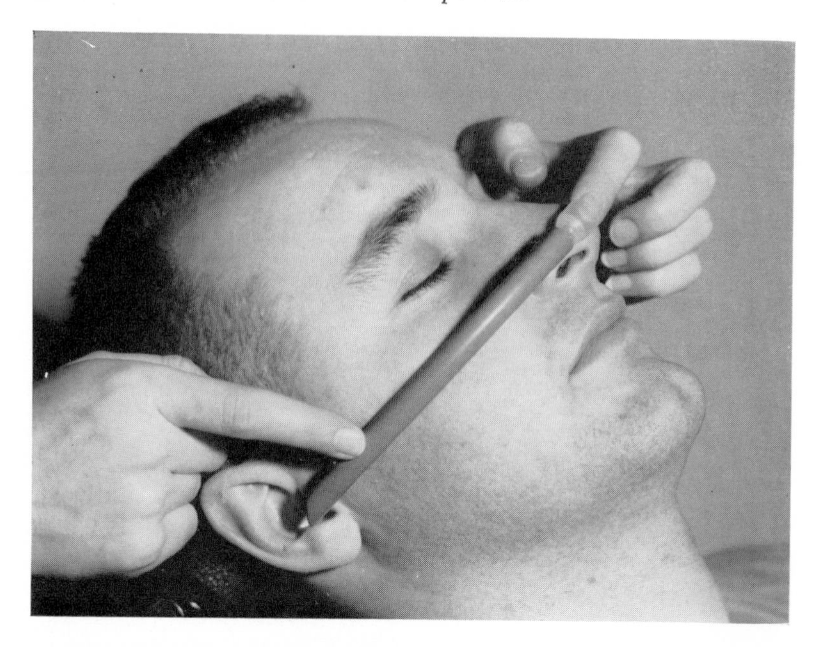

Fig. 10-6. Measuring to determine correct length of nasopharyngeal airway.

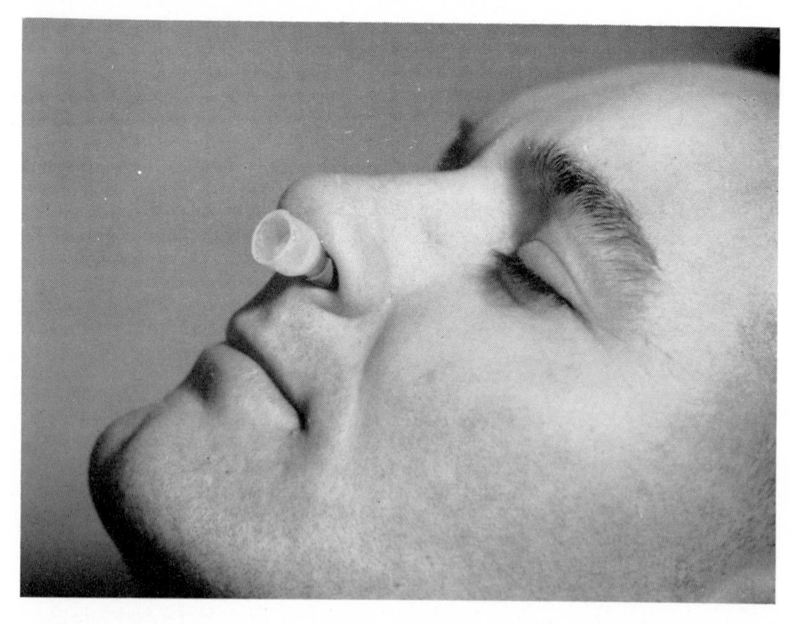

Fig. 10-7. Flange to maintain nasopharyngeal airway in place.

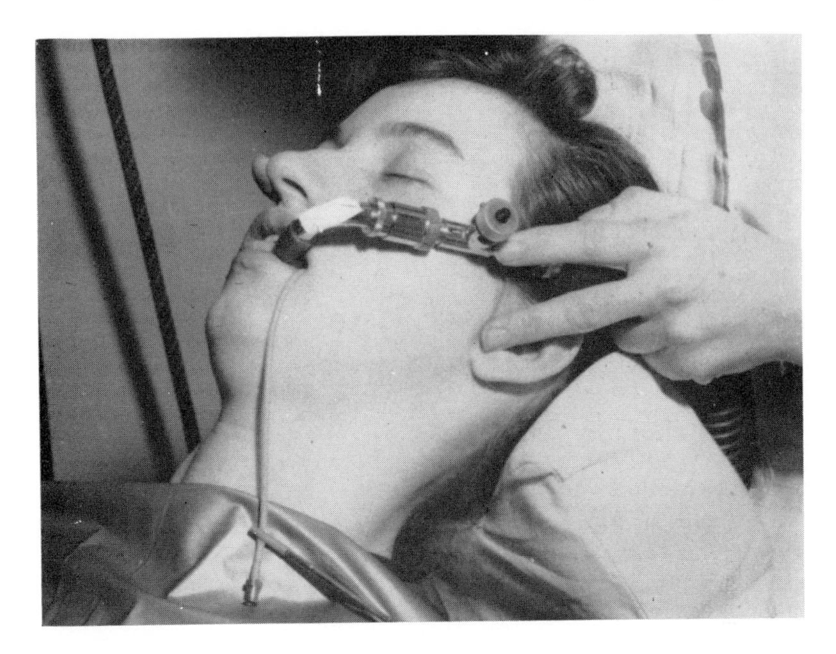

Fig. 10-8. Orotracheal tube in place.

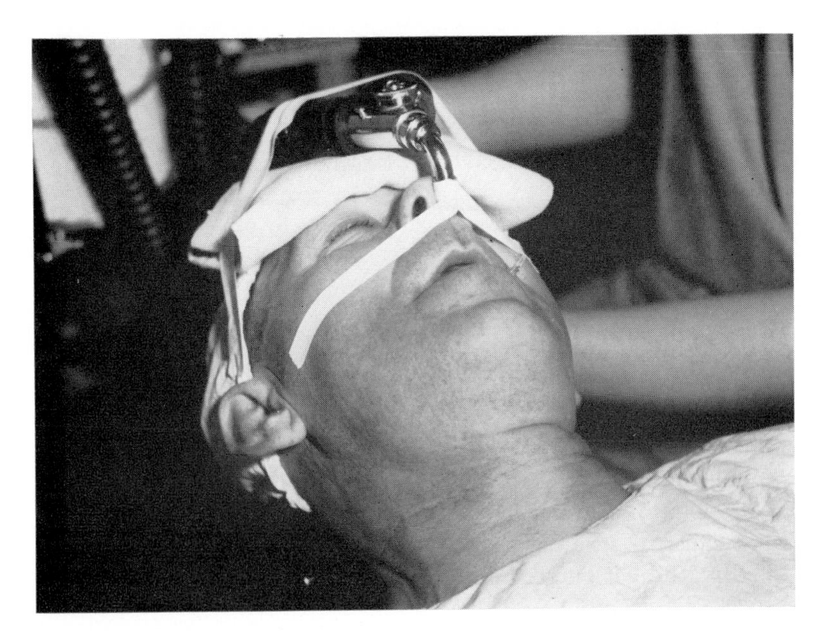

Fig. 10-9. Nasotracheal tube in place.

the use of small doses (20 to 40 mg.) of a short-acting muscle relaxant (succinylcholine chloride) makes it possible to intubate in the very light planes of anesthesia, and thus ensure an unobstructed airway throughout a short or long procedure. The induction time is not increased and the recovery time is actually shortened.

Even when the patient is not intubated, all the necessary equipment should be available to accomplish this maneuver. While it is not necessary to intubate the trachea to ventilate adequately all patients, and at times it may be contraindicated, as a general rule it is the best assurance of a patent airway.

By definition, the term intratracheal anesthesia means the administration of anesthetic vapors or gases or oxygen directly into the trachea by means of a suitable catheter passed through the larynx. For patients with unusual conditions the anesthetic gases may be administered through an opening in the anterior wall of the trachea (tracheostomy). This method should be employed only when the tracheotomy has been performed previously by an otolaryngologist or a plastic or general surgeon. Usually, unless specifically planned otherwise, the inhalations and exhalations may be accomplished through the same tube.

The advantages, disadvantages, indications, and contraindications of intratracheal anesthesia are as follows.

Advantages

1. The intratracheal tube assures a completely unobstructed airway as long as the tube remains patent.
2. Laryngospasm is not a hazard as long as the tube remains in place.
3. Perfect ventilation may be carried out through the intratracheal tube.
4. Tracheal aspirations can be performed without difficulty.
5. Secretions can be prevented from entering the tracheobronchial tree by packing the laryngopharynx or by using an inflatable cuff on the intratracheal tube.
6. Intracheal intubation makes artificial respiration efficient and simple.
7. By the use of the intratracheal technique, the anesthetist need not be in competition with the oral surgeon for the operative field.
8. Breathing is quiet and much more relaxed.
9. A lighter and more even plane of anesthesia can be safely maintained.

10. Respirations can be augmented without fear of gastric distention. This is particularly advantageous when muscle relaxants are used.

Disadvantages

1. Trauma to the anterior teeth, lips, epiglottis, vocal cords, and other tissues is a possibility, particularly by inexperienced operators.
2. The presence of the intratracheal tube may interfere with the oral surgeon's work in a few patients.
3. Bleeding may result, particularly when the tube is inserted roughly or carelessly via the nasal passages.
4. The lumen of the tube may reduce the cross section of the breathing area. This is particularly disadvantageous if exhalations are impeded.
5. Coughing or bucking may be initiated.
6. Adverse reflexes such as vagovagal reflexes or cardiac arrhythmias may be induced.

Indications

1. The primary indication for the intratracheal technique is the anesthetist's doubt of his ability to maintain a patent airway at all times.
2. When it is advantageous for the anesthetist to be completely out of the surgeon's field.
3. When the operation may be prolonged.
4. When excessive intraoral bleeding is anticipated.
5. When there has been previous difficulty in maintaining an airway.
6. When the surgeon desires a particular position that would be difficult without an intratracheal tube in place.
7. When controlled breathing is to be utilized throughout a portion of the procedure.

Contraindications

1. Very short procedures when the hazards of intubation are greater than surgery without intubation.
2. For patients in whom extremely deep anesthesia will be needed to accomplish the intubation.

Intratracheal intubation under ideal circumstances can be a fairly simple maneuver, but at times it may be very difficult. In many instances the skill of the anesthetist may make the difference. For this reason, every dentist who undertakes the administration of a general anesthetic should possess a certain degree of skill with intubation, based on adequate previous training.

Intratracheal intubation has become a much more feasible procedure for dentistry and oral surgery since the introduction of the muscle relaxants. Previously, deep anesthesia with ether or the intravenous agents was necessary to secure a degree of relaxation sufficient to permit intratracheal intubation without difficulty. At present the patient need only be carried into the light surgical plane of anesthesia, and relaxation can be obtained with the muscle relaxants. When using the muscle relaxants, however, the anesthetist should remain acutely aware of the decrease or absence of pulmonary ventilation so that hypoxia or anoxia will not be allowed to occur while the anesthetist is engrossed in accomplishing the intubation. It has been demonstrated by many operators that the mere insertion of an intratracheal tube with light anesthesia will rarely cause arrhythmias in a well-oxygenated patient. They will, however, occur frequently in hypoxic patients.

Methods. There are three commonly used methods of intratracheal intubation: direct orotracheal, direct nasotracheal, and blind nasotracheal. Each must be chosen for its individual merits and by the indications of the individual patient.

In direct orotracheal intubation the glottal opening of the larynx is viewed with a laryngoscope (Fig. 10-10), and then a suitable intratracheal tube is inserted through the glottal opening between the

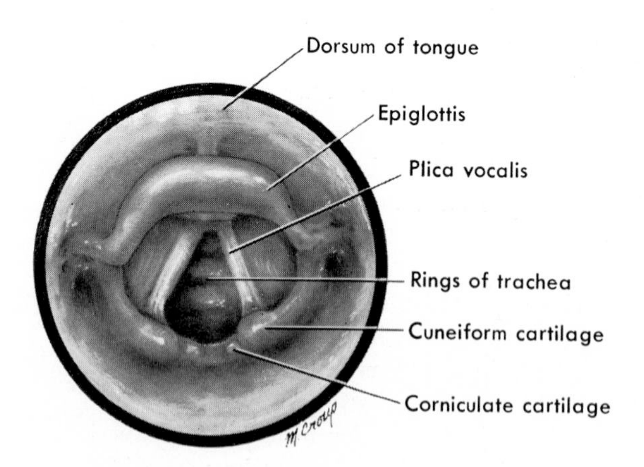

Fig. 10-10. View of glottal opening of larynx with laryngoscope.

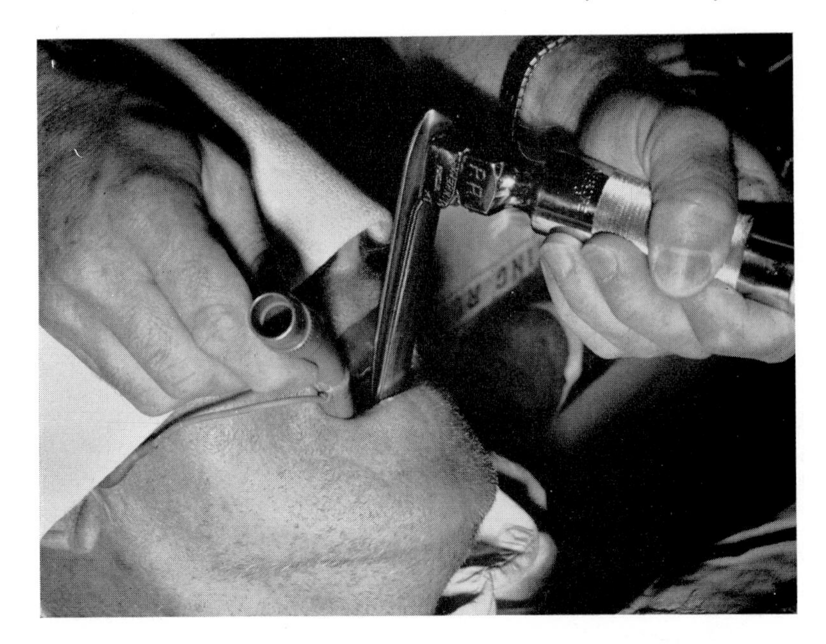

Fig. 10-11. Orotracheal tube is being inserted.

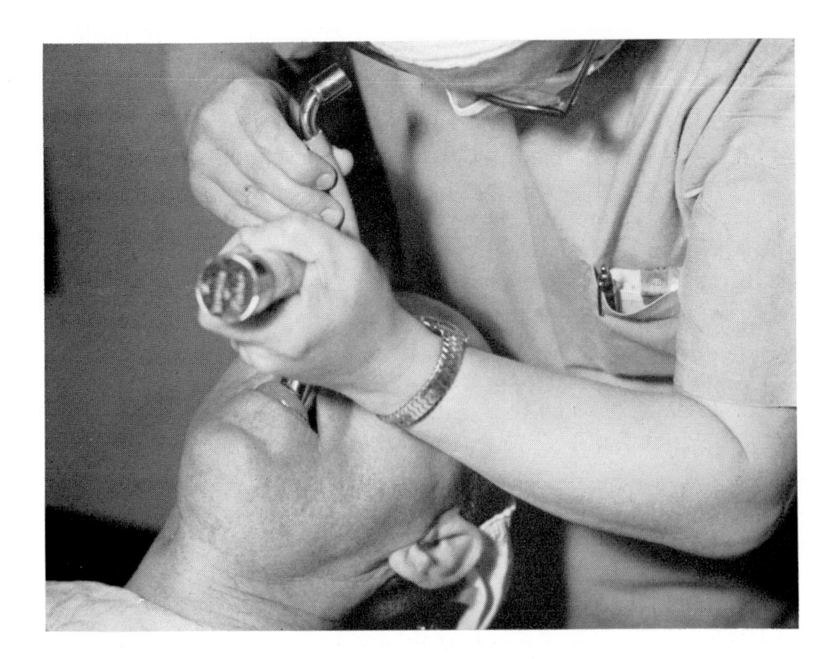

Fig. 10-12. Nasotracheal intubation under direct vision.

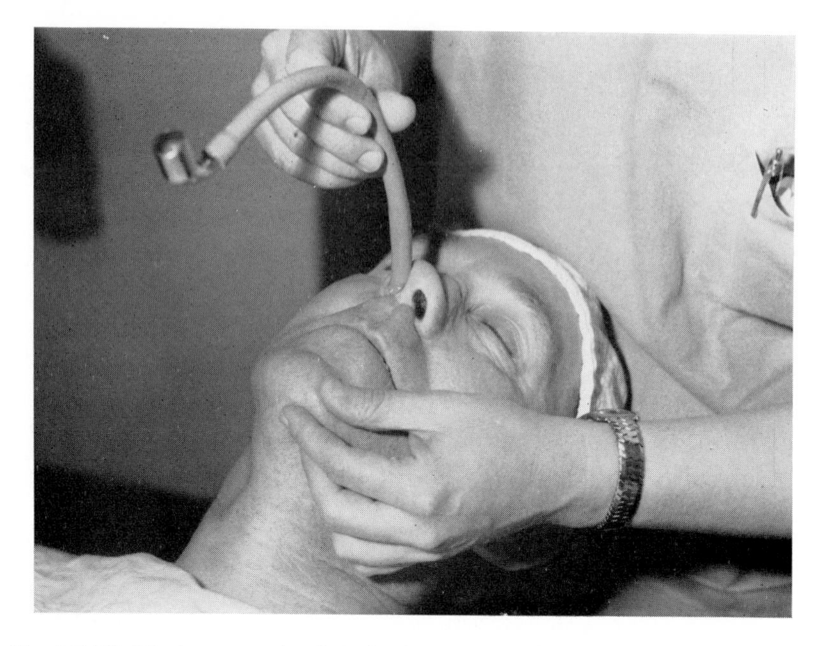

Fig. 10-13. Blind nasotracheal intubation.

vocal cords (Fig. 10-11). In direct nasotracheal intubation the tube is passed through the nasal passage into the laryngopharynx and, under direct vision with a laryngoscope, is guided through the glottal opening (Fig. 10-12). In blind nasotracheal intubation the tube is passed through the nasal passage, and with the exhalations as a guide, the breath sounds are followed through the glottal opening into the trachea (Fig. 10-13).

All three methods can be accomplished with the patient in the dental chair or prone on the operating table. It is, however, of fundamental importance that all necessary equipment be readily available and in good working order so that needless complications may be avoided. It is indeed embarrassing to reach for a suction catheter when none is at hand or to attempt to visualize the glottal opening with a laryngoscope whose bulb will not light. Therefore, the anesthetist who is to perform the intubation should meticulously check all of the equipment himself.

It is also important that the anesthetist closely examine the patient's lips, teeth, and surrounding structures to ascertain their condition before attempting intubation. Any diseased condition should be noted on the patient's chart so that chipped teeth, bruised lips, and so forth can be accounted for. It is also advantageous, when direct intubations under laryngoscopy are done, to examine the vocal cords and surrounding structures and detect any disease that may be present. Preceding blind intubation, the patient's voice should be noted and he should be questioned on his ability to swallow, cough, and so forth without difficulty.

It should be remembered that practically all dental patients will be presenting themselves for an elective operation in that, while it is necessary, it could probably be accomplished at a later date. The presence of any unexplained or previously unnoted disease of consequence warrants canceling the operation until further examination can be made. In one patient, prior to intubation a nodule was noted in the area of the larynx. The lesion was pointed out to the oral surgeon, and the operation was canceled. A later biopsy proved the lesion to be benign. I believe, however, that, if the intubation had been accomplished, the nodule would have been attributed to this maneuver.

When one attempts any form of intubation, three conditions should be assured: (1) that the patient is in proper position in the dental chair or on the table, (2) that the proper plane of anesthesia has been established, and (3) that the proper degree of relaxation has been obtained.

Preparation and precautions. When intratracheal intubation is to be accomplished, definite preparations and precautions should be observed.

Direct orotracheal intubation. When direct orotracheal intubation (see Fig. 10-11) is performed, the following preparations and precautions are advised:

1. As previously stated, all the equipment should be checked and readily available.
2. The patient's lips, teeth, and surrounding structures should be examined.
3. The patient should be properly positioned in the dental chair or on the operating table.
4. If intravenous anesthesia is being used, a satisfactory venipuncture should be made and the needle secured.
5. The patient should be carried to the proper plane of anesthesia.
6. Adequate relaxation should be obtained by the use of muscle relaxants.
7. The patient should be adequately and efficiently oxygenated.
8. The chin should be elevated and the head gently hyperextended.

9. The upper anterior teeth, if present, should be protected by a thin lead covering.
10. The scope should be held in the left hand and the mandible gently pulled over the scope with the right hand.
11. The scope should be placed over the base of the tongue, which should be moved to the left to prevent it from obstructing the view.
12. The scope should be advanced slowly into the laryngopharynx until the epiglottis comes into view.
13. The blade of the scope should be dipped slightly and the epiglottis elevated. The posterior commissure of the larynx should come into view. It is essential that the tip of the epiglottis be elevated by a lifting action and not a prying motion that would use the anterior teeth as a fulcrum. This is one of the prime causes of injury to or dislodgment of the anterior teeth. At this time, before inserting the intratracheal tube, make a survey of the glottal opening and adjacent tissues.
14. A suitable, well-lubricated intratracheal tube held in a pen grasp should be gently directed through the glottal opening and into the trachea. If the patient is breathing spontaneously, the tube should be passed between the cords when they are in the abducted position. However, if the patient is in a state of respiratory paralysis caused by muscle relaxants, the cords will be abducted and motionless.

The tube with the largest gauge that will pass through the larynx should be selected. The length should have been determined previously by measuring the tube from the lips to the area of the cricoid cartilage.

Immediately after the intratracheal tube is properly inserted, the postpharynx should be packed with lubricated gauze if a plain tube is used. If an inflatable cuff tube is used, the cuff should be expanded and clamped. Then the tube should be adequately secured in position and connected to the anesthetic machine by the proper attachments. The anesthetist can now determine the efficiency of the pulmonary ventilations by listening to the breathing tubes during respirations, be they spontaneous or controlled.

In many instances the anesthetist can readily determine whether a successful intubation has been accomplished by applying pressure to the patient's chest and holding his ear to the intratracheal tube immediately after its insertion. Some patients may cough or react to the insertion of the tube into the trachea. In all patients successful intubation can be verified by the characteristic respiratory sounds produced within the breathing tubes of the gas machine.

Watching both sides of the chest rise with each inflation usually assures the anesthetist that the tube not only is in the trachea but is positioned properly short of the right or left main bronchus. An intratracheal tube inserted too far will usually enter the right main bronchus, as it is practically an extension of the trachea. A stethoscope may be used to listen to breath sounds on both sides of the chest and further assure the anesthetist of the proper placement of the tube.

Direct nasotracheal intubation. Basically the same preliminary preparation and precautions hold for direct nasotracheal intubation (see Fig. 10-12) as for direct orotracheal intubation. Exposure of the glottal opening by laryngoscopy is the same. The fundamental differences will be the following:

1. The tube, which was measured previously for length by being placed alongside the face and neck from the anterior nares to just below the cricoid cartilage (Fig. 10-14), is longer than the tube used for orotracheal intubation.

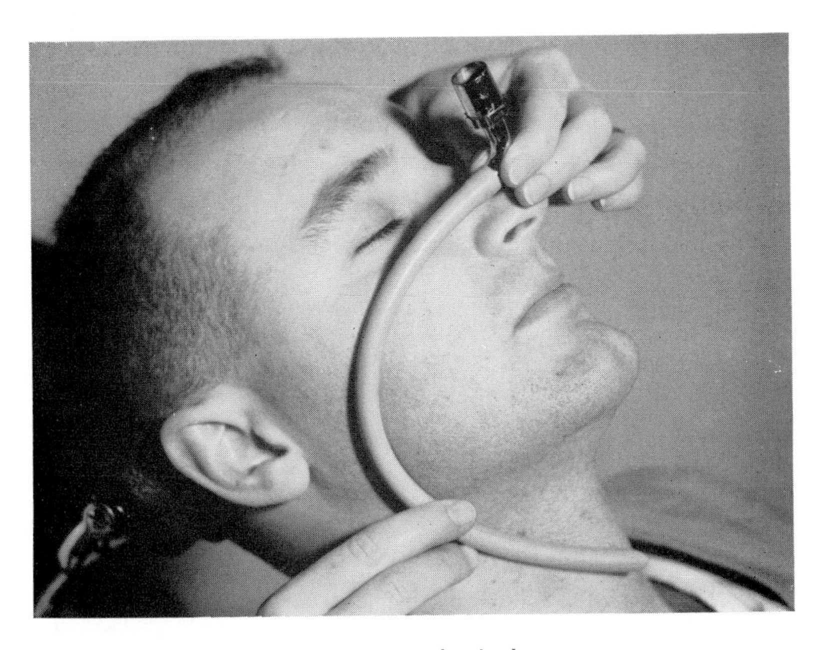

Fig. 10-14. Measuring length of nasotracheal tube.

2. The tube should be of a smaller gauge because it must be passed through the nasal passages.
3. In many patients an easier nasotracheal intubation can be accomplished if the head is slightly elevated after the glottal opening has been brought into view. This makes it possible to direct the curved tube into the larynx.
4. For some patients it is advantageous to insert the tube through the nasal passages and into the laryngopharynx before laryngoscopy is attempted. In this way, the tube is in place and time is not wasted in directing it through the nasal passages. Also, the anesthetist will be aware of any difficulty that may be encountered during insertion of the tube.

Immediately after successful nasotracheal intubation is accomplished, the same steps should be followed as with direct orotracheal intubation.

When direct laryngoscopy has been difficult and the glottal opening is not sufficiently exposed to permit unimpeded direct orotracheal intubation, I have found it advantageous and expedient to insert a nasotracheal tube through the nasal passages into the laryngopharynx and allow the natural curvature of the tube to direct it forward, upward, and through the glottal opening while the larynx is only partly exposed. This maneuver has been especially helpful for patients with protruding upward anterior teeth or a receded mandible.

In these patients, when muscle relaxants have been used, the anesthetist should be acutely aware of the patient's depressed or absent pulmonary ventilation. The inexperienced anesthetist may be so engrossed in the act of intubation that he loses track of both time and the patient's increasing hypoxia. For this reason, I have advocated that the beginner have someone check the pulse, color, and elapsed time while he attempts his first intubations, or that he hold his breath while he attempts the intubation. If intubation is difficult and he himself feels the effects of holding his breath, the patient, who is also not breathing, will no doubt exhibit the effects of hypoxia. When laryngoscopy has been difficult and attempted intubation has consumed valuable time, the anesthetist should not hesitate to withdraw the tube and reoxygenate the patient. Under no circumstances, if hypoxia or anoxia impends, should he gamble on the chance that he will be able to complete the intubation before serious sequelae develop.

Blind nasotracheal intubation. The blind nasotracheal technique (see Fig. 10-13) can at times be very desirable. It is accomplished without the aid of laryngoscopy and, if it is performed gently, can be an atraumatic procedure. Although I prefer to visualize the larynx by laryngoscopy, there are definite indications for the blind technique. It can be accomplished with the patient awake and cooperative, as well as with the patient under anesthesia. When it is accomplished with the patient awake, the nasal and pharyngeal passages should be sprayed with a suitable topical anesthetic and the maneuver explained to the patient. The vast majority of patients are able to cooperate when the topical anesthetic is effective and when they have been previously informed.

Blind intubation is indicated when disease or injury makes laryngoscopy difficult or impossible, or when ankylosis of the mandible makes direct laryngoscopy impossible.

When blind intubation is indicated because of ankylosis of the mandible or when for any reason difficulty in maintaining a patent airway is anticipated. I prefer to perform the procedure with the patient awake after I have previously sprayed the nasal and pharyngeal passages with a suitable topical analgesic. In this technique, once a tube has been directed through the nasal passages, it is mandatory to advance it only on expirations since it is necessary to keep the tube in the air flow. As long as the anesthetist can distinctly hear and feel the expired air coming through the tube, he can be certain that there is proper alignment. If for some reason the expired air cannot be heard or felt coming from the tube, he can be certain that alignment has been lost, and it will be necessary to withdraw the tube partially and redirect it until the expired air can again be heard and felt. It may be necessary to reposition and maneuver the head slightly to keep the tube within the current of the expired air. In some patients, elevating and flexing the head may be advantageous.

Before blind intubation with the patient awake is performed, a satisfactory venipuncture should be made. In addition, the patient should be told that immediately after the intubation has been accomplished he will be unable to speak, but that he will be able to breathe easily and will be in no difficulty whatsoever. He should also be told that within seconds he will go pleasantly to sleep.

The technique for accomplishing this kind of intubation with the patient asleep is identical for that when the patient is awake. However, a satisfactory plane of anesthesia must be maintained, with the patient breathing spontaneously, since the expirations are the only valid guide. It is plain that, while muscle relaxants may be employed, they should not be used to the point of producing respiratory paralysis, since it would then be difficult, if not impossible, to align the naso-tracheal tube accurately with the larynx. Under no circumstances should force ever be used if the advancing tube encounters resistance, since it is possible for it to strike the anterior commissure of the larynx or be guided into either of the piriform fossae.

A frequent cause of failure is guiding the tube into the esophagus instead of into the trachea. This error can be readily detected by the absence of breath sounds through the tube. It is most likely to occur when the curvature of the tube is inadequate or the head is hyper-extended.

Blind nasotracheal intubation can be accomplished with practically every type of anesthetic. However, it is advantageous to undertake it using ether or intravenous anesthesia and thus to obtain a longer period of stable anesthesia. With the gaseous anesthetics, particularly nitrous oxide, the desired plane of anesthesia is of such short duration that, if the intubation is not accomplished on the first attempt, anesthesia must again be reestablished; this may be difficult.

EXTUBATION

When the surgical procedure is completed and the use of the intratracheal tube has terminated, removal of the tube should not be a haphazard or thoughtless maneuver. First, it is important to ascertain the state of the patient's spontaneous pulmonary ventilation. If it is adjudged inadequate, the tube should not be removed.

To look upon extubation as a completely harmless procedure is a mistake and may lead to serious sequelae if proper preparations are not made. The intratracheal tube should be suctioned, if indicated, until clear, without the patient bucking or coughing. The oral cavity and pharyngeal areas should be suctioned of any residual blood, mucus, or debris, and the patient should be hyperventilated with oxygen. In dental or oral surgery the extubation should be accomplished with the patient in as light a plane of anesthesia as possible, but he should still be sufficiently anesthetized to forego stimulating reactions.

If patients have been properly managed during anesthesia and extubation, the vast majority will reacquire the cough reflexes and other protective mechanisms within a short period of time.

If they have been properly managed during the anesthesia, the vast majority of dental patients reacquire the cough reflexes within a very short period and thus can be extubated more safely. When for some reason ether has been used, it may be advisable to extubate while the patient is still in the surgical plane.

Certain precautions should be taken prior to and following extubation:

1. The intratracheal tube should be suctioned until clear.
2. The postpharyngeal area and oral cavity should be suctioned as well as possible.
3. The proper stage and plane of anesthesia should be determined —as light as possible, second stage or lighter, with either anesthesia.
4. The venipuncture should be maintained so that the muscle relaxants can be administered immediately if necessary.
5. The patient should be hyperventilated with oxygen.
6. The intratracheal tube should be withdrawn gently.
7. A full face mask should be attached to the breathing tubes and the patient oxygenated immediately after extubation. When ether has been used, an oropharyngeal airway may be inserted. When intravenous agents have been used, the anesthesia will be too light for the patient to tolerate an oropharyngeal airway.
8. The oral cavity and postpharyngeal area should be resuctioned and the pulmonary ventilation evaluated.

When the nasotracheal technique has been used to maintain a patent airway while fractures of the mandible or maxilla are reduced and wired, it has been my practice to allow the intratracheal tube to remain in place until the patient has reacted completely. If the tube has been properly inserted, just inferior to the larynx and not approaching the carina, the patient will usually tolerate the tube without difficulty. This procedure has been followed with success for treatment of fractured jaws and for patients in whom reentrance into the oral cavity would be difficult.

TRANSTRACHEAL INJECTION

Transtracheal injection is discussed here because, while it is not often used in dental or oral surgery, there are times when it may be advantageous. In patients with complete ankylosis of the mandible in whom blind intubation with the patient awake is indicated, the transtracheal injection of a suitable topical anesthetic (4% Xylocaine) may be used in conjunction with a topical spray of the nasal and pharyngeal passages to enhance the patient's tolerance of the procedure.

To accomplish the transtracheal injection, attach a 2 ml. syringe containing the topical anesthetic of choice to a 20-gauge intravenous needle. The cricothyroid membrane in the midline of the neck is palpated and surgically prepared. The needle with the syringe attached

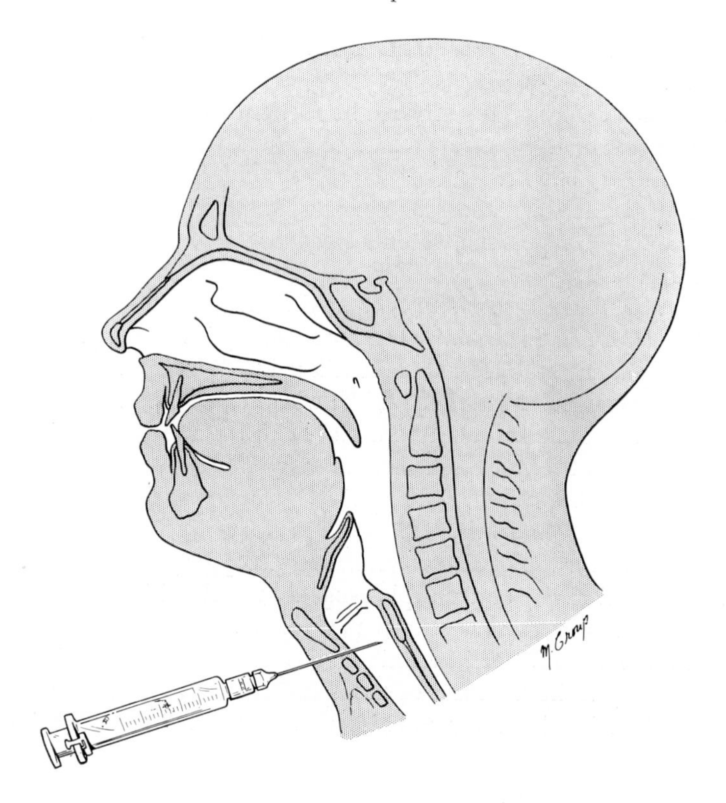

Fig. 10-15. Transtracheal injection.

is inserted through the cricothyroid membrane into the trachea (Fig. 10-15). One can know that this has been accomplished if air can be aspirated freely into the syringe. The contents should be injected rapidly and the needle withdrawn quickly. The patient will, in most cases, cough violently and thus spray the surrounding area with the topical anesthetic.

ARMAMENTARIUM

The proper equipment is essential to assure uniform success with intratracheal intubation, and it should be in perfect working condition. We have found it advantageous to set up individual trays (Fig. 10-16), each complete within itself, so that preparation for the intubation is simplified. If a list of necessary equipment and material is prepared previously and this list is checked against the contents of the tray, the chance of missing necessary items at inopportune times is virtually eliminated.

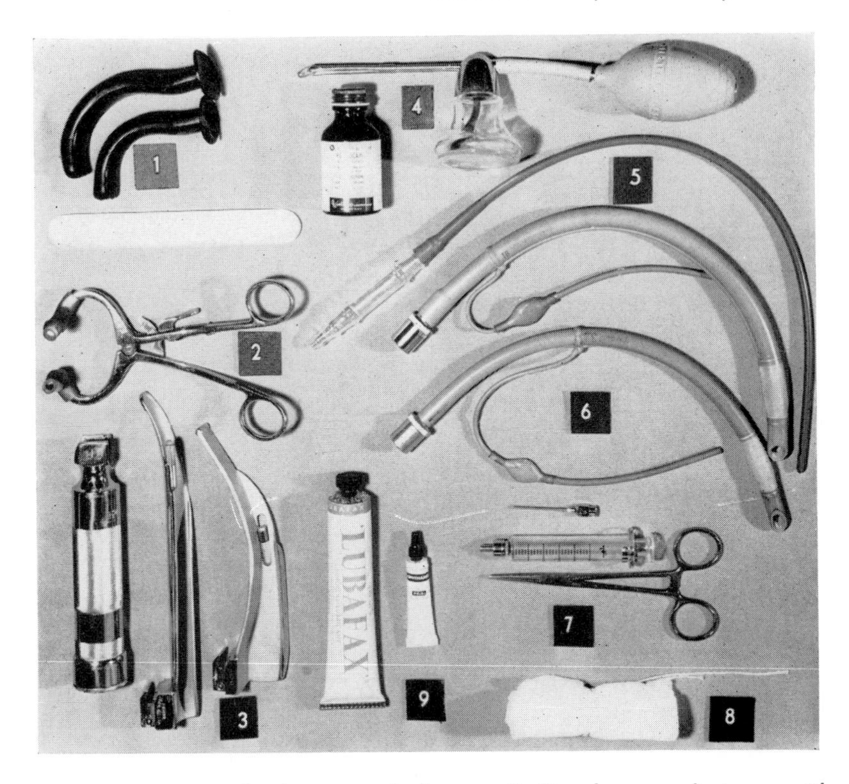

Fig. 10-16. Intratracheal tray ready for use. **1,** Oropharyngeal airway with tongue blade; **2,** mouth prop; **3,** laryngoscope (interchangeable straight and curved blades); **4,** atomizer and solution for spraying vocal cords; **5,** suction catheter; **6,** orotracheal tubes with inflatable cuff; **7,** needle, syringe, and hemostat for inflating and clamping inflatable cuff; **8,** throat pack (note string attached); **9,** lubrication for tube and eye ointment.

The intratracheal tray should contain the following:

- Laryngoscope
  - Handle
  - Blades
    - Interchangeable straight
    - Interchangeable curved
- Intratracheal tubes
  - Orotracheal with inflatable cuff (Nos. 32, 34, and 36)
  - Nasotracheal, with inflatable cuff (Nos. 28, 30, and 32)
  - Nasotracheal, plain (Nos. 29 and 30)
- Mouth prop
- Magil forceps
- Rubber oropharyngeal airway

Lead teeth protector
Needle and syringe for inflating cuff
Hemostat for clamping cuff
Lubricant
Sponges for throat packs
Y adapters and connectors
Pontocaine spray and atomizer
Tongue depressors
Adequate suction apparatus

TECHNICAL CONSIDERATIONS

When preparation for intratracheal intubation is made, the following technical factors should be considered:

1. The length of tube for intubation can be determined by laying it alongside the patient's neck. The trachea begins at the lower border of the cricoid cartilage and bifurcates at the level of the angle of Louis, that of the second costal cartilage. Any tube whose end lies between these two points is long enough for intubation (this method of measuring allows for a margin of error of about 9 cm.). The length is measured either from the incisor teeth or from the nares, according to whether the route of intubation is oral or nasal.
2. If a tube is too long, it will usually enter the right main bronchus because its course is straighter; the left main bronchus makes a more acute angle with the trachea. Either the wall of the tube or an inflatable cuff may obstruct the left bronchus and cause atelectasis on that side.
3. When the trachea has been intubated, the natural air-conditioning apparatus of the upper respiratory tract is suppressed, and vapor enters the trachea at the temperature and degree of humidity at which it is delivered by the apparatus in use.
4. Reflex effects of intubation, such as the following, must be considered:
   a. Intubation in light anesthesia provokes reflex disturbances such as coughing and breath-holding.
   b. Several cases of arrhythmia that occurred at the moment of intubation or of inflation of the cuff have been reported.
   c. Vagovagal reflexes can undoubtedly be caused by the stimulus of intubation, but serious accidents from this cause are extremely rare.
5. The danger to the patient of accidental release of gas at a high pressure is greater when endotracheal anesthesia is in use.

6. It is difficult to compare the circular bore of a round tube with that of a triangular orifice such as the glottis in order to determine the diameter of tube to be used in any given patient. Tuffier has stated that the average adult glottic opening is an isosceles triangle whose sides measure 25 mm. and whose base is 8 mm. wide. The area of such a triangle is 98 sq.mm. (Nos. 10, 9, and 8 Magill tubes are respectively 113, 94, and 80 sq.mm. in size.)
7. Since gaseous exchange does not take place in the dead space of the respiratory tree, it follows that any modification of the volume of the dead space will enhance or diminish the efficiency of respiration. The cubic contents of the mouth, nose, and pharynx varies between 75 and 100 cc. Intubation reduces the dead space by about 25 ml. and therefore enhances the efficiency of respiratory exchange.
8. The relation of endotracheal anesthesia to intrabronchial and intrathoracic pressure should be taken into consideration. The application of intermittent pressure coincident with the normal cycle of respiration is probably less disturbing both to respiration and circulation than the maintenance of constant positive pressure during both phases of respiration. In any intubated subject with the thorax intact, and increase in intrabronchial pressure will of necessity increase the intrathoracic pressure, which means that a back pressure is set up that hinders the return of blood through the vena cava and therefore the filling of the right auricle; as a result, the output of the heart falls.

Intratracheal airways, whether orotracheal or nasotracheal, should be removed with caution and at the proper time. Extubation should be considered an important step and should not be done haphazardly.

The patient should be in a proper plane of anesthesia, and the anesthetist should be reasonably sure that a patent airway can be maintained after the intratracheal tube is removed. Since deeper planes of anesthesia are not required for dental or oral surgery, it has been our policy not to extubate patients until the cough reflex has returned and the danger of laryngospasm has passed. The patient should be closely observed immediately following extubation to make certain that he has reestablished adequate pulmonary ventilation. The oral cavity and the intratracheal tube should be adequately and carefully suctioned so that no mucus or debris remains in the air passages.

Chapter 11

Preanesthetic evaluation and choice of anesthetic agents and techniques

It is inconceivable that any anesthetist would administer a general anesthetic to a patient without first making a physical evaluation. The extent and thoroughness of this preanesthetic evaluation have been much discussed. It should be stressed that in the case of the dentist or oral surgeon, the examination is performed in order to evaluate and not to diagnose or treat any medical condition.

When preanesthetic evaluation is done in a hospital, it is a more or less routine procedure performed by some member of the medical staff. Even then, the dentist or oral surgeon should check the patient's chart closely in order to make certain that this evaluation has been accomplished and that the findings warrant proceeding with the anesthesia and surgery. For patients about whom any doubt exists, the oral surgeon should seek further medical consultation.

On the other hand, the dentist or oral surgeon occupies a unique position among the surgical specialists in that he alone is responsible for the decision to use general anesthesia for patients outside the confines of established and recognized hospitals. This decision should not be regarded lightly and should be arrived at after due consideration. Primary among the considerations is an adequate preanesthetic evaluation.

Before continuing, it may be well to further clarify the term evaluation. In my opinion, to evaluate means to increase one's awareness of a situation or condition. It is not necessary to understand the causes of the condition or the indicated therapy for it. For instance, when an arrhythmic pulse is detected, the dentist or oral surgeon should not attempt to determine the etiology of the arrhythmia, nor should he attempt to treat it. Also, when a patient gives a history of dyspnea, the dentist should not necessarily attempt to ascertain the causes of the dyspnea, but again should be aware of its presence. If the overall evaluation indicates the need for further examination, the patient should be sent to a physician for more thorough examination, diagnosis, and treatment. The dentist's main concern will be his awareness of any physiological deviation that may affect the patient's reaction to the anesthetic, and whether or not this condition deserves further study by a physician or internist.

The preanesthetic evaluation should encompass the more important physiological systems basically involved in the administration of the anesthetic and should be an aid in determining (1) whether the patient should be ambulatory, an outpatient, or a hospital patient, (2) whether the patient should be given a general anesthetic, (3) the choice of anesthetic agent and technique, (4) the optimal duration of anesthesia and surgery, (5) whether premedication should be employed, and (6) what preoperative preparation, if any, is necessary. In addition to the above six determinations, the preanesthetic evaluation is important (1) to achieve a more complete understanding of the patient to prevent unpleasant experiences, morbidity, or a fatality, (2) to fulfill medicolegal requirements, and (3) to aid in the prompt recognition and treatment of emergencies.

In determining whether a patient should be considered ambulatory, an outpatient, or a hospital patient, we have found the following classification very helpful:

1. Ambulatory patients—classified Class A, whose surgical procedure will not consume more than about 30 minutes. These patients should recover and be able to leave the office, escorted by a responsible adult, within approximately the time used for the operation.
2. Outpatients—classified Class A or Class B, who meet certain qualifications for anesthesia and surgery to be done in a hospital. Anesthesia is not to exceed 60 minutes. These patients should be able to leave the hospital, escorted by a responsible adult, within 1 to 2 hours after the operation.
3. Hospitalized patients—classified Class C, and includes those patients whose condition requires hospitalization and those who must be hospitalized because of surgical intervention.

Preanesthetic evaluation may be divided into three parts: subjective history, objective observations, and laboratory examination.

As previously stated, it is assumed that the hospitalized patient will be given a routine physical examination as specified for all surgical patients. This discussion, therefore, is confined to the preanesthetic evaluation indicated for ambulatory, or office, patients. This evaluation, in many respects, may fulfill the requirements for outpatients and hospitalized patients.

SUBJECTIVE HISTORY

The subjective history should be brief thorough and should be outlined in such a fashion that the office nurse or assistant can obtain a portion of the necessary information without difficulty or undue loss of time. This information will, of course, be checked by the dentist himself. The questions should be so stated that they are concise, easily answered, and not confusing to the patient. The subjective history should be conveniently recorded on a card or examination sheet that can be filed with the patient's permanent record for future reference.

Patients may be classified as A, B, or C. The classification should not depend on the preanesthetic evaluation alone but should take into consideration other factors involved, which will be enumerated later. The primary classifications, based on the preanesthetic evaluation alone before the other factors are considered, are the following:

Class A: Patients between the ages of 6 and 60 years who are free from organic disease or patients in whom ordinary physical activity does not cause undue fatigue or dyspnea belong in this category. This could include patients with well-compensated valvular heart disease except when it is associated with hypertension or syphilis.

Class B: Patients under 6 and over 60 years of age, even if in good condition otherwise, must be placed in this category. Also, patients with an impairing organic disease, but who compensate well and thus do not manifest more than first-degree circulatory depression. belong in this classification.

Class C: Patients in whom organic disease or circulatory depression causes them to be a calculated risk for anesthesia are placed in this classification.

Again, it should be stressed that other factors such as the nature of the surgery, the time involved, and the anesthesia technique will influence the classification of patients. For instance, a patient who is to have one or two anterior teeth extracted may be graded Class A, whereas the same patient with fourteen or fifteen teeth to be extracted may be graded Class B. A suggested examination sheet is given below.

The questions of the subjective history and the data of the objective observations for the ambulatory patient should be directed primarily toward the status or presence of (1) the cardiovascular system, (2) the respiratory system, (3) any nervous system disorders, (4) metabolic deficiencies, (5) endocrine imbalances, (6) allergies, and (7) iatrogenic diseases.

Patients with sufficiently impaired function of the liver and kidneys so that they are unable to metabolize or eliminate the small doses of anesthetic drugs given to outpatients will hardly be ambulatory. If they are, their general condition will surely be in evidence enough to contraindicate the use of a general anesthetic.

If a person is able to indulge in moderate activity without untoward symptoms, no concern need be felt about the ability of the heart to sustain the extra work entailed by anesthesia and surgery, provided the anesthetic is properly chosen and administered. The subjective questions plus the objective observations may reveal symptoms that forecast impending difficulties if the patient is subjected to undue stress. The questions and observations are therefore not only a guide as to the advisability of the use of general anesthesia but also a clue to the precautions to be taken during its management.

The preanesthetic evaluation may reveal the presence of previously undisclosed or overlooked diseases of the heart or lungs.

Loss_____
Name_______________________ Age___ Height_____ Weight_____ Gain_____
Occupation_______________________________ Race__________ Class________

Subjective history

1. **Are you presently, or within the past year have you been, under the care of a physician?________ If answer is yes, give circumstances______________**
____
2. **Are you now taking, or within the past six months have you taken, any drugs or medication?___________________________ Why?________________**
3. **Do you require frequent rest periods when engaged in normal activity?_____**
4. **Do you become unduly fatigued after walking up a flight of stairs or walking faster than usual?____**
5. **Do you routinely experience shortness of breath?_________________________**
6. **Do you now experience or have you even experienced any chest pains?_____**
____
7. **Do your ankles swell?____**
8. **Do you ever have dizzy spells?______________________________________**
9. **Do you require pillows for sleeping or reclining?_______________________**
10. **Are you ever conscious of your heartbeat?_____________________________**
11. **Do you have a cough?____**
12. **Does heat or a warm room bother you?________________________________**
13. **Do you sweat excessively?____**

14. Do you have any known allergies?______________________
15. Are you now or have you ever been subject to asthmatic attacks?__________
16. Are you diabetic?______________________
17. Do you void frequently?______________________
18. Have you even been anesthetized?______________________
19. As briefly as possible state your daily habits (use of tobacco, alcohol, etc.)___
____

Objective data

1. Pulse__________ Rate__________ Volume__________ Rhythm__________
2. Blood pressure ______________________
3. Respirations: Rate__________ Depth__________ Character__________
4. Temperature ______________________
5. General appearance
   Skin: Jaundice________ Petechiae_____ Ecchymosis_____ Cyanosis_____
   Eyes: Pallor__________ Jaundice__________ Exophthalmos__________
   Hands: Clubbing_____ Pigmentation_____ Tremor_______ Temp._______
   Neck: Thyroid________ Enlarged glands________ Neck veins__________
   Chest: Shape______________ Respiratory movements______________
   Abdomen ______________________
   Legs: Edema______________ Ulcers____________ Cyanosis____________
6. Any other obvious physical defects that may interfere with the anesthesia?
____

Laboratory examination

1. Bleeding time (normal, 1-3 min.)______________________
2. Coagulation time (normal, capillary tube method, 3-5 min.)______________
3. Microhematocrit (female, 35-45; male, 40-50)______________________
4. Urinalysis ______________________
5. Time-volume vital capacity test______________________
6. Henderson's breath-holding test______________________

PATHOLOGY OF THE HEART

The most frequent diseases of the heart of concern to the anesthetist are congenital heart disease, coronary artery disease, valvular heart disease, arrhythmias and defects of the conductive system, and congestive heart failure.

Congenital heart disease. Congenital heart diseases are due to developmental defects of the heart. Their interest to the dentist evaluating a patient for general anesthesia will depend on the degree to which they impair cardiac function. It is very unlikely that persons with severe congenital defects would present themselves as ambulatory patients without some previous knowledge of their own condition. On the other hand, minimal defects may permit normal activity.

The dentist should suspect a congenital defect if there is general retardation of growth and maturation, accompanied by cyanosis of the lips and nail beds. The fingers may or may not be clubbed, depending on the severity of the defect.

Coronary artery disease. Coronary artery disease is usually the result of a narrowing of the lumen of the coronary vessels (atherosclerosis). The most common clinical manifestations of coronary artery disease are angina pectoris, coronary thrombosis, and myocardial insufficiency.

The usual symptoms are substernal or precordial pain, anginal attacks, and dyspnea. The most frequent early symptom is dyspnea, which may be present without other demonstrable signs. Although anginal pain on exertion may be an early symptom, it is entirely possible for a patient with an occlusion of a coronary artery to have no pain but to experience dyspnea, weakness, or dizziness. If a coronary occlusion develops over a prolonged period, there may be very few, if any, demonstrable signs other than gradual impairment of activity.

Angina pectoris is in itself a symptom rather than a disease. It is the result of local ischemia due to coronary artery disease or coronary spasm.

Valvular heart disease. Valvular heart disease is usually the result of a disease of long standing that causes obstruction or stenosis of the valvular opening. Not only may this interference with normal valvular function inhibit the normal flow of blood in its proper direction, but it also may permit a return of the blood against the normal flow.

Valvular defects are usually recognized by the presence of characteristic murmurs. As a general rule these defects, unless accompanied by other symptoms, do not contraindicate the administration of a general anesthetic.

Rheumatic fever is in itself responsible for a high percentage of valvular defects, and any patient giving a previously history of this disease should be thoroughly questioned as to his ability to carry on normal activities without undue stress.

Arrhythmias and defects of the conductive system. An arrhythmia is any deviation from the normal rhythm of the heartbeat. As a general rule, an arrhythmia accompanied by no other symptoms does not preclude the administration of a general anesthetic. However, it will, in most instances, be advantageous to seek further consultation when an obvious arrhythmia exists.

Arrhythmias arising in the sinoatrial node, such as sinus tachycardia (pulse rate, 100 or over), sinus bradycardia (pulse rate, 60 or less), or sinus arrhythmia (pulse rate varies with respirations), are not necessarily significant unless present to a marked degree. Other arrhythmias may have their origin in the atria or ventricles and deserve further consideration.

Defects of the conductive system arising in the A-V bundle or the Purkinje fibers may result in bradycardia due to partial heart block or other arrhythmias. Although these arrhythmias may be compatible with a relative degree of cardiac efficiency, they also warrant further consultation.

Congestive heart failure. In congestive heart failure the functional capacity of the heart is greatly impaired. Cardiac output is diminished and circulation time is increased. The most common symptoms are dyspnea on mild exertion, prominent and distended neck veins due to increased venous pressure, short spells of coughing due to pulmonary congestion, and possibly edema of the ankles.

It should be considered that borderline congestive failure may be aggravated by the administration of a general anesthetic, particularly if any difficulty is encountered during anesthesia.

Hypertension. High blood pressure, like angina, is not a disease but a symptom of some underlying disease. The blood pressure is a variable factor in normal persons, and the systolic pressure, particularly, varies greatly with emotional stress, position, exercise, and so forth.

Hypertension may produce cardiac changes due to strain on the heart muscle and subsequent hypertrophy. It is therefore reasonable to assume that patients manifesting hypertension may have some degree of cardiac disease. It should also be remembered that the hypertension, particularly the systolic pressure, may be transitory, because of emotional stress or apprehension. Whenever this situation is suspected, the patient should be put at ease and the pressure should be taken under the most favorable conditions possible.

The dentist performing the preanesthetic evaluation should always be cognizant of the importance of the patient's cardiac status. A large percentage of the fatalite that occur during anesthesia in the dental office could well be the result of some underlying cardiac disease. In these particular patients, the margin of acceptable error and safety is greatly reduced. Whereas a normal patient may withstand some degree of physiological insult, one with already impaired cardiac function may react poorly to the unknown deviation.

PATHOLOGY OF THE VENTILATORY MECHANISM

Diseases of the lungs are of the utmost importance to the anesthetist because oxygen is taken into the body and carbon dioxide given off through this organ. Also, any mild diseases of the ventilatory mechanism (nasal passages, pharynx, tracheobronchial tree, or lungs) may alter the smooth course of anesthesia.

The most commonly encountered conditions of the ventilatory mechanisms are upper respiratory infections, bronchitis, bronchiectasis, obstructions, asthma, and pulmonary emphysema.

Upper respiratory infections. Patients manifesting any symptoms of acute upper respiratory infection should be considered unsatisfactory candidates for elective general anesthesia and surgery. The increased secretions, together with possible fever and increased metabolic rate, may produce hazardous conditions that would warrant postponing the procedure.

Bronchitis. Bronchitis is an infection in the lower trachea and bronchi and may be acute or chronic. It is characterized by increased secretions, probably secondary to congestion and edema of the mucous membranes. These conditions usually interfere with, and decrease the efficiency of, the gaseous exchange.

The earliest symptom is usually a slight cough, which may or may not be productive. Other accompanying symptoms may be low-grade fever, anterior chest pains, and a generalized feeling of malaise. Dyspnea may or may not be present, depending on the severity of the symptoms. When these symptoms are manifested, medical consultation should be sought in an attempt to alleviate them if possible, since the administration of a general anesthetic may produce severe coughing spasms, laryngospasm, or bronchiospasm.

Bronchiectasis. Bronchiectasis is a chronic infectious disease in which there is pronounced dilation and thickening of the terminal bronchi. The infection may be localized in a single area or involve as much as an entire lobe. As would be expected, the severity of symptoms will depend on the area of involvement.

A persistent productive cough is the earliest symptom and in many patients may be the only one. When larger areas are involved, a fetid breath, chest pain, and anoxia are usually present. In most severe chronic conditions there is clubbing of the fingers and cyanosis.

Patients with bronchiectasis usually present an anesthetic risk because of the presence of large amounts of mucopurulent secretions in the tracheobronchial tree. These secretions may so increase or accumulate during anesthesia as to produce a partial or complete obstruction.

Obstructions. During the preanesthetic evaluation, the anesthetist should observe the patient closely for any signs or symptoms of respiratory obstruction. These obstructions may be due to existing disease outside the tracheobronchial tree or air passages. Enlarged thyroid gland may so impinge on the trachea as to produce a partial obstruction. When the patient is awake, he may be able to compensate, but when he is anesthetized, the interference may be in evidence.

Any pronounced deviation in the nasal septum should be noted, since nasal breathing is essential for the maintenance of adequate oxygenation and sometimes anesthesia when the mouth is open and the oropharyngeal partition is in place.

Patients with severe asthmatic conditions may manifest a type of respiratory obstruction that most often interferes with expiration rather than with inspiration. Medical advice should be sought to improve the condition to whatever extent possible. Anesthetic agents that will not aggravate the condition should be chosen. Vinethene, which has definite bronchodilating properties, may be advantageous.

During the administration of a general anesthetic, when so much depends on a patent airway, the anesthetist or dentist—whoever makes the preanesthetic evaluation—should be keenly alert to observe the presence of any condition that may interfere with the airway. It is well to bear in mind that obstructions are usually exaggerated while the patient is undergoing general anesthesia.

Asthma. Bronchial asthma produces a constriction of the bronchi that interferes with the free flow of air into and out of the lungs. The condition is usually caused by a specific allergen or by nonspecific irritative stimuli.

Asthma is a somewhat common condition that occurs in both sexes and all ages. The most frequent symptoms are periodic attacks of wheezing, dyspnea, etc. The degree may range from very mild to very severe. The asthmatic patient can be extremely difficult, and any patient with an asthmatic history should be closely evaluated as to the frequency of attacks and their severity.

Pulmonary emphysema. Pulmonary emphysema is a condition in which there is marked distention and inelasticity of the pulmonary alveoli. This condition, like other pulmonary diseases, may be either localized or general. The most common symptom is dyspnea, but the symptoms may vary since this condition is usually associated with other underlying disease.

As previously stated, the ability of the patient to perform efficiently an exchange of gases (oxygen and carbon dioxide) with the external atmosphere or gas machine is so important to the conduct of a satisfactory anesthesia that evaluation of the ventilatory mechanisms is of major importance.

DYSPNEA AND COUGH

Dyspnea and cough are symptoms of such importance in the evaluation of both the cardiac and pulmonary status of the patient that a thorough discussion of these symptoms is required.

Dyspnea. Dyspnea is usually present to some degree in diseases of the heart and lungs. There is nearly always an increase in the severity of this symptom in direct proportion to the severity of the disease.

The most common cause of dyspnea is the interference with adequate oxygenation, which results in oxygen want. This demonstrates the importance of dyspnea as a symptom and further stresses the fact that it cannot be accepted as a cardiac or pulmonary symptom since it may also be present with circulatory, metabolic or nervous disorders. Surely it is evident that any patient exhibiting dyspnea deserves an especially thorough medical examination.

Cough. A cough in a normal person must be considered a protective reflex since it clears the tracheobronchial tree of foreign material. When the cough is persistent, however, it must be considered a symptom of some underlying disease, usually cardiac or pulmonary in origin. As with dyspnea, persistent cough is an important diagnostic symptom and should not be overlooked or minimized. It, too, deserves medical consultation and further study.

OBJECTIVE OBSERVATIONS

In many instances various subjective questions or objective observations may reveal the presence of cardiac or pulmonary disease, or both. A cough may indicate interference with normal respiratory function (bronchiectasis), or it may be a symptom of congestive heart failure. Cyanosis and clubbing of the fingers may indicate either cardiac or pulmonary disease of long standing.

The inability of a person to withstand heat, together with excessive sweating, exophthalmos, tremor, anterior enlargement of the neck, tachycardia, and so forth, and an increased metabolic rate may indicate hyperthyroidism.

It is equally important that the oral surgeon be aware of any known allergies or susceptibility to allergies that an asthmatic person may manifest. Furthermore, a diabetic patient may present a problem, particularly if the diabetes is severe, in which event control is borderline and timing and management are important.

It is most advantageous to know of any medication the patient is currently taking or has taken, inasmuch as many modern drugs may seriously alter the course of the anesthetic, even to the extent of creating hazardous complications. Some of these drugs are adrenal steroids and ACTH, tranquilizers, antihypertensives, digitalis, quinidine, or Pronestyl, anticonvulsants, thyroid and antithyroid drugs, sedatives, insulin, and narcotics.

It is also advantageous to be informed of the excessive use of tobacco or alcohol.

If the oral surgeon understands previous unpleasant anesthetic experiences, he may be able to alter the technique or to employ premedication or psychotherapy to the fullest extent and thus eliminate the possibility of the recurrence of a similar situation.

An important part of preanesthetic evaluation is the objective observations. A tremendous amount may be learned by observing each patient closely. It is not enough merely to look at the patient; the examiner should observe each area of interest closely.

In addition to the pulse, blood pressure, respirations, and temperature, there are many visible clues to underlying disease. When the oral surgeon sees these outward manifestations, it is not within his realm to attempt an accurate diagnosis. These symptoms, by their presence, should definitely point out the need for a more careful medical evaluation. In many instances the oral surgeon may render the patient a great service and save himself embarrassment by referring the patient to his own physician or internist for a more thorough examination and diagnosis. The oral surgeon should then work closely with the examining physician to give the patient the benefit of the professional skills of both examiners.

As a possible guide only, but not as authentic diagnostic criteria, the following visible clues may be useful.

Skin

Jaundice—impairment of liver function, hepatitis, and carcinoma
Petechiae—subacute bacterial endocarditis, blood dyscrasias, and physical trauma
Cyanosis—cardiac disease, venous congestion (congestive failure), pulmonary disease, argyria, and polycythemia
Pallor—anemia, hypotension
Redness (flushing)—hypertension, fever, alcoholism, and drug toxicity

Eyes

Pupils:
- Constricted—narcotics
- Dilation—belladonna drugs and fear
- Unequal—lesion of the central nervous system

Exophthalmos:
- Bilateral—toxic thyroid and leukemic infiltration
- Unilateral—inflammatory or neoplastic lesion involving the orbit of the affected side

Hands

Clubbing of fingers—chronic cardiovascular pulmonary lesions
Pigmentation—blood dyscrasis
Tremor—toxic thyroid
Temperature—toxic thyroid and infections

Neck

Enlarged glands—Infections (local or systemic) malignancies, and secondary allergic reactions
Veins—right-sided congestive cardiac failure and obstruction of vena cava

Chest

Barrel chest—chronic obstruction of air passages, emphysema, and dyspnea

Tongue

Enlargement—cretinism, and severe myxedema
Atrophy of papillae—primary pernicious anemia
Coloring—pallor, anemia; redness or cyanosis, polycythemia; deep red, vitamin deficiency

Obesity

Obesity is a very important consideration for the anesthetist. These patients should be observed closely since the degree of obesity will be an important factor in the management of the anesthesia. Extremely obese persons, because of their excess weight, should be classified Class B. Obesity superimposed upon other pathological conditions almost certainly forbids anesthesia in the office.

Pulse

Normal adult—60 to 80 per minute
Normal child—80 to 100 per minute
Tachycardiac adult—100 or over per minute
Bradycardiac adult—60 or below per minute

Blood pressure

Normal adult male (20 to 40 years of age)—approximately 120/80; may vary within reasonable limits
Normal adult female (20 to 40 years of age)—5 to 10 points lower than male

Respirations

Normal adult—16 to 18 per minute
Normal child—24 to 28 per minute
The respirations should be observed closely for rate, depth, and character since the respiratory pattern may be significantly altered by many abnormal states. Primary among these are chronic pulmonary disease, cardiac disorders, cerebral arteriosclerosis, increased intracranial pressure, acidosis, alkalosis, and severe anemia.

Temperature

Normal oral—98.6° F.
Normal rectal—0.5 to 1 degree above normal
Temperatures may vary from 0.5 to 1.5 degrees during a 24-hour period, with the lowest temperature occurring during sleep and the early morning hours. Higher temperatures are recorded in the late afternoon.

LABORATORY EXAMINATIONS

Preanesthetic laboratory examination for the ambulatory patient is a distinct aid in the successful management of both anesthesia and surgery. The bleeding and coagulation times should be known prior to surgery, rather than prior to anesthesia, since they have a much greater bearing on the indications or contraindications for surgery than those for anesthesia. However, it has been decided to include these two tests in the preanesthetic evaluation since they can be so easily accomplished at the same time.

Bleeding time. Bleeding time does not necessarily parallel coagulation time. Bleeding time may be used with coagulation time but should not replace it.

The bleeding time depends on the efficiency of the tissue fluid to accelerate clotting, on the elasticity of the skin, and on the mechanical and chemical actions of the thrombocytes. The normal range is 1 to 3 minutes.

Bleeding time is prolonged in the following conditions: thrombocytopenic purpura, pernicious anemia, aplastic anemia, infectious mononucleosis, acute leukemia, chronim lymphatic leukemia, Hodgkin's disease, and multiple myeloma.

Contrary to common belief, the bleeding time is usually not prolonged in hemophilia.

Technique. Make a slight cut in the earlobe, just deep enough to produce bleeding without pressure. At half-minute intervals blot the blood with a piece of absorbent paper. The decrease in the size of the blot indicates the decrease in bleeding. The blood should be blotted without touching the skin. About six blots on the average are required.

Coagulation time. Coagulation consists essentially of the transformation of fibrogen into fibrin by means of a ferment called thrombin. The coagulum is made up of a mesh of fibrin fibrils with entangled corpuscles and platelets. The straw-colored fluid that remains is called blood serum.

The theory of the coagulation of blood is not completely understood. According to Howell's theory (one of the best known), five coagulation factors are assumed to take part in this process. Four of these, fibrinogen, calcium salts, prothrombin, and antiprothrombin, are normal and constant constituents of the blood plasma. The fifth factor, thromboplastin, a coagulation accelerator, is not present in the tissue fluids outside the blood vessels.

When blood is obtained by an ordinary skin puncture, coagulation takes place in 2 to 6 minutes (average, 4 minutes). Clotting may be more rapid after meals and when the blood is squeezed from a wound. A more accurate test is obtained when blood is taken from a vein.

The normal range of coagulation time is as follows:

Capillary tube method, 3 to 5 minutes
Lee and White method, 5 to 10 minutes
Howell method, 20 minutes

Technique. The capillary tube method is by no means the most accurate, but it is the most adaptable to office use. The other methods may be resorted to when more accuracy is desired.

For the capillary tube method, a length of capillary tube is filled with blood from an incision. A small section of the tube is then broken off every 30 seconds. The appearance of a thin line of fibrin signifies completion of the test.

Coagulation time is prolonged in hemophilia, prothrombin deficiency due to a diseased liver, vitamin K deficiency, inability to absorb vitamin K, fibrinogenopenia, and afibrinogenemia.

Microhematocrit. Hematocrit measures the relative volume of cells and plasma in the blood. Anemias and hemorrhage lower the hematocrit reading; polycythemia and dehydration raise it. The normal range is 35 to 45 for females and 40 to 50 for males.

Technique. Previously, the hematocrit reading required the use of venous blood and was a comparatively difficult and time-consuming test. Since the introduction of the microhematocrit apparatus, venous blood is no longer necessary, and the test may be accurately and easily completed in 2 to 3 minutes.

Urinalysis. Urine is formed by the kidneys. The glomeruli allow a filtrate of the blood plasma to pass into the tubules. The cells lining the tubules selectively reabsorb most of the filtrate. The tubule cells may also excrete certain substances into the urine being formed. During a 24-hour period about 200 liters of fluid are filtered through the glomeruli and about 199 liters are reabsorbed by the tubules. The difference represents the urine excreted. Urine varies widely in composition from time to time; such variations are indicative of good function and are not abnormal. These differences may be the results of changes in the ionic balance, acid-base balance, or water balance of the body.

Specific determination of urine. Data on the specific determination of urine are given in Table 11-1.

Specific gravity. The specific gravity of the urine depends on the concentrating ability of the kidneys. The normal range is 1.010 to 1.030. It is elevated in diabetes mellitus, acute glomerulonephritis, fever, sweating, vomiting, and diarrhea. It is low in diabetes insipidus and chronic nephritis.

Technique. Place a urine sample in a graduated cylinder and with a float determine the specific gravity.

pH. This is a measure of the degree of acidity or alkalinity of the urine. The kidneys maintain the blood at the correct pH by excreting into the urine any excesses that might alter the pH of the blood. The urinary pH, therefore, varies widely, and changes do not indicate abnormality. In some situations it is advantageous for the urine to be acid or alkaline, and in these cases the pH measurement is important.

The normal range is 4.8 to 8.0.

Technique. To determine the pH of the urine, the technician dips a strip of Nitrazine into the urine specimen. The pH is indicated by the color of the urine when it is compared to a standard color chart.

Acidic states are produced by acidosis, diabetes mellitus, gout, lithiasis, acute articular rheumatism, chronic nephritis, leukemia, and scurvy.

Alkaline states are produced by debility, resorption of alkaline transudates, transfusion of blood, frequent vomiting, and prolonged cold bath.

Sugar. Sugar is present in the urine in some disorders. This occurs most often in diabetes mellitus, but it may also occur in other metabolic disorders of varying importance. Because of its simplicity the sugar test is usually employed as a screening procedure to discover

Table 11-1. Specific determination of urine by color

Color	*Cause*
Orange-yellow to green-brown	Bilirubin due to obstructive jaundice
Clear red to red-brown	Hemoglobinuria due to (1) incompatible blood transfusion, (2) severe burns, or (3) intra-abdominal bleeding
Smokey red to brown	Unhemolyzed red cells due to bleeding in urinary tract
Port wine color	Hemochromatosis; hemolytic jaundice
Dark brown	Urobilin due to liver infections, pernicious anemia, or acute infection

Color
- Normal urine is yellow or amber colored
- Depth of color depends on concentration:
  - Large fluid intake, pale urine
  - Low fluid intake, highly colored urine
- Certain pathological processes and the administration of drugs affect the color of urine

diabetes. If sugar is found, other tests then may be ordered to determine the type of sugar. The presence of sugar in the urine is called glycosuria. This may be benign or transitory or pathological.

Technique. The more complex tests of a few years ago have now been replaced with more simplified procedures.

1. Clinitest
   - 0.5 ml. water; add 5 drops of urine and drop a Clinitest tablet in tube containing the mixture
   - Blue—negative
   - Blue to yellow—positive
2. Tes-Tape (sugar)
   - Insert Tes-Tape in urine specimen
   - Yellow—negative
   - Light green to blue—positive

Benign or transitory glycosuria includes the following: alimentary glycosuria—temporary presence of glucose or other carbohydrates in urine, which is shown after large amounts of carbohydrates have been ingested; emotional glycosuria—a temporary hypoglycemic state, which will exist when a patient is angry or is under nervous tension; renal glycosuria—a condition in which the fasting blood sugar is normal and which appears to be due to lowering of the renal threshold, at which stage the kidneys will begin to excrete glucose.

Pathological glycosuria includes diabetes mellitus, hyperthyroidism, hyperpituitarism, increased intracranial pressure, hypertension, chronic liver disease, and acidosis of anesthesia.

Albumin. Ordinarily the albumin in the blood does not pass through the glomerular wall into the urine. However, in several conditions, such as kidney disease, hypertension, severe heart failure, and drug toxicity, albumin appears in the urine. It may also occur in orthostatic albuminuria, which is not a disease. Therefore, the test is not specific but indicates that a more precise examination is needed.

The normal range is negative (trace).

Albuminuria may be physiological or pathological. The former includes high protein intake, hemoglobinuria, methemoglobinuria, transient albumin during pregnancy, mental strain, exercise or prolonged exposure to cold, and orthostatic albuminuria, found when the patient is in an upright position. The latter disappears on a change in position. This condition must be considered early renal disease since it occurs in early nephritis.

The causes of pathological albuminuria are as follows:

- Renal diseases
  - Nephritis
  - Nephrosis
  - Nephrosclerosis, associated with hypertensive states
  - Kidney infections, such as the following:
    - Tuberculosis
    - Pyelonephritis
    - Septic emboli
- Noninfectious states
  - Polycystic disease
  - Bleeding
  - Incompatible transfusion
  - Amyloidosis
- Other systemic diseases
  - Diabetes mellitus
  - Hyperthyroidism
  - Jaundice
  - Fever
  - Certain blood diseases
- Extrarenal diseases
  - Prostatitis
  - Urethritis
  - Cystitis
  - Pyelitis

Technique. First, place two drops of sulfosalicylic acid in a test tube of urine. A positive reaction will cause a white precipitate. Second, apply heat, and if the precipitate does not disappear, it indicates a positive test for albumin or protein. The amount of precipitate is designated +, ++, +++, and ++++.

Vital capacity tests. The following tests are used to determine vital capacity.

Time-volume test. The vital capacity test previously used to determine cardiac reserve and cardiopulmonary impairment has proved to be inadequate. With this in mind, we use a time-volume vital capacity test that has proved more accurate in evaluating the patient as a cardiopulmonary risk. In this procedure, the patient is asked to expand the bellows six times in 30 seconds. The evaluation thus obtained is based on the average of the six readings and is more reliable than the reading obtained when the patient blows into the mechanism only once.

Henderson's breath-holding test. Henderson's breath-holding test provides an approximate measure of the vital capacity. It depends on the size and age of the patient, his athletic habits, and the condition of the lungs.

To take the test, the patient lies absolutely quiet for 5 minutes; he then draws a moderately deep breath and holds it as long as possible, with the lips closed and the nostrils pinched. A normal subject should be able to hold his breath under these conditions for 45 seconds; 30 seconds indicate good vital capacity. The strength of the vital capacity decreases progressively with periods of breath-holding of 12 to 10 seconds. Below 10 seconds, gravely impaired vital capacity is indicated, with possible cardiac involvement, and such a patient should be classed as a poor or subnormal risk.

Moot's index. Moot's index provides an approximate indication of the cardiac reserve. It is apt to be unreliable for patients with thyrotoxicosis because of the high pulse pressure. This index is derived by multiplying the pulse pressure by 100 and dividing by the diastolic pressure. Normal subjects have an index of about 50. Patients showing an index ranging from 25 to 75 probably have an adequate cardiac reserve, with 40 to 60 as the optimum figures. If the index is below 25 or above 75, the reserve is gravely inadequate.

Energy index. The energy index gives an approximate measure of the circulatory reserve, which is a product of cardiac energy and diastolic vascular resistance. The energy index is equal to the systolic blood pressure plus the diastolic blood pressure multiplied by the pulse rate. The first two figures of the product are expressed in millimeters of mercury per minute. For example, a product of 17,300 gives an energy index of 17.

Values between 6 and 24 indicate probable satisfactory circulatory energy; values of 12 to 18 are the optimum or more nearly normal. Values below 6 or above 24 indicate a grave deficiency in circulatory energy, and a patient with such an energy index is a correspondingly poor risk for anesthesia. If this test is given soon after an operation, it frequently will furnish an accurate clue to the prognosis.

CLASSIFICATION OF PATIENTS

It has long been my contention that only patients with an A classification should be considered ambulatory patients for anesthesia and surgery in the office. This does not mean, however, that patients are classified by the preanesthetic evaluation alone. The final classification of any patient must come about by grouping all the factors involved and arriving at an unbiased conclusion. These factors should include preanesthetic evaluation, surgery to be done, experience of the operator, experience of the anesthetist, and the physical setup.

Without a doubt a patient who is to undergo a single, uncomplicated extraction may be classified Class A, whereas a patient who must receive multiple extractions or has difficult impactions may be classified Class B. Also, if an experienced, well-trained anesthesiologist is used, some patients who should be classified Class B if an inexperienced anesthetist is used are considered Class A. Furthermore, it would be wise for an inexperienced oral surgeon with a newly functioning organization to hospitalize some patients whom an older, more experienced oral surgeon with a smoothly functioning organization might treat as ambulatory office patients.

It should be kept in mind, particularly for ambulatory patients, that long procedures may be accomplished in two stages, and thus a patient who might be in Class B could be changed to Class A.

The ability to recognize certain signs as manifestations of physiological deviations from the normal may emphasize for the examining dentist the need for a more thorough examination of the patient by a physician or internist. By obtaining an adequate preanesthetic evaluation before any general anesthesia is administered, the dentist renders a service to his patients commensurate with his advanced training, his background, and the place he occupies in his profession.

CHOICE OF ANESTHETIC AGENTS AND TECHNIQUES

To a great degree the choice of an anesthetic agent or agents and the techniques of administration should depend on the results of the preanesthetic evaluation. In all cases, one should choose the agents and techniques to fit the individual patient, not the patient to suit the agents and techniques. There is no doubt that some agents and techniques are superior in the hands of certain operators. This, of course, should be taken into consideration, but it should by no means be the only deciding factor.

The dentist who wishes to utilize general anesthesia and make available to his patients the advantages of this method of pain control should be well versed and proficient in the use of various agents and techniques. He should not, as is so often the case, limit himself to one or two agents at the most and follow the same routine for all patients. The dentist who is to administer the anesthetic should view each patient as an individual and tailor the anesthetic to that individual.

At present, the dentist has a wide variety of anesthetic agents and techniques at his command, and while he may favor particular ones, he should not fail to make use of the others when they are specifically indicated. For instance, I do not advocate the routine use of the intratracheal technique for ambulatory patients. When, however, it is definitely indicated, this method should be employed. Also, while many dentists may prefer intravenous induction for their patients, certain circumstances such as difficult venipuncture or extreme fear of a needle puncture may warrant the use of oral premedication and inhalation anesthesia. Also, the patient may give a history of allergy to particular intravenous or intraoral agents. These agents, of course, should not be used. On the other hand, a patient may have a particular fear, such as the fear of a mask being placed over his face. For such a patient, intravenous induction and then use of a mask are indicated.

A variety of techniques may be employed for children, depending on the age of the child, his size and physical condition, his cooperation, and the anticipated length of the procedure. Also, the decision whether or not to employ premedication must be made on an individual basis.

The dentist should always be prepared to supplement nitrous oxide with one of the volatile anesthetic agents such as divinyl ether, ethyl ether, trichloroethylene, ethyl-vinyl ether, or fluothane. The agent may enable the anesthetist to stabilize what would otherwise be a difficult anesthesia and to maintain adequate oxygenation at all times.

An important question to be considered in the choice of an anesthetic agent or technique is whether the patient is a hospital patient, an outpatient, or an ambulatory patient. For a hospitalized patient, the reaction time from the anesthetic is less important than it is for an ambulatory patient. Therefore, it is necessary to choose an agent or agents for ambulatory patients that will not retard the reaction time. The technique of administration will also differ for the hospital patient, the outpatient, and the ambulatory patient. Rarely, if ever, will an ambulatory patient be deliberately carried beyond the light surgical plane of anesthesia. In fact, the techniques of anesthesia for ambulatory patients are characteristically different from those used for most hospital patients and outpatients.

As previously stated, the agents and technique selected for ambulatory patients should afford rapid, pleasant induction, satisfactory maintenance, rapid recovery, and a high safety factor. These four factors are essential for the successful management of these patients, particularly when a large number of patients are to be anesthetized and dismissed within a comparatively short time. Since no one anesthetic agent, at the present time, will fulfill all these requirements, it is necessary to combine two and sometimes more agents to achieve the desired results. In essence, this means combining agents in such a manner as to utilize their desirable qualities and eliminate their undesirable ones. For instance, the intravenous agents, when used alone, afford rapid, pleasant induction and satisfactory maintenance, but they may not ensure a rapid recovery or carry as high a safety factor as desired. It is advantageous, therefore, to induct the patient with an intravenous agent and then maintain anesthesia with nitrous oxide and oxygen. This combination possesses the advantage of the intravenous agents and nitrous oxide and eliminates their disadvantages to a great extent.

The same pattern of logical sequence for the use of the anesthetic agents should be utilized with every patient so that the patient and dentist alike will benefit from a more nearly ideal anesthetic management. This desirable results will be achieved when the dentist takes into consideration all the factors involved, such as the age and physical condition of the patient, the duration and nature of the surgery, the skill of the anesthetist, and the skill of the surgeon.

Chapter 12

Preanesthetic preparation and medication

The preanesthetic preparation of any patient who is to receive a general anesthetic is an extremely important part of the overall procedure and contributes immeasurably toward its success. There are no means by which the preanesthetic preparation can be circumvented without increasing the risk to the patient.

PREANESTHETIC PREPARATION

The preanesthetic preparation will differ somewhat for the ambulatory patient as compared to the hospitalized patient. However, it should not be neglected for either patient since thorough preparation is just as necessary for one as for the other. The degree of thoroughness will vary from patient to patient, whether the anesthetic is administered in the hospital or in the office. For instance, for some patients it may be deemed advisable to have various consultants and many laboratory tests, whereas in others the routine physical examination and evaluation may be sufficient. For most patients, the results of the usual routine preanesthetic examination and evaluation will determine the need for further consultation.

As stated previously, only Class A patients should be considered candidates for office procedures. Others should receive the benefits of a more thorough evaluation by an internist, and the procedure should be completed in a hospital.

HOSPITALIZED PATIENTS

The hospitalized patient should be admitted at least 24 hours prior to anesthesia and surgery in order to permit an adequate preanesthetic examination and evaluation by a member of the medical staff, as required by all accredited hospitals. After the preanesthetic examination and evaluation are completed, it would be very advantageous for some member of the anesthesia department to visit the patient in his room and explain the anesthetic procedure as concisely as possible. This helps to instill confidence in the patient and makes him a better subject for smooth induction. This psychological approach should never be overlooked because the benefits to be derived from it are enormous. In many instances, gaining the patient's confidence and cooperation is as important as the premedication, if not more so.

Specific orders governing the intake of food and water before anesthesia should be written. If the anesthesia is scheduled for the following morning, the patient should take nothing by mouth after midnight. This will ensure an empty stomach and eliminate the possibility that vomitius may occude the airway or otherwise interefere with or interrupt the administration of the anesthetic. If the anesthesia and surgery are scheduled for the afternoon, the patient may be permitted a liquid breakfast, with nothing by mouth afterward.

The patient should be instructed to remove dentures, partial dentures, or removable bridgework. Also, rings, watches, or anything else that may be broken, lost, or cause injury to the patient should be removed. Both general and private-duty nurses should make certain that these instructions are complied with. Before beginning the induction, the anesthetist should also recheck to make certain that the patient does not have anytihng loose in his mouth that may cause respiratory obstruction. The patient should be instructed to void on awakening and to defecate if possible. An enema or a cathartic prior to anesthesia for a dental procedure is not necessary unless the patient is to receive Avertin or some other type of rectal anesthetic.

AMBULATORY PATIENTS

The ambulatory patient will, by necessity, require certain alterations in the preoperative preparation. Ideally, the dentist should see the patient 24 to 48 hours prior to his appointment for anesthesia and surgery so that the preanesthetic evaluation can be completed. For the majority of patients the dentist assumes responsibility for the anesthesia, and he is thus obligated to complete the preanesthetic evaluation or have it completed. Under no circumstances should this procedure be eliminated or slighted because the patient is ambulatory, since this is an essential part of the preanesthetic preparation. In fact, many subsequent decisions will be based on this portion of the preparation.

Prior to the appointed time for anesthesia and surgery, the patient can be given further instructions as to the intake of food and water. If anesthesia and surgery are to be performed in the morning, the patient should not have food or water after midnight. If they are planned for the afternoon, a liquid breakfast is permissible. It is mandatory, however, that at least 6 to 8 hours elapse after the intake of any food or liquid before a general anesthetic is administered.

It is very doubtful that any condition that can be treated in the office is of sufficient urgency to risk the administration of an anesthetic to an unprepared patient, particularly one who has eaten within 6 hours. The danger of the unprepared patient's vomiting and aspirating, with resultant respiratory obstruction, hypoxia, or anoxia with cardiac arrest, is even imminent. No elective surgery warrants such a risk. The patient can be relieved of pain by analgesics or narcotics, and a later appointment can be made for the anesthesia. In all too many cases this risk is taken for the convenience of either the doctor or the patient.

It is absolutely essential that the ambulatory patient be told that he must be accompanied by a responsible adult. No patient should leave the office unescorted after having received a general anesthetic. This also holds true for patients who have been premedicated, even though they do not receive a general anesthetic.

Ambulatory patients should be instructed as to what type of clothes to wear. They should be advised aaginst wearing extremely tight-fitting garments or clothing that encroaches on the neck. Whether or not intravenous anesthesia is contemplated, the patient should be advised to wear a short-sleeved shirt or some other clothing that leaves the arms readily available for venipuncture.

All patients should be instructed to void immediately prior to induction of the anesthetic. Children who are to be premedicated should be told to visit the bathroom prior to the medication.

PREANESTHETIC MEDICATION

Preanesthetic medication is a vital factor in the preparation for general anesthesia. Its value has been proved over and over again. Indeed, medication can be considered an integral part of the anesthesia. However, it may vary from patient to patient, and for this reason the preanesthetic medication should be tailored to the individual patient rather than established on a routine basis.

The basic purposes of premedication are as follows: (1) to afford a restful night before the anesthesia and surgery, (2) to allay apprehension or produce amnesia immediately preceding the anesthesia, (3) to depress reflex irritability, (4) to lessen metabolic activity, (5) to check excessive salivation, and (6) to raise the pain threshold when indicated.

1. The patient should be well sedated so as to assure a satisfactory night's rest. It is not uncommon for an unsedated or inadequately sedated patient to remain awake because of worry about the following day's procedure. Experience has shown that patients who have spent a restless night come to surgery more apprehensive, more irritable, and less cooperative and are thus more difficult to manage.

2. The chief reason that patients are premedicated is to allay their fears. The patient becomes quiet and relaxed so that the metabolic activity more nearly approximates normal. Amnesia is particularly advantageous for children and extremely apprehensive persons.

3. Depression of reflex irritability is *essential* for a hyperactive person. The premedication should be sufficient to reduce markedly reactions to both external and internal stimuli. Otherwise the nervous system may be unable to compensate adequately for extreme reactions, resulting in severe physiological derangements.

4. Metabolic activity during anesthesia is an extremely important factor because it denotes the energy needed to maintain the chemical processes vital to body function. This energy is derived from the utilization of oxygen and glycogen and eventually results in the formation of carbon dioxide. Directly related to the utlization of oxygen is the production of body heat. The basal metabolic rate represents the amount of oxygen consumed and the heat produced by a conscious patient who, in a fasting state, is at complete rest. When the calories produced per square meter of body surface are normal for a particular patient, the metabolic rate is considered zero. Any increase or decrease in caloric production and oxygen utilization is expressed as plus or minus, depending on the percentage of calories produced above or below the normal level.

During anesthesia it is essential that sufficient oxygen be administered at all times to fulfill the patient's metabolic requirements. Adequate premedication will, in most patients, depress metabolic activity sufficiently to permit a satisfactory induction and lessen the possibility of hypoxia.

It is important to point out the dangers of overpremedication since it is possible to depress metabolic activity below functional levels or to depress vital functions (respiration and circulation) so that hypoxia will occur. For this reason the vital signs (pulse, respiration, blood pressure, and color) must be closely observed so that any manifestations of overdepression may be quickly recognized.

Many factors influence metabolic activity. Among them are age, sex, emotions, pain, disease, and temperature. At birth and during early infancy this activity is low, but from the early months to about 2 years of age it rises precipitously. The basal metabolic rate is correspondingly high to about the age of 14 or 15 years, when a slow, gradual decline begins and continues until the early twenties. From then on, the basal metabolic rate declines slowly until middle age, and more rapidly as old age is approached. It should be understood that each patient is to be judged on an individual basis according to physiological rather than chronological age.

Females have, as a rule, a lower basal metabolic rate than do males of a corresponding age group. Emotion plays a distinct part in elevating metabolic activity and is no doubt one of the major fatcors to be considered preceding anesthesia and surgery. The importance of pain and its effect on the basal metabolic rate should not be overlooked. When pain is present the patient should definitely be given narcotics preoperatively to raise the pain threshold and to decrease metabolic activity correspondingly.

Various diseases alter the metabolic activity. Hyperthyroidism, diabetes, and infections raise the basal metabolic rate, whereas hypothyroidism, certain glandular diseases, and obesity may lower it.

The patient's temperature should be noted, particularly when there is high fever, since there will be about a 7% increase in metabolism for each degree (Fahrenheit) his temperature rises. For the vast majority of dental patients, the anesthetist does not know the basal metabolic rate. For this reason the patient's vital signs must be closely observed. The metabolic activity may vary greatly during induction and maintenance as compared to that brought about by the premedication alone. During the lighter stages of anesthesia, which are required for most dental procedures, the stimulation and manipulation during surgery greatly increase the metabolic activity; this should be constantly taken into consideration so that the oxygen requirements are always satisfied.

The use of premedication as an antisialogogue depends on the anesthetic agent or agents to be employed. Atropine and scopolamine are widely adopted for this purpose, but we do not routinely advocate them for outpatients, particularly when nonstimulating or nonirritating agents are to be administered. However, the value of these drugs to depress parasympathetic activity and for their vagotonic effect should not be underestimated.

Analgesics or narcotics are particularly indicated for premedication when the patient is experiencing moderate or severe pain. Raising the pain threshold will significantly reduce metabolic activity and make possible smoother induction.

The type of anesthesia to be employed should always be considered when premedication is ordered. For instance, premedication should be given in larger doses when nitrous oxide is to be employed as the primary anesthetic. Smaller doses may be employed advantageously when the barbiturates are to be used for induction or as a primary anesthetic.

As stated previously, the importance of evaluating each patient as an individual and planning the premedication accordingly cannot be overstressed. Furthermore, the dentist should consider the type of anesthetic to be used, the length of the procedure, the skill of the anesthetist, and the patient's status as an ambulatory patient, an outpatient, or a hospital patient.

CHOICE OF DRUGS

The drugs used for premedication should be administered for a definite purpose and not as a routine procedure. The dosages as well as the individual drugs should be varied to suit individual patients and circumstances.

The drugs in the following list are by no means the only ones used for premedication. However, they are by far the most widely employed ones and will, in varying doses, fulfill the preanesthetic requirements for a vast majority of patients.

- Barbiturates
  - Secobarbital (Seconal)
  - Pentobarbital (Nembutal)
- Narcotics
  - Morphine
  - Meperidine (Demerol)
- Psychosedative drugs
  - Promethazine (Phenergan)
  - Hydroxyzine (Vistaril)
- Belladonna derivatives
  - Atropine
  - Scopolamine

Barbiturates. In recent years the barbiturates have been more commonly used for preanesthetic medication. These drugs, more than any others, tend to allay apprehension and fear and bring pronounced psychic sedation. The short-acting barbiturates (Nembutal and Seconal) are preferable for ambulatory patients and outpatients. In the prescribed dose, they should have no great effect on circulation or respiration but should make the patient drowsy and receptive to anesthesia.

Secobarbital (Seconal) or pentobarbital (Nembutal) may be administered orally, intramuscularly, or intravenously in doses ranging from $\frac{3}{4}$ to 3 grains (50 to 180 mg.), depending on the individual patient. For maximum effect they should be given 60 to 90 minutes preoperatively by mouth or intramuscularly. For controlled premedication, they may be given intravenously and the induction completed with other agents. For ambulatory patients or outpatients, the oral route is often preferred. For pediatric patients, rectal administration may be advantageous.

Patients premedicated with barbiturates should be observed for hypersensitivity to the drug. On rare occasions the premedicating dose may produce some degree of respiratory depression or affect the central nervous system more than is usually expected. For these patients, additional barbiturates should be given with extreme caution. The patient should also be observed for allergic manifestations, and if they are in evidence, barbiturates should not be administered.

Narcotics. The narcotics (morphine and Demerol) are more commonly used for hospitalized patients than for ambulatory patients or outpatients. Meperidine (Demerol), however, is being more widely used for ambulatory patients. Recent research has proved to us the value of the narcotics administered preoperatively for dental outpatients since the pain threshold may be substantially raised and the procedures accomplished with much lighter planes of anesthesia. We have used meperidine administered by intravenous drip most advantageously for controlled premedication and its supplemental effect.

Psychosedative drugs. The term psychosedative is used in preference to the term tranquilizer or ataractic. As previously reported, we have continued to use this class of drugs for premedication. The drugs have been used primarily in conjunction with the barbiturates and the narcotics. Significant cortical depression is not produced by the drugs alone, as patients receiving these drugs alone can be aroused by sufficient stimuli and then become drowsy again after the stimuli are removed. Their prime site of action is thought to be on the brain stem reticular formation. Promethazine (Phenergan) is used in 25 to 50 mg. doses and hydroxyzine (Vistaril) in 50 to 100 mg. doses. Both drugs can be given orally, intramuscularly, or intravenously. However, the intravenous route is by far the most effective.

Belladonna derivatives. Atropine and scopolamine are more frequently used for premedication for hospitalized patients than for office patients. For short office procedures, we do not routinely administer them since in the vast majority of patients the anesthetic agents employed are nonirritating to the mucous membrane and do not induce increased salivation.

It is my opinion that the use of atropine or scopolamine to prevent or reduce the incidence of laryngospasm is overrated unless sufficient amounts are given (1/100 to 1/75 grain). As previously stated, the depressing effect of these drugs on parasympathetic activity and their vagotonic effect should not be underestimated when sufficient doses are administered.

The chemistry and pharmacology of these drugs are discussed in Chapter 8

Chapter 13

Charting and evaluation of patient during anesthesia

Accurate charting and adequate evaluation are essential factors that are often overlooked during the administration of a general anesthetic for ambulatory dental patients and are sometimes neglected for hospitalized dental patients. Perhaps the reason is that dental procedures are often considered to be minor and consequently to involve only slight risk for the patient. This may be particularly true if the surgical procedure is a short one requiring extremely light anesthesia. Even then, the patient should be closely observed during the anesthesia for manifestations of minor complications. Close observation of the patient is extremely important during all general anesthesias because even a seemingly minor complication, if it is unrecognized and untreated, may rapidly develop into a severe complication or an emergency.

The anesthetist should understand that he has two specific obligations: to maintain the patient in the proper plane of anesthesia and to keep him in as nearly normal a physiological condition as possible. This being so, he must be well trained and should be entrusted with these duties and no others. The successful administration of an anesthetic is a full-time endeavor requiring the utmost skill and attention.

Time and time again, dentists (both general practitioners and oral surgeons) tell me that they constantly check the patient while engrossed in their surgical or operative procedures. To me, this is an unreasonable practice, because the operator can be aware of the signs of impending danger only after they have become obvious, which is much later than they should be recognized. Also, I have known of many occasions when the operator has become so engrossed in his work that he has missed important manifestations.

A person who devotes his entire time to administering the anesthetic and who is trained to recognize quickly the earliest signs of an impending complication will take steps to remedy the situation at once. These steps should be taken, in most cases, before the operator is aware that all is not well. In fact, as far as the operator is concerned, all has been well because the trained anesthetist with no other duties has fulfilled his fundamental obligations by alertly preventing the impending complication rather than belatedly treating it.

In addition to observing the signs of anesthesia closely, the person administering the anesthetic should constantly watch the signs denoting the condition of the patient. As previously mentioned, the signs of anesthesia are the respirations, the eye signs, and the degree of muscle relaxation. The signs denoting the physiological status are the pulse, blood pressure, and color.

The maintenance of a free and patent airway is another essential. Event persons possessing a minimum of experience will soon learn that without airway, no patient can be kept in good physiological condition. For all patients, the anesthetist should do all within his means to see that there is an unobstructed intake of oxygen of adequate volume and an efficient elimination of carbon dioxide by means of unimpeded expirations.

It is granted that during anesthesia for ambulatory patients blood pressure readings are not taken routinely. It is my contention, however, that the blood pressure should be recorded preoperatively, and in procedures lasting longer than 10 or 15 minutes, the cuff should be in place for a periodic check. The pulse should be constantly checked during anesthesia since it renders much valuable information and forecasts early hypoxia and the presence of body stress and physiological deviations. While color is a valid sign of a physiological condition, if at all possible, the anesthetist should never allow cyanosis to develop.

It is thus evident that the alert anesthetist who constantly observes the patient is in a much more favorable position than anyone else to monitor the patient's condition during the anesthesia.

It is equally necessary to chart or otherwise record these observations. Adequate charting is a constant reminder of the patient's condition and immediately shows any variations that may occur.

To rely on one's memory is a shortsighted practice and has many disadvantages.

In addition to affording a ready appraisal of the patient's physical status during the anesthesia, the anesthesia chart or record is of inestimable value for future reference. It may serve as the basis for clinical research or may be a ready source of information about a patient requiring subsequent anesthesia. The record may bring to mind difficulties experienced during the previous anesthesia. This knowledge will undoubtedly be an aid in planning the next anesthetic procedure to eliminate the complications experienced previously.

Much valuable clinical information is lost to both the anesthetist and the profession when inadequate records or no records are kept. It is impossible to discuss or write from memory when a series of cases is involved. Certain incidents may be retained in the mind, but as a rule this information is neither sufficient nor accurate enough to be of real value.

Accurate anesthesia records are desirable also from a medicolegal point of view and are a valuable source of information in case of litigation. A recent book states that malpractice suits are rare in cases in which the records of the anesthetic course are complete.

The authors of this book also point out that, while anesthesia records are very important, the patient should not be neglected for their sake. They state:

> A fine record is not much good if the anesthesia is poor; in other words, the patient should never be sacrified for the record. There are times during difficult procedures when the patient demands complete attention. It would be foolish at such times to withdraw attention from him in order to complete the record. In the majority of cases, however, one should be able to keep a full and detailed account of the entire procedure.*

The anesthesia record (Fig. 13-1) should contain all necessary information pertinent to the case. Included should be the following:

1. Name, race, age, and sex
2. Address
3. Date of preanesthetic evaluation and classification
4. Adherence to preoperative instructions
5. Date and time of administration of anesthetic
6. Preoperative medication, if any

---

*Dripps, R. D., Eckenhoff, J. E., and Vandam, L. D.: Introduction to anesthesia, Philadelphia, 1957, W. B. Saunders Co.

Anesthesia chart

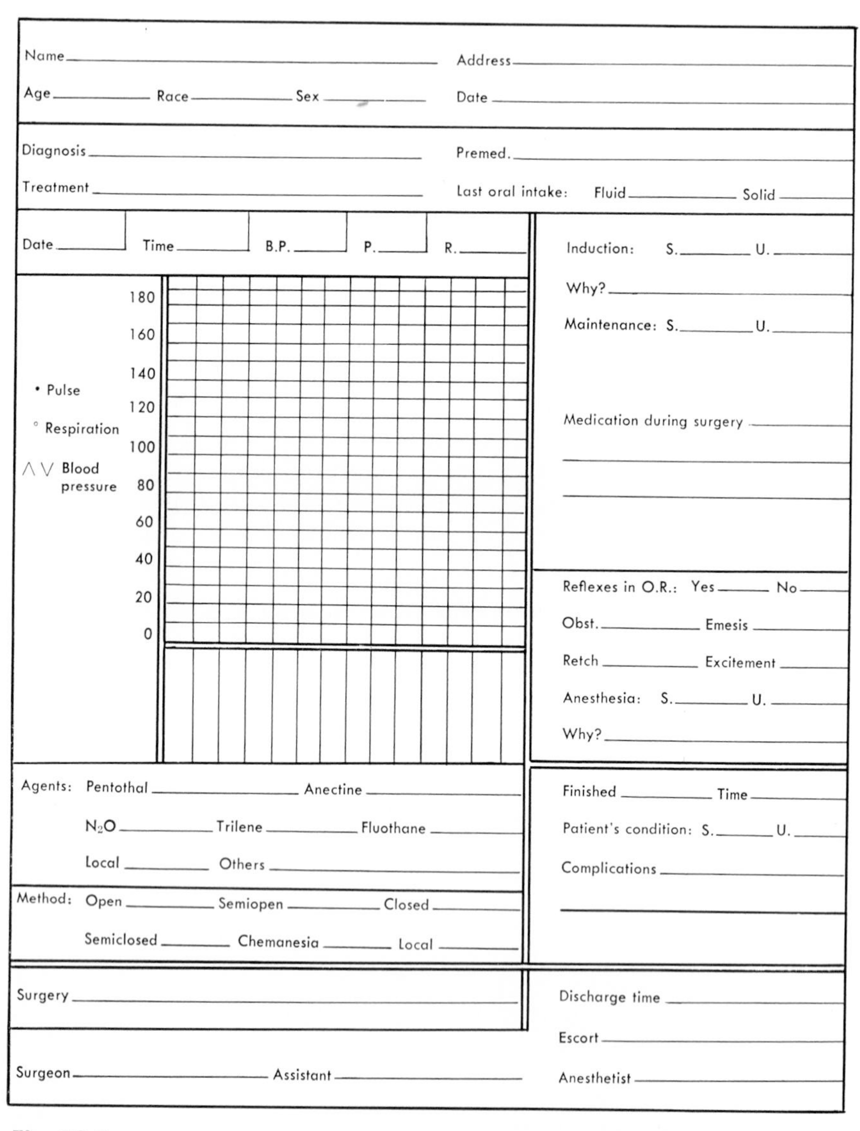

Name ______ Address ______

Age ______ Race ______ Sex ______ Date ______

Diagnosis ______ Premed. ______

Treatment ______ Last oral intake: Fluid ______ Solid ______

Date ______ Time ______ B.P. ______ P. ______ R. ______

180
160
140
120
100
80
60
40
20
0

• Pulse

° Respiration

∧ ∨ Blood pressure

Induction: S. ______ U. ______

Why? ______

Maintenance: S. ______ U. ______

Medication during surgery ______

Reflexes in O.R.: Yes ______ No ______

Obst. ______ Emesis ______

Retch ______ Excitement ______

Anesthesia: S. ______ U. ______

Why? ______

Agents: Pentothal ______ Anectine ______

N_2O ______ Trilene ______ Fluothane ______

Local ______ Others ______

Method: Open ______ Semiopen ______ Closed ______

Semiclosed ______ Chemanesia ______ Local ______

Finished ______ Time ______

Patient's condition: S. ______ U. ______

Complications ______

Surgery ______

Discharge time ______

Escort ______

Surgeon ______ Assistant ______ Anesthetist ______

Fig. 13-1

7. Preoperative (immediate) pulse, blood pressure, and respirations
8. Anesthetic agents employed, and doses
9. Status of induction
10. Status of maintenance
11. Artificial airways, if any
12. Time of completion of surgery, and patient's condition at completion
13. Status of recovery
14. Anesthesia time
15. Description of complications, if any
16. Time of discharge and name of escort

The anesthesia record serves as a checklist to ascertain that all necessary preanesthetic instructions have been given and followed, as well as to verify that the preanesthetic evaluation was completed. It should also give as graphic a picture as possible of the progress of the anesthesia. Since we deem it mandatory that all ambulatory patients subjected to a general anesthetic be escorted from the office or hospital by a responsible adult, the name of that person is included. If an unforeseen complication were to arise postoperatively, this information could be valuable.

The keeping of an accurate chart for an ambulatory dental patient is understandably difficult since the anesthetist, in practically all instances, has both hands fully occupied supporting the chin, stabilizing the head, and often augmenting the respirations. It is therefore advisable that all possible information be charted before the anesthesia is started and that the record be completed as soon after its termination as possible. Fortunately, anesthesia for ambulatory patients is a reasonably short procedure and can be recorded without difficulty.

In addition to the patient's preanesthetic evaluation, the completed anesthesia chart should be filed as part of the permanent record.

Chapter 14

Postanesthetic care

Every general aneshesia, as previously stated, is divided into three phases (induction, maintenance, and recovery), regardless of its duration. The induction and maintenance phases are under the scrutiny of the anesthetist, and in all instances the recovery phase is initiated under his guidance. However, it is not unusual for the recovery phase to be supervised by someone else. While this stage is often considered a postanesthetic period, it is, in reality, an integral part of the anesthetic procedure. For this reason, the anesthetist should maintain a close watch over the patient and turn him over to ancillary personnel only when he is certain that the patient's condition and status warrant it.

The period immediately following the termination of the surgery (maintenance phase) and the beginning of the recovery phase may be fraught with danger. During this time residual blood and mucus in the oral cavity may be aspirated if the patient is not under close supervision.

Even though the surgery is completed and the patient seems to have withstood the procedure well, the anesthetist should not take this opportunity to wash the mask and tubing (Fig. 14-1), prepare for the next patient, or do anything else that takes him away from the patient, no matter for how short a time.

The dental patient requiring intratracheal intubation to maintain an adequate airway may present a postoperative problem if he does not receive the proper treatment. The intratracheal tube should be removed by the anesthetist when the patient is in a proper plane of anesthesia. Patients, particularly younger ones, should be closely observed after extubation, and, if by chance the intubation was a trau-

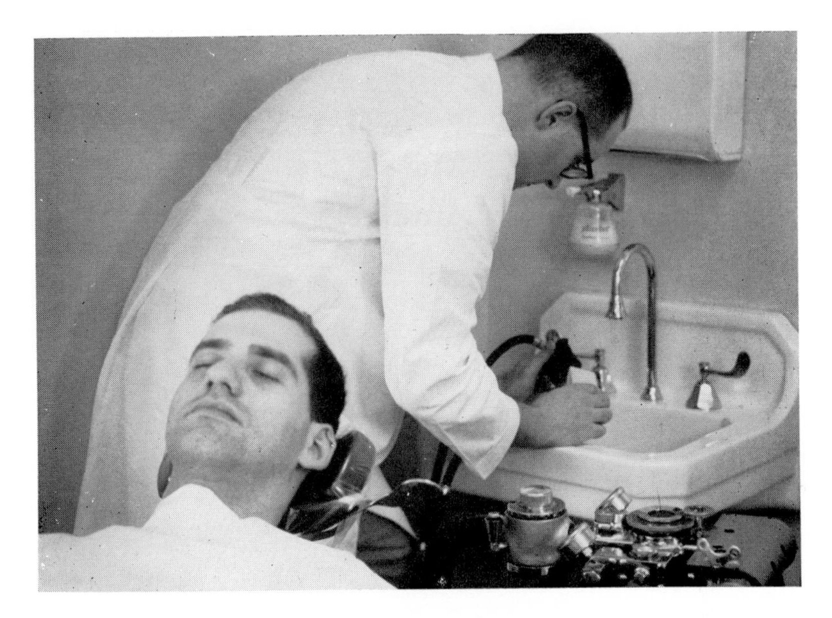

Fig. 14-1. Anesthetist should not turn from the patient until he has recovered completely.

matic one, the possibility of glottal edema should always be considered and prepared for.

The anesthetist should supervise moving the patient from the dental chair or operating table to the recovery suite and should not leave him until he is completely satisfied as to his condition and the competence of the person who is to take over the immediate care of the patient. Sudden movements or abrupt changes of position may drastically alter the circulatory physiology of an anesthetized patient. For this reason the anesthetist should make certain that the patient is moved gently and slowly and has withstood the movement without undue alteration of blood pressure or pulse.

During recovery from anesthesia for oral surgery the patient should not be placed in a supine position, since this position may cause blood or mucus to gravitate to the pharynx and create a respiratory hazard. The patient should be placed in a side or prone position so that any residual material in the oral cavity will gravitate away from the pharynx rather than toward it.

The patient should be constantly checked while in the recovery room and not left alone until he is in full command of his reflexes and well oriented to his surroundings.

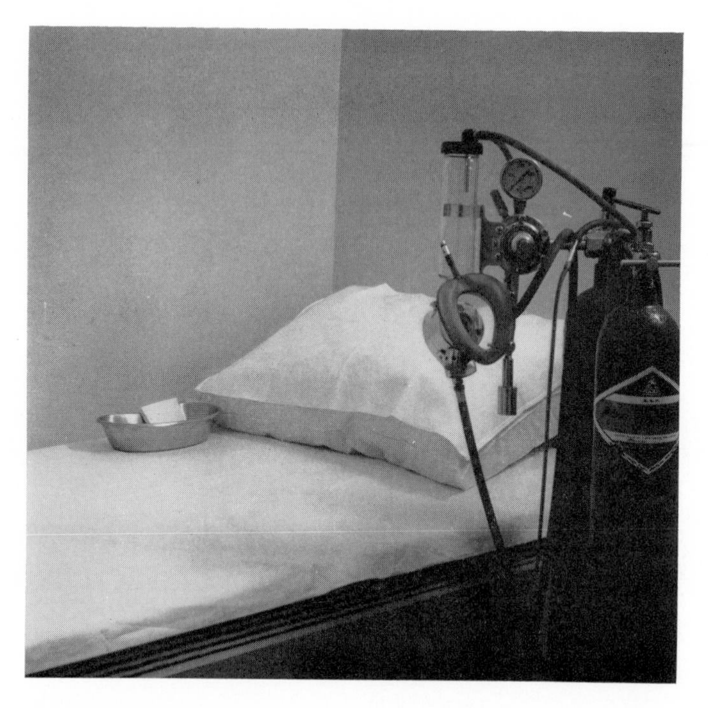

Fig. 14-2. Oxygen for emergency use and suction catheter should be available in recovery rooms.

Oxygen and suction apparatus and all other necessary equipment should be readily available for use in the recovery room (Fig. 14-2), and the personnel should be well trained in their use. However, the vast majority of office patients will be sufficiently recovered so that the protective reflexes have returned before they leave the operating room. Even then, they should be closely checked for impending hypoxia since this danger is always present during the immediate postoperative period.

Respiratory obstructions of any degree should not be tolerated during the recovery period since the onset of hypoxia can be insidious. For this reason, the airway should be kept free and patent, which will assure an adequate intake of oxygen and elimination of carbon dioxide. Oxygen should be administered at even the slightest provocation (Fig. 14-3). Many persons believe that it should be given routinely during the recovery period. Patients should be observed very closely during this phase for respiratory obstruction secondary to vomiting or for seepage of blood and mucus into the pharynx. Proper

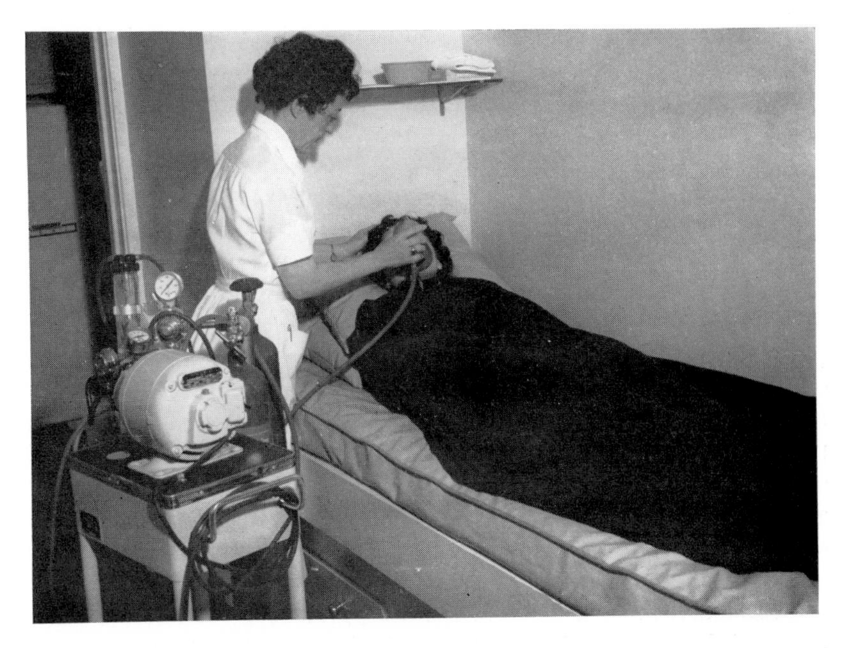

Fig. 14-3. Patient should be under observation in the recovery room, and oxygen should be administered at the slightest provocation.

positioning during recovery will help to prevent these conditions. Nevertheless, suction and oxygen apparatus should be readily available.

Many patients experience severe pain during the immediate postanesthetic period. This manifestation of pain may seem out of proportion to the surgical procedure. However, it should be considered that during this period of being half awake and half asleep, pain reaction may be exaggerated, particularly if the barbiturate–nitrous oxide sequence was employed. In these cases the nitrous oxide is eliminated in 2 or 3 minutes, whereas the action of the barbiturates persists. Since the barbiturates alone in hypnotic doses tend to lower rather than raise the pain threshold, the exaggerated manifestation of pain is not difficult to understand. Narcotics can be administered either intravenously or intramuscularly to raise the pain threshold and thus eliminate or decrease the conscious manifestation of severe pain. The dose should be carefully calculated in order not to depress the patient unduly, because he may be depressed already from the residual effect of the previously given barbiturates. If the patient is ambulatory and is to leave the office or hospital, a miscalculated dose may prolong the recovery period. For this reason it is suggested that the narcotic dose for such patients be underestimated rather than overestimated.

Emergent delirium, while uncommon, may create a postanesthetic problem. This is most frequent in younger patients and, in my opinion, is brought about to a great extent by the presence of persisting pain. The use of the narcotics or other sufficiently potent analgesics may alleviate this condition. However, here also they should be used with caution in order not to prolong the recovery time unduly or severely depress the patient. During the recovery period, particularly while they are in the recovery room, patients should be observed to prevent them from injuring themselves. All potential hazards should be removed. Usually, recovery rooms in hospitals are planned with special carriages that have side rails and other necessary arrangements to aid in protecting the patient. This same standard of protection for the patient should be maintained in the recovery room of an office. I know of a postanesthetic patient who was placed in an office recovery room in which a white porcelain hopper was located next to a built-in, bunk type of bed. While he was unattended, he attempted to lean over the hopper to spit or vomit and either misjudged the distance or lost his balance. As a result, his chin was badly lacerated, and the injury was more serious than the original operation. This is just one example of what can occur when there is improper supervision and hazardous conditions are not eliminated.

The postanesthetic care of ambulatory patients involves one major consideration that rarely applies to hospital patients. These patients, being ambulatory, must leave the office within a reasonable length of time. They should be permitted to depart only after the person responsible for the anesthetic is completely satisfied that they have sufficiently recovered to be in no danger whatsoever.

The pulse and blood pressure should be stable, and the postanesthetic drugs should be sufficiently broken down or eliminated that the patient is in complete harmony with his surroundings and has a sufficient degree of muscle coordination to permit unaided ambulation. No patient who has undergone general anesthesia should be permitted to leave the office unless escorted by a responsible adult. I have reached this conclusion since two cases were brought to my attention in which completely unexpected, unfortunate incidents occurred to patients permitted to leave the office unescorted following the administration of a general anesthetic.

In summary, both the dentist and the anesthetist are cautioned that the postanesthetic phase of the procedure should not be neglected since it is during the emergent period that unexpected complications can occur. Complete preparations for the proper care of the patient should be made by having adequate and efficient personnel available in the recovery room. This area should also be completely equipped with all the necessary armamentarium for both routine and emergency treatment.

Chapter 15

Anesthetic complications and emergencies

General anesthesia is a procedure that should never be taken lightly, for a complication or an emergency may occur at any time. Any person administering an anesthetic should be fully aware of this possibility. The anesthetist will be in a better position to prevent complications if he understands the conditions that might create them and then does his best to see that these conditions do not occur. It has been stated that the best treatment for any complication is prevention.

An anesthetic complication may be defined as any deviation from the normally expected physiological pattern during or following the administration of an anesthetic. An anesthetic emergency may be defined as any unforseen combination of circumstances requiring immediate attention. It should be stressed that not all emergencies are necessarily life endangering, but, since an element of doubt may exist as to the final outcome, some immediate treatment is indicated.

In general anesthesia as compared to regional analgesia, a much greater percentage of the complications are emergency in nature in that they require immediate treatment. A seemingly minor complication may become a serious emergency if it is neglected.

Complications may be considered immediate or secondary, mild or severe, and permanent or transitory. Systemically, they may be classified respiratory, circulatory, nervous, gastrointestinal, metabolic, cosmetic, or technical.

A complication or emergency affecting any one of these systems may eventually encompass or affect the others. For example, if a respiratory complication creating a hypoxic or anoxic condition is allowed to continue, it may eventually affect the nervous and cardiovascular systems, even to the point of causing cerebrocortical damage or cardiac arrest.

A *primary* complication is one that occurs and manifests itself at the time the anesthetic is administered. A *secondary* complication is one that is manifested later, even though it may have been caused during the actual administration of the anesthetic.

A *mild* complication is one that exhibits a slight change from the normally expected pattern and reverses itself without any specific treatment other than correcting its cause. A *severe* complication manifests itself by a pronounced deviation from the normally expected pattern and requires a definite plan of therapy to reverse it.

A *transitory* complication is one which, even though severe at the time of occurrence, leaves no residual effect. A *permanent* complication will, of course, leave a residual effect, even though mild.

RESPIRATORY COMPLICATIONS

The vast majority of complications that occur during anesthesia for dental or oral surgery are primarily respiratory in nature and may induce varying degrees of hypoxia or even anoxia. Such a complication may be termed an emergency in that some immediate treatment is necessary. Respiratory complications can usually be classified as primary, mild, and transient in that they manifest themselves during the administration of the anesthetic and, as a rule, can be readily reversed by removing the cause; thus they leave no residual effect. If they are allowed to continue untreated, these same respiratory complications may create emergencies involving the circulatory or nervous system. On the other hand, while vomiting is primarily a gastrointestinal complication, when it occurs during anesthesia it may interfere grossly with respirations and create a respiratory complication and emergency that could result in hypoxia, which would cause complications of the cardiovascular and nervous systems.

Since all respiratory complications produce some degree of hypoxia, it will be well to discuss this entity thoroughly.

Hypoxia. Hypoxia may be defined as a decrease in the normal level of oxygen in the tissues. It may be divided into five types—hypoxic, anemic, stagnant, histotoxic, and metabolic.

Hypoxic hypoxia. In hypoxic hypoxia there is decreased oxygenation of the arterial blood, which results in decreased oxygen tension and causes the hemoglobin to fall below its normal oxygen saturation. The most frequent causes are a low percentage of oxygen in the inspired air, obstruction of the airway, depression of respiration, and breathing of inert gases.

Anemic hypoxia. In anemic hypoxia the arterial blood contains oxygen at normal tension, but there is a shortage of functioning hemoglobin. The most frequent causes are anemia (primary or secondary), hemorrhage (acute or chronic), and alterations in the hemoglobin.

Stagnant hypoxia. In stagnant hypoxia the arterial blood contains oxygen at normal tension, with an adequately functioning hemoglobin, but there is a diminution in the circulatory rate. The most frequent causes are circulatory failure (probably cardiac in origin), impairment of venous return, and shock.

Histotoxic hypoxia. In histotoxic hypoxia the arterial blood contains oxygen at normal tension, there is no shortage of functioning hemoglobin, and the circulation is adequate. However, the tissue cells are poisoned or depressed to such a degree that they are unable to utilize the available oxygen. The most frequent cause is some agent that markedly depresses cellular respirations.

Metabolic hypoxia. The four types of hypoxia just discussed are those listed by Barcroft, Peters, and Van Slyke. I have added metabolic hypoxia to take into account the following condition. Although the arterial blood contains oxygen at normal tension, the functioning hemoglobin is adequate, the circulation is adequate, and the tissue cells are not conspicuously depressed, the metabolic rate and oxygen consumption are sometimes elevated beyond the ability of the existing mechanisms to supply the increased need for oxygen. The outstanding causes of this condition are a pronounced increase in body temperature (fever), extreme fear or apprehension, and a stormy induction that results in excitement and struggling. It has been my experience, particularly with children, that a combination of these factors may produce hypoxia that is just as insidious and dangerous as the hypoxic, anemic, stagnant, and histotoxic types.

Hypoxia may be an insidious complication; because of its gradual onset, it may defy early recognition. Certain manifestations, however, are usually evident. The earliest manifestation of oxygen want is an increase in pulse rate and a slight increase in respiratory rate. If the want is allowed to continue, the pulse becomes slow and bounding, with a rise in systolic pressure and a normal diastolic pressure. If the oxygen lack is permitted to continue further, the heart muscle begins to show the effect of hypoxia. The heartbeat becomes weak, and the systolic pressure falls. Further continuance will be manifested by a slow, weak pulse and possible arrhythmia, with eventual circulatory collapse and cardiac arrest.

With the possible exception of the early increase in the respiratory rate, the character of respirations may vary little until relatively late. The effect on the central nervous system will be manifested by early rigidity, muscular tremors, twitching, and eventually convulsions. Cyanosis will not always be present, especially in an anemic patient. When it does occur, it will be noticed first in the lips, nail beds, earlobes, and face. On the other hand, a plethoric type of patient may show cyanosis very early.

To summarize, the clinical manifestations of hypoxia are an increase in pulse rate, a slight increase in rate of respiration (depending on the anesthetic agent used), an increase in systolic pressure with normal diastolic pressure, a slow, bounding pulse, a weak, thready pulse, a drop in blood pressure, a weak, slow arrhythmic pulse, and cardiac arrest.

The most frequent respiratory complications are mechanical obstructions, pathophysiological responses, depression of respiration, and excessive stimulation of respiration.

Mechanical obstructions. Without a doubt, most respiratory complications are caused by obstructions within the air passages. These obstructions may be partial or complete. The anesthetist should be

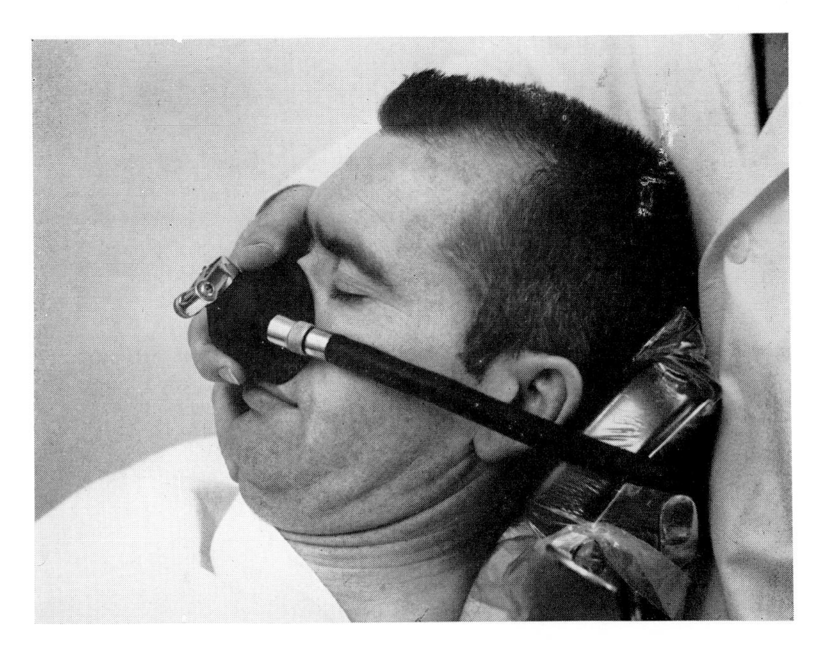

Fig. 15-1. Improper head position, with lower jaw unsupported.

constantly on guard against any interference whatsoever with normal respiratory function because even a slight obstruction may create a serious problem.

Mechanical obstruction of the airway, which results in respiratory complications, can be caused by various conditions. Improper position of the head (Fig. 15-1) is a common cause. A misplaced oropharyngeal partition (Fig. 15-2) would cause respiratory complications. A misplaced nasal inhaler exerting pressure against the nares (Fig. 15-3) would most certainly cause a respiratory complication. If the tongue is relaxed posteriorly (see Fig. 10-3), the airway will be obstructed. The more common causes, symptoms, and prevention and treatment of mechanical obstructions are summarized in Table 15-1.

Pathophysiological responses. There are certain physiological responses that may have an effect on the air passages. When these

Table 15-1. Common causes, symptoms, and prevention and treatment of mechanical obstructions

Cause of obstruction	*Symptoms*	*Prevention and treatment*
Improper head position	Stertor; inadequate respiratory volume	Proper head position to facilitate respiration
Overdepressed mandible	Stertor; inadequate respiratory volume	Lift mandible upward and forward; support mandible
Foreign material in oral cavity and pharynx	Stertor with characteristic gurgling sound; decreased respiratory volume; may induce laryngeal irritation	Proper use of oropharyngeal partition; adequate suction to remove blood, mucus, and tooth particles
Misplaced oropharyngeal partition	Stertor; markedly decreased respiratory volume; may induce gagging or laryngeal irritation	Use proper partitions with protruding strings attached; correctly place partition and change when necessary
Misplaced facial mask or nasal inhaler	Stertor; decreased respiratory volume; absence of respirations	Choose proper mask to fit patient; place mask properly
Posterior relaxation of tongue	Stertor; depression or absence of respiratory volume	Maintain tongue in forward position; proper use of mechanical airways; tongue suture if necessary

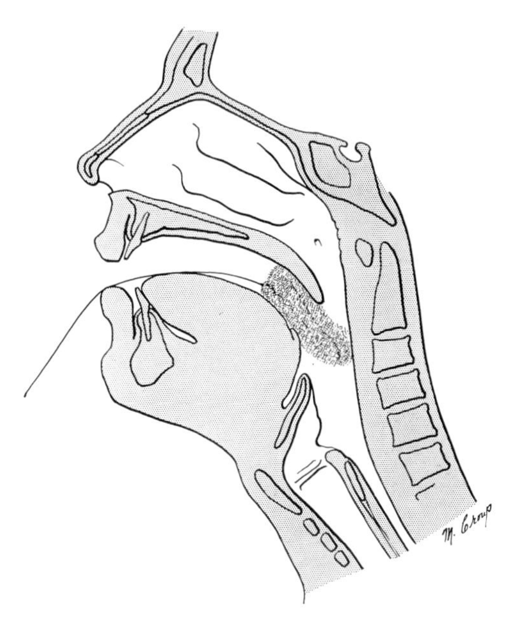

Fig. 15-2. Misplaced oropharyngeal partion. Partition has slipped into pharynx, causing respiratory obstruction.

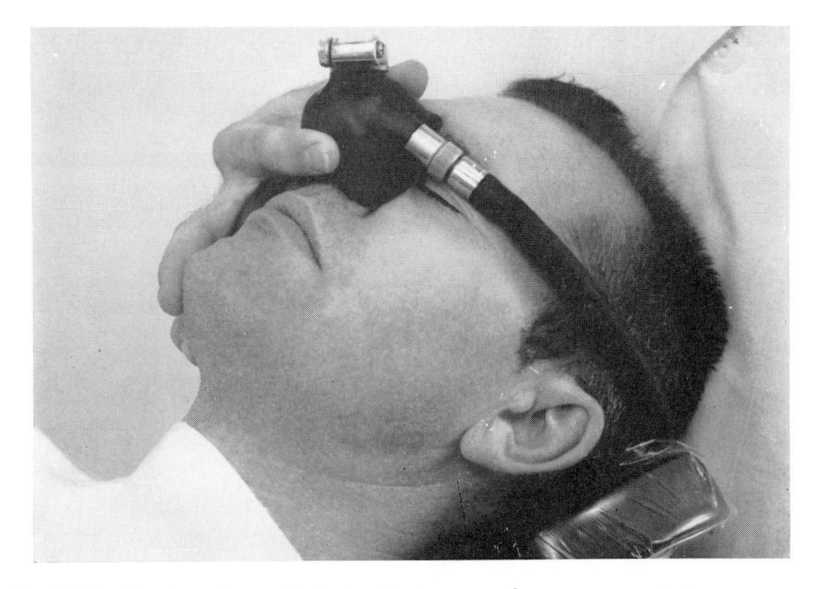

Fig. 15-3. Misplaced nasal inhaler. Note upward pressure against nares.

Table 15-2. Common complications, symptoms, and prevention and treatment of pathophysiological responses

Complication	*Symptoms*	*Prevention and treatment*
Coughing and gagging	Characteristic manifestations	Keep foreign substances from pharynx; avoid early, strong concentrations of irritating gases and too early stimulation; use suction equipment properly
Vomitus	Characteristic manifestations; stertor or gurgling	Proper instructions about food and water intake before anesthesia; smooth induction; during vomiting, rapidly lower head and use efficient suction
Laryngospasm	Characteristic manifestations; patient makes a determined effort to inspire without success; may be wheezing, crowing type of inspiration; abdominal muscles active	Achieve proper plane of anesthesia before permitting painful stimulation; proper premedication; keep pharynx clear of foreign substances postanesthetically; use topical anesthetics when indicated; administer oxygen under pressure with muscle relaxants; use intratracheal techniques

responses occur during anesthesia, they usually interfere with the respirations or affect them sufficiently to create an anesthetic complication—hence the term pathophysiological responses. Table 15-2 summarizes the more common complications, symptoms, and prevention and treatment of pathophysiological responses.

Laryngospasm. Since the introduction of intravenous anesthetic agents, laryngospasm has been a much discussed complication, and rightly so since it may have dire consequences. Actually, the laryngeal reflex is a protective one since it permits the egress of air into the tracheobronchial tree and the lungs and prevents the entrance of foreign substances. This protective reflex may be abolished in deeper planes of anesthesia; on the other hand, in the lighter planes its occurrence may be so enhanced that spasm of the involved muscles is a distinct possibility. The muscles of the larynx are divided into extrinsic and intrinsic groups; the intrinsic muscles cause laryngospasm as they produce motion of the vocal cords.

The motor and sensory nerve supply of the larynx are from the superior and recurrent branches of the vagus. The superior branch supplies the larynx in the area above the vocal folds and the cricothyroid muscle, whereas the recurrent branch supplies the intrinsic muscles and sensation to the intrinsic muscles and the area below the vocal folds.

Adduction of the vocal cords with closure of the laryngeal aperture is not always spastic or complete and may occur in the following ways: apposition of the vocal cords (adduction), apposition of the false vocal cords, and closure of the aryepiglottic folds. These conditions may occur separately or in combination and will determine the degree of laryngospasm. It should be kept in mind that adduction of the vocal cords is necessary for normal respirations, phonation, and so forth. When adduction of the vocal cords alone is manifested, inspiration is usually impaired to a much greater degree than expiration.

Apposition of the false vocal cords (ventricular ligaments) usually occurs during coughing and may cause "crowing" during anesthesia. When spasm of both the vocal cords and false vocal cords occurs, both inspiration and expiration are affected.

Laryngospasm is more complete and difficult when the aryepiglottic folds come into apposition to close the superior laryngeal aperture in a sphincterlike manner. Both inspiration and expiration are strongly affected, and laryngospasm is complete.

Whereas laryngospasm was previously a frightening complication and did at times terminate fatally, this complication has been reduced to a minor status since the introduction of the muscle relaxants. It has also been my observation that the incidence of laryngospasm is greatly decreased when the concentration of the intravenous agent (Pentothal) is reduced to 2%.

If the intravenous needle is in place and a muscle relaxant is readily available, there is not only a means for successful treatment of laryngospasm but also an ideal method for preventing this complication.

Bronchial spasm. Bronchial spasm is a not uncommon respiratory complication. It may occur simultaneously with laryngospasm and, if not managed properly, may lead to severe consequences.

The lungs consist of a large amount of smooth muscle that controls the diameter of the bronchioles. This is particularly true around the smallest bronchioles, where minute sphincters are formed around the alveolar sacs. Any constriction of these smooth muscles will reduce ventilation. When this constriction and reduction of pulmonary ventilation occur, the patient is said to have a bronchial spasm.

Like other smooth muscles in the body, the bronchioles are thus believed to be under autonomic control. The sympathetics dilate the bronchi and constrict the bronchial arteries, whereas the parasympathetics constrict the bronchi and dilate the bronchial arteries. The sympathetic supply is from the first through the fifth thoracic segments, and the parasympathetic innervation is from fibers of the vagus nerve.

Bronchial spasm is most likely to occur in asthmatic persons or when any degree of vagus stimulation is created. Patients suffering from chronic disease of the lungs are also prone to develop bronchial spasm.

Bronchial spasm may be exhibited first by a coughing spell and a wheezing type of expiration. It is possible for the condition to continue, and expiration becomes extremely difficult, if not impossible. Thus, inspirations are seriously impeded secondarily to the difficult expirations.

The best treatment for bronchial spasm, as for laryngospasm, is prevention. Patients who are to undergo anesthesia, especially those with chronic disorders of the lungs, should be carefully chosen after an adequate preanesthetic evaluation. Induction should be slow and atraumatic, with nonirritating agents if possible. Aminophylline given intravenously in doses of 3½ to 7 grains is a useful bronchial dilator and has proved effective when used clinically to treat this condition.

Depression of respiration. When all general anesthetic agents are administered, the rate and volume of the respirations must be constantly observed to prevent any decrease in pulmonary ventilation, which may eventually induce a degree of hypoxia. Respiratory depression should be differentiated from decreases in respiratory volume secondary to obstructions. Respiratory depression may occur either centrally or peripherally.

Central respiratory depression. Central respiratory depression is usually the result of an overdose of the anesthetic agent, secondary depressive effects of increased carbon dioxide levels, or depression of the respiratory center due to hypoxia.

Overdose of the anesthetic agent. The signs of anesthesia should be understood and closely observed to prevent an overdose of the anesthetic drug. It is rarely if ever necessary to carry a patient beyond the light surgical plane of anesthesia for dental or oral surgery.

Secondary depressive effects of increased carbon dioxide levels. Although carbon dioxide may be an early respiratory stimulant, it can markedly depress respirations if allowed to accumulate. Also, the depressing effects of the anesthetic agent on the respiratory center will not only prevent its stimulation by the initial increase of carbon dioxide but will also, by a decrease in respiratory ventilation, permit a further buildup of carbon dioxide within the body, which may further depress the respiratory center.

Respirations should be augmented to assure not only adequate oxygenation but also efficient elimination of carbon dioxide. Carbon dioxide absorbers should be used when a closed system of induction is used.

Depression of respiratory center due to hypoxia. It should be kept in mind that hypoxia never stimulates the respiratory center but only depresses it. It is true that when arterial oxygen falls below 92% of saturation, the depth of the respirations is increased by the stimulating effect of the chemoreceptors. This level, however, could not be considered hypoxic. The anesthetist should make certain, therefore, of adequate oxygenation so that the respiratory center will respond to any afferent stimuli.

Peripheral respiratory depression. The most frequent cause of peripheral respiratory depression is the use of muscle relaxants, which by their paralyzing effects on the respiratory muscles decrease pulmonary ventilation. It is therefore mandatory that whenever the muscle relaxants are used, the volume of pulmonary ventilation be accurately observed so that augmentation or controlled respiration may be utilized to assure adequate oxygenation and efficient elimination of carbon dioxide. It is essential that the muscle relaxants never be used unless means and methods of augmenting or controlling respirations are available, along with personnel adequately trained in these maneuvers.

Excessive stimulation of respiration. While excessive stimulation of respiration in itself may not be a serious situation, it must nevertheless be considered a complication. Also, it may be the forerunner of complications of a more serious nature if it is not corrected. The most frequent causes of excessive stimulation of respiration are painful stimuli in light stages of anesthesia, strong concentrations of irritating anesthetic gases, and early excess of carbon dioxide.

Painful stimuli in light stages of anesthesia. Excessive stimulation of respiration (hyperpnea) may result if a patient is subjected to painful stimuli before an adequate depth of anesthesia is reached or if he is not properly conditioned to the stimuli. The insult of an ill-timed, painful stimulus may create a forceful inspiration and sometimes laryngospasm. Also, an unwanted depth of anesthesia may be obtained, particularly with pediatric (pedodontia) patients when potent inhalation agents, such as ethyl chloride, vinyl ether, trichloroethylene, or fluothane, are used.

Strong concentrations of irritating anesthetic gases. Strong concentrations of irritating anesthetic gases may on occasion produce early hyperpnea followed by apnea. When irritating gases are used, the concentration should be increased slowly. Wherever possible induction should be performed with nonirritating agents.

Early excess of carbon dioxide. An early excess of carbon dioxide results in an increased rate and depth of respiration. This in itself may be of no major importance as far as complications are concerned since the increase in rate and depth of respiration will blow off the excess carbon dioxide and restore carbon dioxide to normal levels. However, when a patient is under anesthesia, the respiratory center may not respond sufficiently to prevent the early buildup of carbon dioxide, with the result that increasing levels of carbon dioxide may depress secondarily rather than stimulate. It is therefore essential to prevent an initial buildup of carbon dioxide if possible.

CIRCULATORY COMPLICATIONS

It is my opinion that the vast majority of circulatory complications that occur during anesthesia for dental or oral surgery are secondary to respiratory complications. However, circulatory complications may occur as a separate entity unrelated to respiration. The most common circulatory complications are tachycardia, bradycardia, arrhythmias, hypertension, hypotension, shock, and cardiac arrest.

Tachycardia. Tachycardia may be defined as a marked increase in the heart rate. The term is usually applied to a rate above 100. The principal causes of tachycardia and their prevention and treatment are summarized in Table 15-3.

Bradycardia. Bradycardia is a marked decrease in the heart rate, usually a rate below 60. Bradycardia, or even cardiac arrest, is a possibility when cardiac depression caused by overstimulation of the vagus nerve occurs. It is more likely to occur from strong vagal stimulation while a patient who was not previously conditioned to the stimuli is in the lighter plane of anesthesia. The term vagovagal reflex is usually used to indicate a powerful afferent vagal stimulus that causes a vagal depression of the heart.

Table 15-4 gives a summary of the principal causes of bradycardia and their prevention and treatment.

Arrhythmias. An arrhythmia is any variation from the normal rhythm of the heartbeat.

The most common arrhythmias that occur during anesthesia for dental and oral surgery are extrasystoles and premature beats. However, other arrhythmias (dropped beats, pulsus bigeminus, and so forth) may occur. The vast majority of arrhythmias may go unrecognized unless there is some gross disturabnce of the peripheral pulse. It

Table 15-3. Principal causes of tachycardia and their prevention and treatment

Causes	*Prevention and treatment*
Fear and apprehension	Use of adequate premedication; choice of proper anesthetic agents to prevent prolonged induction; psychotherapy
Excitement during induction	Psychotherapy; avoid disturbances and loud noises during induction; proper premedication; choose proper agents for smooth, rapid induction; prevent too early stimulation
Overdose of atropine or sympathomimetic drugs	Careful, judicious use of drugs; oxygenation; barbiturates if necessary.
Hypoxia	Maintain free, patent airway with adequate oxygenation
Direct effect of anesthetic agents	Avoid use of irritating agents for induction; choose proper agents for rapid, smooth induction
Painful stimulation	Do not stimulate patient until proper plane of anesthesia is achieved; condition patient to painful stimulus; use analgesics to raise pain threshold; supplement with regional analgesia
Atropine	Vagotonic effect of atropine may produce tachycardia; avoid overdose of atropine; use when indicated
Blood loss	Proper hemostasis; replace blood loss
Hypotension	Avoid sudden pressure drops if possible; use vasopressor drugs to elevate pressure; use Solu-Cortef if drop is due to adrenal insufficiency

Table 15-4. Principal causes of bradycardia and their prevention and treatment

Causes	*Prevention and treatment*
Hypoxia	Maintain patent airway with adequate oxygenation
Vagal stimulation	Avoid early moderately severe or severe stimulation in light planes of anesthesia

is my opinion that when the dentist or anesthetist recognizes an obvious arrhythmia that did not previously exist, and it does not respond to oxygenation and reduction in concentration of anesthetic agent, the procedure should be discontinued and further medical evaluation of the patient sought. If subsequent appointments are required, the anesthesia technique may be varied accordingly. It is of interest to note the use of intravenous lidocaine (Xylocaine) to correct ventricular arrhythmias. The drug, injected in amounts from 50 to 100 mg. of 1 or 2%, is rapid in its action and possesses a seemingly low degree of toxicity. Its action is of short duration and may be repeated.

The principal causes of arrhythmias and their prevention and treatment are summarized in Table 15-5.

Hypertension. Whether a patient has hypertension during or following anesthesia depends upon the pressure readings (arterial, venous, capillary, etc.) taken during the preanesthetic evaluation. These readings indicate the extent to which a patient can withstand increases in pressure. It is necessary, therefore, to determine in advance of the anesthesia how much of an increase in pressure a patient can be expected to tolerate.

The principal causes of hypertension and their prevention and treatment are summarized in Table 15-6.

Hypotension. As with hypertension, the pressure readings taken

Table 15-5. Principal causes of arrhythmias and their prevention and treatment

Causes	*Prevention and treatment*
Hypoxia	Hypoxia from any cause may produce varying arrhythmias and therefore should never be tolerated
Carbon dioxide increase	Carbon dioxide accumulation may cause various arrhythmias, and therefore efficient carbon dioxide elimination is essential
Anesthetic agents	Anesthetic agents (trichloroethylene, cyclopropane, ethyl chloride, etc.) should be used with caution and adequate oxygenation; avoid overdoses or prolonged deep anesthesia
Sympathomimetic drugs	Use sympathomimetic drugs only when indicated and with caution; avoid overdosage

during the preanesthetic evaluation determine whether a patient is hypotensive. It is necessary, also, to determine in advance of the anesthesia how much of a drop in pressure a patient can be expected to tolerate before specific action is needed.

Table 15-7 gives a summary of the principal causes of hypotension and their prevention and treatment.

Shock. Shock is of the utmost concern to anyone who administers general anesthesia because it may occur with startling rapidity. The anesthetist is in a position not only to recognize its onset but also to prevent it or to initiate successful treatment once it has occurred. Failure to understand its mechanisms, its conditions of occurrence, its early recognition, and its prevention and treatment will result in failure to cope with it. This means that the anesthetist must thoroughly understand the physiology of shock and be familiar with its symptoms and treatment.

Table 15-6. Principal causes of hypertension and their prevention and treatment

Causes	*Prevention and treatment*
Apprehension and fear accompanied by excitement during induction	Proper premedication and choice of agents and methods for smooth induction; psychotherapy when indicated
Painful stimuli	Proper plane of anesthesia before beginning surgery; adequately condition patient to stimulus when operating in light planes of anesthesia; use high potency analgesic agents when indicated; supplement with regional analgesia (local anesthesia)
Carbon dioxide accumulation	Adequate respirations to assure efficient carbon dioxide elimination; avoid deep stages of anesthesia with respiratory depression; use carbon dioxide absorber with fresh soda lime when indicated
Hypoxia	Rise in systolic pressure may accompany early hypoxia; hypoxia should not be tolerated at any time; maintain patent airway and adequate oxygenation
Drugs	Injudicious use of vasopressors may produce hypertension and should be used with caution; amyl nitrite or sympathetic blocking agents may be used to lower pressure if specifically indicated

Table 15-7. Principal causes of hypotension and their prevention and treatment

Causes	*Prevention and treatment*
Deep anesthesia	Maintain light planes of anesthesia
Adrenal insufficiency	Secure adequate preanesthetic history; patients previously one tsroids should receive maintenance doses and medical consultation; intravenous Solu-Cortef may be used when necessary
Blood loss	Blood loss should be closely observed and replaced when necessary; radical or extensive surgery should never be attempted unless adequate preparations are made
Carbon dioxide excess	While carbon dioxide may produce an early rise in systolic and diastolic pressures, it is not uncommon to have the hypertensive episode followed by gradual hypotension; usually the diastolic pressure begins to fall first, followed by a drop in systolic pressure; follow steps described in Table 15-6 to prevent accumulation of carbon dioxide

Shock is defined by Moon as "a circulatory deficiency, not cardiac nor vasomotor in origin, characterized by a decreased blood volume, a reduced volume flow and by a hemo-concentration."* Cullen defines shock as simply "a circulatory insufficiency caused by a disparity between the circulating blood volume and the vascular capacity."†

The causes of shock are many and varied and may range from psychological or emotional reactions (neurogenic shock) to trauma and hemorrhage (traumatic or hemorrhagic shock).

Neurogenic shock. Neurogenic shock is the result of the body's reaction to an unpleasant experience or situation; this causes a loss of nervous control of the peripheral vessels and permits dilation of and a distinct increase in the vascular bed. This increase creates a marked disparity between the effective circulating volume and the vascular bed, which results in hypotension.

Neurogenic shock is usually characterized by a sudden hypotensive episode, a comparatively weak pulse, and pallor. There is no pro-

*From Moon, V. H.: Shock and related capillary phenomena, London, 1938, Oxford University Press.

†From Cullen, S. C.: Anesthesia—a manual for students and physicians, Chicago, 1957, Year Book Medical Publishers, Inc.

nounced loss of blood or increase in blood volume, and the pulse rate is usually unchanged.

As a rule neurogenic shock can be readily reversed if the cause is removed and treatment is instigated without delay. The hypotensive episode must not be allowed to continue, for it may predispose the patient to a coronary attack, acute renal failure, or hypoxia, each of which in itself may perpetuate shock.

The removal of the cause together with giving oxygen will alleviate the condition in a fair percentage of patients. Lowering the head to facilitate venous return will usually be advantageous, particularly when the patient is sitting up in a dental chair. If these maneuvers fail to produce the desired results, vasopressors should be given intravenously. In indicated cases, hydrocortisone sodium succinate may also be used to advantage.

Traumatic or hemorrhagic shock. Traumatic or hemorrhagic shock is usually the result of an ineffectual circulating volume due to loss of plasma or whole blood. Blood volume usually is a matter of balance between the fluids within the vessels and in the tissues. When conditions arise that tend to lower or raise the volume of blood, counterforces come into play that restore the normal level. When circulating fluid is lost, the vessels replenish themselves from the extravascular space. On the other hand, any tendency for the blood volume to rise is met by a discharge of the excess fluid into the tissues or along the excretory routes. Thus a balance is struck, and normally the blood volume is maintained in a remarkably constant balance.

The clinical signs of shock are well known. The patient is profoundly depressed. Metabolic and functional activities are low. Normal tissue turgor is absent, the flesh has a lifeless, doughy feel, and the superficial veins are collapsed and bloodless. The respirations are shallow and interspersed with deep sighs. The pulse is rapid and weak and may be imperceptible in the peripheral arteries. In the late stages, the blood pressure declines progressively. Following surgical operations or severe trauma, low temperatures are common, but following burns and in shock from certain other causes, the temperature may be increased. The patient is usually restless and may become delirious. Stupor or coma develop and may lead to death.

A decline in arterial blood pressure has been overemphasized as a cardinal feature; low pressure is not regularly present. Often increased blood pressure is observed in the early stages, and other signs of shock may manifest themselves while the blood pressure is at its highest level. Cowell (1919) noted that no immediate fall in arterial pressure occurred in severely wounded men, but moderate increases were frequent; in such cases the decline occurred several hours later. Blalock stated that the blood pressure was an inadequate guide to the state of the circulation in incipient shock. There is no doubt that a progressive decline in the arterial pressure occurs in the late stages of shock. It appears that, so long as the mechanism of compensation is adequate, there is no prolonged hypotension; when the latter develops, it indicates ineffective compensation or decompensation. Often the first indication of impending shock is a rising systolic pressure and a normal or decreasing diastolic pressure.

Changes in the rate and quality of the pulse vary with the stage and degree of shock. In incipient shock the pulse may be slow and strong. It usually increases in rate just before the blood pressure declines; when decompensation occurs, it becomes very rapid, thready, and weak.

During the course of an operative procedure under general anesthesia, various conditions may occur, any one of which is sufficient to cause an increase in the permeability of the capillary walls. Some of these conditions are under the control of the anesthetist, but others are not.

The causes which the anesthetist may control or eliminate are lack of oxygen in the anesthetic mixture, obstruction of the airway, prolonged deep anesthesia, and psychic factors. The last-named factor can be controlled by proper premedication. Causes beyond the anesthetist's control are hemorrhage, manipulation of tissues, prolonged surgical procedures, and the patient's preoperative condition.

Anoxia probably is the chief factor tending to increase or perpetuate the circulatory deficiency. Once the lack of oxygen in a large area of tissues reaches the point at which capillaries and venules lose their tonus and become permeable, the condition tends to become self-perpetuating. Plasma escapes into the tissues, and the minute vessels become jammed with corpuscles. This further impedes the circulation, decreases the volume flow, lowers the blood volume, and increases the anoxia. With increasing anoxia, the reestablishment of circulatory efficiency becomes progressively more difficult.

The evidence therefore indicates that there are three major factors in the development of shock. They are atony and dilation of capillaries and venules in an extensive visceral area, anoxia, and hemorrhage.

It is self-evident that any one of these factors brings the others into action—a self-perpetuating mechanism that operates as a vicious cycle (see diagram on p. 273).

The diagram illustrates the mechanism by which various agents and conditions affect the circulation. When circulatory deficiency is such that anoxia develops in the tissues, that effect itself causes atony of capillaries and introduces the self-perpetuating quality into the mechanism. The diagram illustrates how this mechanism may originate elsewhere than in the capillaries. When reduced blood volume, reduced volume flow, or asphyxia causes anoxia in the tissues, the anoxia causes atony of the capillaries and thereby initiates the operation of the same cycle.

The vicious cycle of shock*

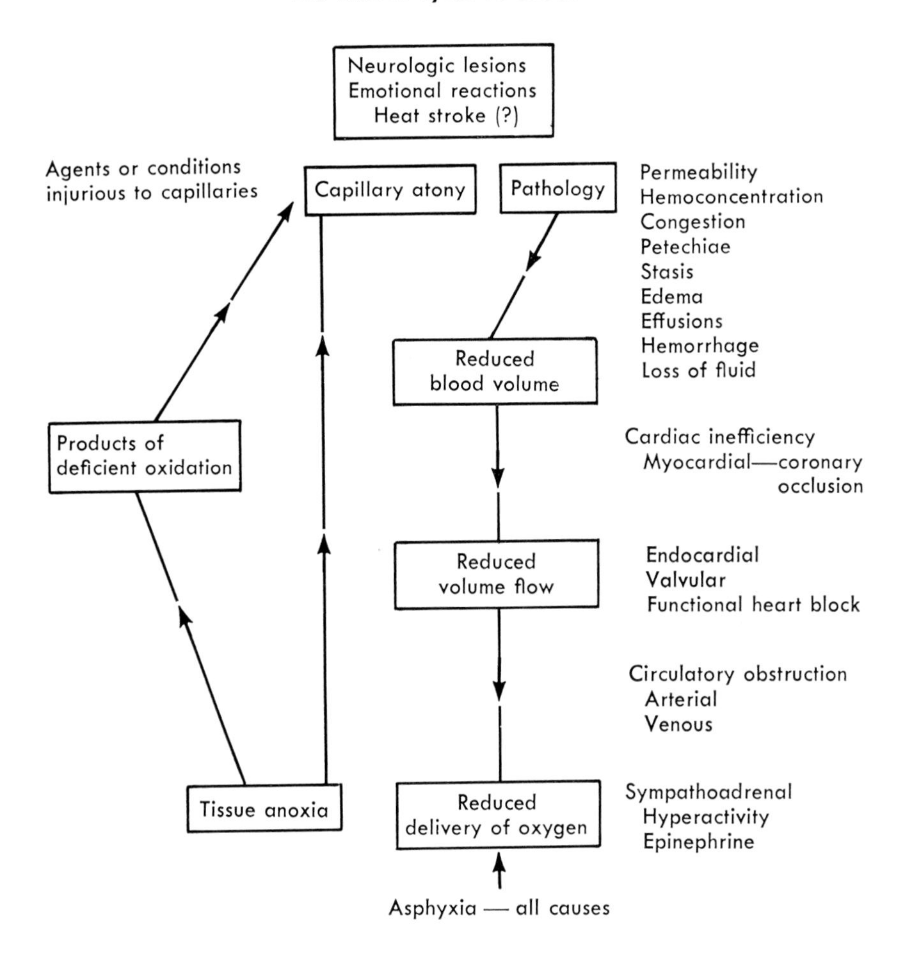

University Press.

*From Moon, V. H.: Shock and related capillary phenomena, London, 1938, Oxford

Treatment. The successful management of shock depends on its early recognition and on the removal of the causative condition or the alleviation of its effects. An understanding of the conditions under which the development of shock may be expected and the ability to detect the signs of its approach are therefore necessary.

At no time is watchful waiting more disastrous than during the development of shock. The anesthetist who waits until the pulse is rapid, weak, and thready, the blood pressure progressively declines, and the face becomes ashen in color and moist with cold sweat will seldom treat the patient successfully. By then the vicious cycle is in motion and can easily result in death.

The preventive treatment of shock may be summarized in the following manner:

1. Perform a careful preanesthetic examination and choose the premedication carefully.
2. Select the anesthetic agent or agents best suited to a particular patient.
3. Do not rush the induction period, and avoid external stimuli during this period.
4. Avoid continued deep narcosis and maintain an efficient airway at all times.
5. Consider the importance of the time factor during surgery, which is frequently overlooked in the prevention of shock.
6. Check carefully the minute-to-minute restoration of the circulating blood volume.

If the active treatment is to be effective, it must precede the development of the clinical manifestations just described. It must anticipate the complicated interplay of the various agencies whose combined effects culminate in failure of the circulation. Measures to prevent shock should be taken when a steadily increasing pulse rate, together with a rise in systolic pressure and a drop in diastolic pressure that increases pulse pressure, is noted. If the rise in the systolic pressure occurs, it may be due to the vasoconstrictor action of a histamine-like substance that is released by body tissues in an attempt to maintain a satisfactory pressure, but this in no way increases the blood volume.

The initial treatment should be restoration of the blood volume. This is the most logical and beneficial measure and should be started while the vascular system is still able to benefit by the fluids used. The use of the vasopressor drugs in an attempt to maintain an adequate pressure should be on a temporary basis until adequate replacement of fluid is made. Steroids have proved of value in the treatment of shock. Patients who have not readily responded to the vasopressors alone have reacted very favorably to a combination of vasopressor and steroids.

Because of the type of surgery and the shallow depth of anesthesia required, shock is infrequent during anesthesia for dental procedures. When it does occur, it is likely to be secondary to hypoxia.

Cardiac arrest. Cardiac arrest is one of the most serious of all anesthetic complications. Although this term is widely used, it is not completely accurate since it does not describe in physiological language the complication as it occurs during anesthesia. According to Jacoby and co-workers, the term cardiac arrest has created much confusion and is nothing more than "a statement that death has occurred."* On many occasions respiratory obstruction, traumatic shock, or an overdose of the anesthetic may have resulted in a fatality attributed to cardiac arrest. In such cases cardiac arrest is the result of hypoxia and other pathological conditions, and is not sudden and unexpected, as the term implies. Jacoby further states: "Either the term must be completely discarded, or its use must be limited to those patients for whom no cause of death can be found."* Others feel that the term asystole is more descriptive because it denotes a sudden, unexplained failure of the heart to initiate a stimulus.

Cardiac arrest, or asystole, may occur under varying circumstances and during local, as well as general, anesthesia. Most authorities, however, agree that hypoxia, to some degree, is an underlying factor. It is my opinion that while other causes such as vagovagal reflexes, overdose of premedication, and lack of premedication (insufficient atropine) may contribute, it is the accompanying hypoxia that triggers the mechanism. While fulfilling the requirements for a Master of Science degree and with the help and guidance of Dr. Adolphus Koenig, cardiologist at the Presbyterian and Woman's Hospitals, Pittsburgh, I observed electrocardiographic tracings of patients during intubation and stimulation. Cardiac arrhythmias were demonstrated in practically all patients when the intubation or stimulation was accompanied by some degree of hypoxia. The intubation or stimulation did not produce demonstrable arrhythmias in well-oxygenated patients. This is particularly applicable to anesthesia for dental or oral surgery because other harmful reflexes (traction reflex and so forth) are not present in these particular patients. Also, since dental surgery is always elective, poor-risk patients need not be subjected to the additional hazard of general anesthesia.

However, because of their academic interest, the causative factors are listed: (1) underlying cardiac or cardiopulmonary disease, (2)

---

*Jacoby, F., and others: Safety in surgery, Anesth. Analg. **34**:346, 1955.

overdose of premedication, (3) insufficient premedication, (4) decreased vital capacity, (5) improper position, (6) high fever with increased metabolic rate, (7) undue anxiety and apprehension, (8) harmful reflexes (vagovagal, painful stimulation in light anesthesia, and so forth), (9) direct effect of anesthetic agents, (10) increased carbon dioxide retention, (11) shock, and (12) respiratory obstruction.

In addition to respiratory obstruction, other, previously listed causative factors may in themselves induce a degree of hypoxia.

Cardiac arrest, or asystole, must be recognized immediately, and this can be accomplished only when the person administering the anesthetic is well trained and has no other duties. The dentist operating within the oral cavity and engrossed with other duties will undoubtedly lose valuable time before he realizes that cardiac arrest has occurred. The most important factor, however, is that a well-trained anesthetist who closely observes the patient can take definite steps to prevent this calamity.

Once there is a possibility that cardiac arrest has occurred, there are things to do and things not to do. According to Hosler, the following things should not be done:

1. Do not listen for faint heart sounds. If there is no palpable pulse and no measurable blood pressure and if respiration has ceased, the surgeon can be certain that any slight movement of the heart is of no consequence.
2. Do not wait for an electrocardiogram.
3. Do not inject epinephrine through the chest wall into the heart.
4. Do not dilate the rectal sphincter.
5. Do not give a blood transfusion.
6. Do not undertake to administer artificial respiration by compression of the thoracic cage.*

Following is an outline of the procedures to be executed by the anesthetist and surgeon and the necessary drugs and equipment should cardiac arrest occur.

Cardiac resuscitation: program of action†

Anesthetist

1. *Notify surgeon immediately* when pulse and blood pressure disappear.
2. *Do not waste time.*
3. *Deliver 100% oxygen immediately*—breathing bag and mask.
4. *Ask surgeon* to check pulses. Palpation of the aorta, heart, carotid, or other major artery to palpable pulse excludes ventricular fibrillation or cardiac standstill.

---

*From Hosler, R. M.: A manual on cardiac resuscitation, ed. 2, Springfield, Ill., 1958, Charles C Thomas, Publisher.

†From the outline prepared by the Los Angeles County Heart Association as modified after the program of the Cleveland Area Heart Society.

5. *Endotracheal intubation.* When feasible, tracheobronchial aspiration.
6. *Keep time* from onset. Notify surgeon when 3 minutes have elapsed.
7. *Instruct nurse* to get drug tray and sterile instrument package.

Surgeon

1. *Cardiac standstill* (spontaneous function may recur at any step)
   a. *Cardiac compression*—Direct thoracotomy incision, fourth or fifth interspace, compress ventricles 50 to 60 times per minute
   b. *Atropine,* 1/50 grain, in 10 ml. of normal saline solution, in ventricular cavity (if of reflex or vagal origin)
   c. *Calcium chloride,* 2 to 4 ml. of 10% solution, injected directly into ventricular cavity
   d. *Epinephrine,* 0.3 ml. of 1:1,000 diluted in 10 ml. of normal saline, injected directly into right or left ventricular cavity
   e. *Isopropylnorepinephrine,* 0.2 to 0.4 mg. diluted in 10 ml. of normal saline solution, injected directly into ventricular cavity.
2. *Ventricular fibrillation* (spontaneous function may recur at any step)
   a. *Cardiac compression*—Direct thoracotomy incision, 4th or 5th interspace, compress ventricles 50 to 60 times per minute
   b. *Electroshock* directly to heart, 2.5 amperes, 110 volts, for one full second (repeated shock if necessary)
   c. *Procaine hydrochloride,* 5 or 10 ml. of 1% solution injected directly into right or left ventricular cavity
   d. If asystole occurs after defibrillation or procaine, epinephrine, 0.3 ml. of 1:1000 diluted in 10 ml. of normal saline, may be necessary, injected directly into ventricular cavity.

Oxygen is the fuel of the heart

3. Trendelenburg position, 5 to 10 degrees
4. Electrocardiogram for definite diagnosis if available—but do not wait
5. Cautious use of pressor drugs, intravenous fluids, and blood after restoration of heartbeat
6. Close observation in the operating room

Cardiac compression must continue throughout the entire procedure. (The above program must be executed with the precision of a fire drill.)

Drug tray

1. Epinephrine, 0.3 ml. of 1:1000
2. Isopropylnorepinephrine, 0.2 mg., only if it is not available in 0.4 mg. (Isuprel, Aleudrine, Norisodrine)
3. Calcium chloride, 10% solution
4. Atropine, 1/50 grain
5. Procaine HCl, 1% solution
6. Normal saline, 100 ml.

Sterile instrument package

1. Electrical defibrillator apparatus
2. Rib spreader (1)
3. Hemostats (3)
4. Medicine glasses (1 oz.) (4)
5. Scalpel with blade
6. Scissors (1)
7. Forceps (2)
8. Syringes, 10 ml. (4)
9. Sponges
10. Hypodermic needles, 18 × 1½ (2), 22 × 1½ (4)

The cardiac resuscitation program of action as outlined by the Los Angeles County Heart Association was and still is an exceptionally good plan. However, since the introduction and acceptance of external cardiac compression for the treatment of cardiac arrest, this method is by far the method of choice for the treatment of cardiac arrest in the office.

As soon as it is determined that cardiac resuscitation is necessary, the heel of one hand should be held over the lower half of the sternum and the heel of the second hand should be placed on top of the first hand (Fig. 15-4). The hands should then be pressed forcefully downward on the sternum about once every second. The pressure should be sufficient to produce a carotid or femoral pulse.

If the sternal cardiac compression is to be successful, the patient should be on a surface that is sufficiently firm to permit the sternal pressure to compress the heart between the sternum and the vertebral column when downward force is applied on the chest, and the legs should be slightly elevated to aid in venous return. Also, it is assumed that whenever a general anesthetic is given, a capable individual who will continue to ventilate the lungs with oxygen during the closed chest compression is administering the anesthetic.

No attempt should be made to intubate a patient unless intubation can be accomplished rapidly without loss of time. The lungs should be inflated with oxygen once for every five compressions of the chest. Care should be taken to make certain that the ventilations are timed between the fifth and sixth compressions, the tenth and eleventh, and

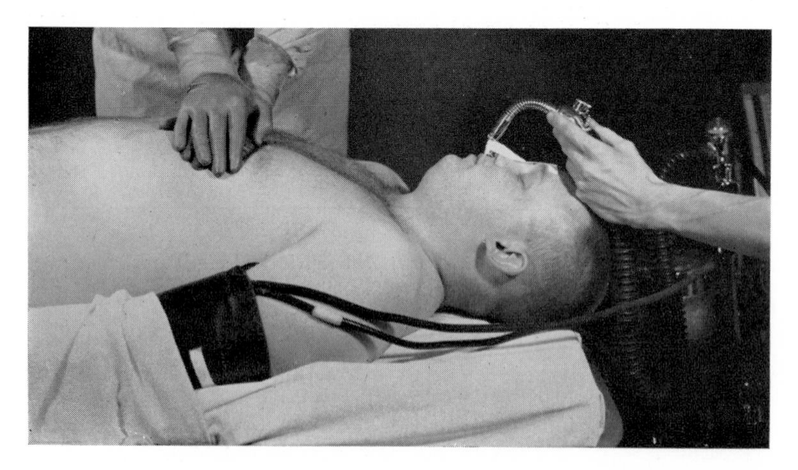

Fig. 15-4. Position of hands for closed chest compression.

so forth, so that the chest is not being compressed as an attempt is being made to inflate the lungs. The carotid pulse should be felt for at intervals to determine the status of the circulation.

If, after 1 to 2 minutes of external cardiac compression, a spontaneous pulse is not felt, epinephrine 1 mg. (1 ml. of 1:1,000) should be given intravenously. The intravenous needle should be kept in place, and intravenous fluids should be started. If the pulse does not return after 4 or 5 mintues, 3 to 4 Gm. of sodium bicarbonate should be given intravenously to combat existing acidosis.

Ventricular fibrillation should be suspected if, after proper resuscitative procedures plus epinephrine and sodium bicarbonate, a spontaneous pulse is not felt. With cardiopulmonary resuscitative procedures continuing, the patient should be moved to a hospital where an ECG can be obtained and the heart can be defibrillated if necessary (Fig. 15-5).

The resuscitative procedures should be continued until the patient's pulse and respirations return. If they do not return, the operator should discontinue only on the advice of a knowledgeable physician. If the pulse and respirations return, the patient should be moved to a hospital for medical monitoring and care.

Cardiac arrest or asystole during anesthesia for dental or oral surgical procedures is a rare occurrence, for the following reasons:

1. Only light planes of anesthesia are required.

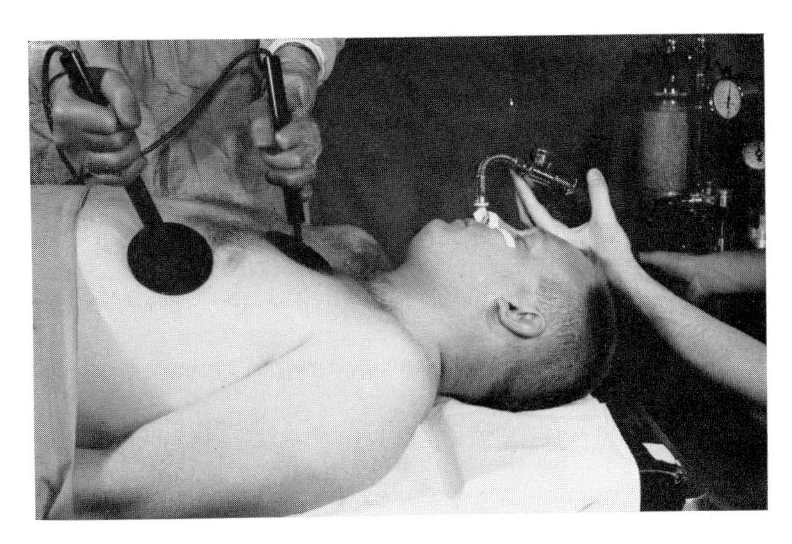

Fig. 15-5. External defibrillation.

2. All procedures are elective, and the patient is usually properly prepared.
3. Preanesthetic evaluation should be completed and techniques altered (chemanesia plus analgesia) to increase the safety factor for poor-risk patients.
4. The vast majority of procedures are of comparatively short duration.
5. The procedures can be terminated at any time.
6. Harmful reflexes are not usually initiated.

COMPLICATIONS OF THE CENTRAL NERVOUS SYSTEM

Practically all complications of the central nervous system occur as a result of hypoxia or anoxia and are usually secondary to respiratory or circulatory complications.

The most common complications of the central nervous system are delayed or prolonged recovery, cerebral cortical damage, convulsions, and emergent delirium.

Delayed or prolonged recovery. Delayed or prolonged recovery from anesthesia for dental procedures is infrequent but by no means rare. Many patients respond to painful stimuli but fail to regain complete control of cerebral faculties until much later. In some patients this may be due to a retarded breakdown and elimination of the anesthetic, with resultant prolonged cortical depression. However, it is possible that an episode of hypotension or hypoxia may greatly prolong the recovery time.

Cerebrocortical damage. The occurrence of cerebrocortical damage during anesthesia has been a much discussed complication. Courville considered it at length, with particular reference to nitrous oxide and accompanying hypoxia. There is no doubt that the cerebral cortex is highly susceptible to hypoxia, and what may seem to be a minor hypoxic episode can have grave consequences. Personality changes, deterioration of mental ability, headaches, and so forth have resulted from hypoxia during anesthesia. It is possible that the hypoxia may not be of the hypoxic type, which results from low concentration of oxygen. Stagnant, histotoxic, anemic, or metabolic hypoxia may be the underlying cause.

Cerebral edema may occur secondarily to hypoxia. Thus, the edema may persist even after the preliminary hypoxia has been corrected. The persisting edema may seriously interfere with cerebrocortical circulation and function. Serum albumin administered intravenously will aid in alleviating the edema since the solution is markedly hypertonic and thus will cause the edematous fluid to diffuse from the cerebral tissues into the vascular bed.

It should be kept in mind that cerebrocortical damage has occurred as a result of a fat embolus or cerebral degeneration coincidental with, but not necessarily attributed to, the anesthetic. However, it behooves anyone administering a general anesthetic to maintain as normal a physiological state as possible and thus eliminate any degree of cerebrocortical damage that might be remotely attributed to the anesthetic.

Convulsions. The incidence of convulsions during anesthesia does not seem to be so great as it once was. Undoubtedly this is due to a more thorough understanding of the causes and means of prevention. In my experience, convulsions have occurred in children during induction with the semiopen drop method when ether, Vinethene, or ethyl chloride was used. Hypoxia, even though slight, and carbon dioxide and heat retention were undoubtedly contributing factors.

It has been some time since I last saw a convulsion during anesthesia. This may be due to better premedication, more adequate oxygenation, and more efficient elimination of carbon dioxide. Barbiturate induction and better control of elevated temperatures have no doubt played an important part.

Emergent delirium. Emergent delirium occurs most often in healthy young (teen-age) persons. This entity is usually related to the barbiturate anesthetics and occurs during the recovery phase and in the second stage (chemanesia) of anesthesia. In the majority of patients a painful experience is associated with the delirium. As is well known, the barbiturates possess no analgesic properties and therefore are unable to dull the pain of the recent surgery. At the same time, the lingering effects of the anesthetic continue to depress cortical function, with the result that the patient is unable to cope with the pain, and thus the emergent delirium occurs. Narcotics in conservative doses are very helpful in controlling this condition.

COMPLICATIONS OF THE PERIPHERAL NERVOUS SYSTEM

Complications of the peripheral nervous system are usually the result of faulty position or undue pressure over areas where nerves lie close to the surface. The most frequent injuries are those of the branchial plexus and ulnar nerve.

Brachial plexus. With intravenous anesthesia, one arm or the other is often extended on an arm board to expose the antecubital fossa or the dorsum of the hand to facilitate the venipuncture and subsequent administration of the anesthesia. Particularly in anesthesia for dental or oral surgery, the operator or assistant often extends the patient's arm upward for greater convenience. Also, if the patient is being operated on in a dental chair, the chair may be raised without the arm board's being elevated; this permits the arm to hang, which causes hyperextension of the brachial plexus. This may also occur when an operating table is used.

This complication is comparatively rare in procedures of short duration. I have seen only one instance of injury of the brachial plexus, and it occurred after a 3-hour dental procedure. The patient complained of weakness and tingling and was unable to raise the arm completely. Full function returned in about two months.

Ulnar nerve. Complications of the ulnar nerve are usually the result of undue pressure at the elbow, which usually results in the paralysis of the flexor corpi ulnaris, with numbness of the little finger. This complication can be easily prevented by placing a pad beneath the elbow to prevent undue pressure.

GASTROINTESTINAL COMPLICATIONS

The gastrointestinal complications that occur during anesthesia for dental or oral surgery consist principally of vomiting and gastric dilation.

Vomiting. Vomiting occurs most often during the induction phase of anesthesia and before surgical anesthesia has been obtained. It can be a serious complication, for the vomitus may obstruct the airway, creating a severe primary respiratory complication, or the gastric contents may be aspirated, producing a severe secondary complication, as well as a primary one. The resulting hypoxia secondary to obstruction of the airway by vomitus may then lead to complications of the circulatory or nervous system. The primary cause of vomiting is the ingestion of food or water prior to administration of the anesthetic. For this reason, at least 6 hours should elapse after the ingestion of food before an anesthetic is administered.

Since dental and oral surgery must be classified as elective in that it can be done on a prearranged schedule, there is no reason to administer a general anesthetic for such surgery to a patient who has eaten within a 6-hour period. As stated previously, pain can be controlled by analgesics, which will allow the stomach sufficient time to empty. Under no circumstances is the anesthetist or dentist justified in risking the occurrence of a severe complication for expediency or convenience.

If vomiting does occur unexpectedly, the anesthetist should quickly

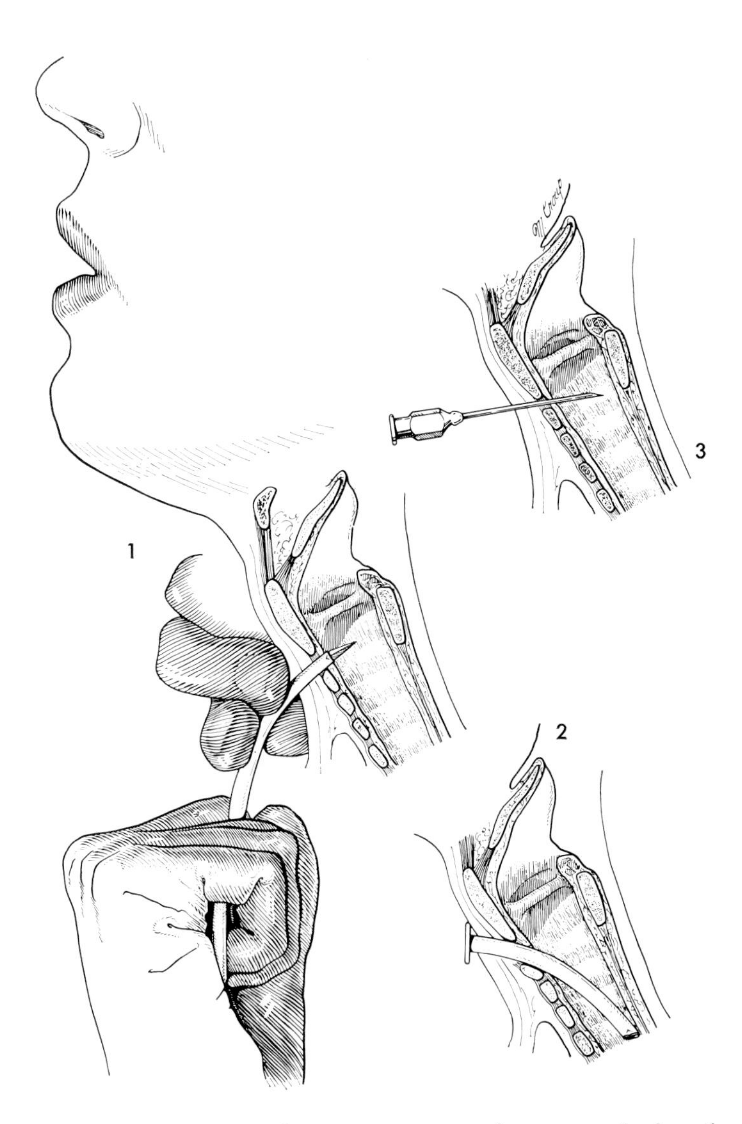

Fig. 15-6. Cricothyrotomy for emergency tracheostomy. **1,** Insertion of cricothyrotomy trocar; **2,** cricothyrotomy tube in place; **3,** 13-gauge needle inserted for minimal emergency airway.

recognize the occurrence of the complication and immediately take steps to correct it. The head should be lowered quickly so that the risk of aspiration is reduced and the postpharynx is efficiently suctioned. The anesthetic should be discontinued, and the patient should be allowed to recover until a cough reflex has returned. After this reflex has been restored and the tracheobronchial tree as well as the pharynx has been cleared, the decision of whether the patient should be reanesthetized is made.

When a full face mask is used, oxygen should not be administered until the pharynx is reasonably clear of vomitus because, if such positive pressure is applied without clearing the pharynx, vomitus may be forced into the tracheobronchial tree, creating a complete obstruction or setting the stage for a secondary lung abscess. If the patient has aspirated any quantity of vomitus, direct tracheal aspiration should be instituted and continued long enough to afford oxygenation. Bronchoscopy and a medical regime are then indicated.

If vomitus in the postpharynx creates a severe occlusion of the air passages in the area of the larynx, and it is felt that the condition cannot be corrected by intratracheal intubation and oxygenation in time to offset rapidly increasing anoxia, tracheotomy is indicated (Fig. 15-6, *1* and *2*). In such a serious emergency, a No. 13 needle should be inserted into the trachea in the midline through the cricothyroid membrane (Fig. 15-6, *3*). Sufficient oxygen can then be administered to sustain life until more positive measures can be taken.

A smooth induction in a well-prepared patient will practically never cause vomiting, but a difficult or stormy induction with bouts of hypoxia may induce small amounts of fluid vomitus in a patient who is apparently adequately prepared. The improper insertion of an oropharyngeal partition in a lightly anesthetized patient may produce gagging and vomiting.

The injudicious preoperative use of narcotics produces nausea and attempted vomiting in about 15% of the patients. Overpremedication with barbiturates may also induce nausea and vomiting in a few patients.

Gastric dilation. Gastric dilation may occur secondarily to augmentation or controlled respiration, particularly if muscle relaxants are used. It is therefore important that the respirations be augmented or controlled with calculated pressures in order not to force air into the stomach and create acute dilation.

It is also advisable to use the intratracheal method of administration if the muscle relaxants are used and the respirations are depressed to a degree that constantly requires augmentation. By this means the anesthetist can be certain that the gases are being forced into the tracheobronchial tree and lungs and not into the esophagus and stomach.

METABOLIC COMPLICATIONS

Metabolic complications may produce liver or kidney damage. It is extremely doubtful that a patient with a serious degree of liver or kidney damage would be considered an outpatient. It would be well to use regional analgesia or a combination of regional analgesia and chemanesia for all hospitalized patients with serious liver or kidney damage who require dental procedures.

It must nevertheless be kept in mind that liver or kidney damage may be produced during anesthesia. The primary cause of liver damage during anesthesia is hypoxia superimposed on the administration of anesthetic agents such as chloroform, Vinethene, and ethyl chloride. These agents may cause liver damage when administered over a period of time (10 or 15 minutes), with a minimal degree of hypoxia. Therefore, when these agents are administered for dental procedures, it is mandatory that the anesthesia time be short (15 minutes or less) and that oxygen in excess of metabolic requirements be given. If an excess of oxygen is available for the patient, the possibility of hypoxia in any degree will be eliminated.

Caution should be exercised in handling patients with a fever. The anesthetist should be cognizant of the fact that for every 1° increase in temperature the metabolic rate is increased approximately 7%. He should therefore make certain that the increased metabolic rate is compensated by an increased supply of oxygen.

Kidney damage may be induced during anesthesia when a hypotensive episode is allowed to continue untreated. This should not be a problem for outpatients since the procedures are of comparatively short duration. On the other hand, the blood pressure and pulse of hospitalized patients undergoing longer procedures should be constantly checked and recorded at intervals during the anesthesia so that the possibility that a hypotensive episode may persist untreated can be eliminated.

Kidney damage may occur as the result of reaction to a blood transfusion. This possibility also presents no problem for the dental outpatient. A hospitalized dental patient may on occasion require a transfusion. If so, at least two persons should check and recheck the typing and cross matching of the blood prior to its administration. Also, the first 50 or 75 ml. should be administered slowly and the patient should be observed closely. At the first sign of reaction, the transfusion should be discontinued. If a dental patient needs blood transfusions, every attempt should be made to give the blood before or after surgery with competent medical supervision.

COSMETIC COMPLICATIONS

Cosmetic complications usually result from external trauma or irritation. The most frequent ones are chipped or loosened teeth, cuts or bruises about the lips, and corneal abrasions or irritation of the eyes.

The word cosmetic has been arbitrarily chosen to classify this group of complications because they usually mar the patient's appearance, temporarily or even permanently. Care should be taken to protect the patient from abrasions or bruises caused by restraining straps and so forth.

Chipped or loosened teeth. This complication usually occurs in the upper anterior teeth and is generally caused by the handle of the laryngoscope during intubation (Fig. 15-7). The anterior teeth should be protected by a thin lead strip (Fig. 15-8) during intubation, and the scope should be used properly—lifting, not prying the mandible and not using the maxillary arch as a fulcrum. In edentulous patients, the maxillary ridge may be bruised or injured by undue prying pres-

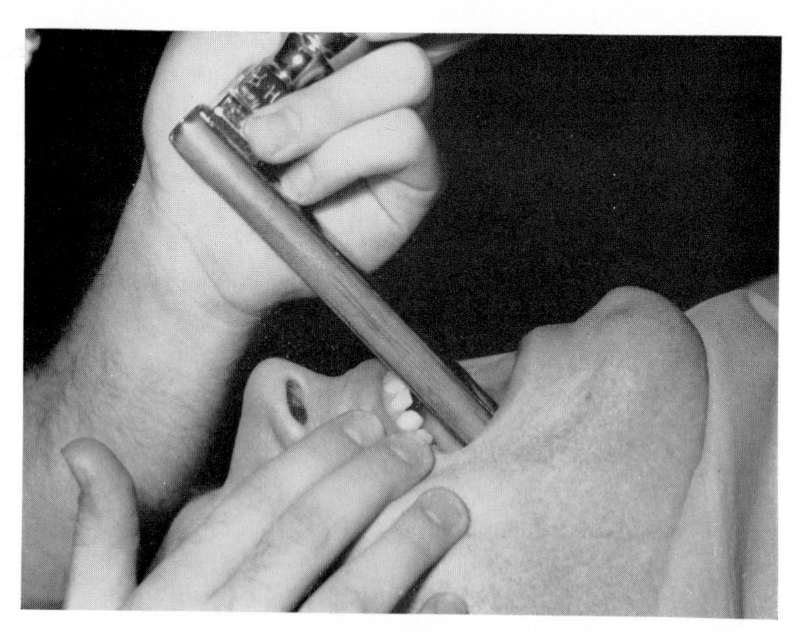

Fig. 15-7. Pressure of laryngoscope against upper anterior teeth.

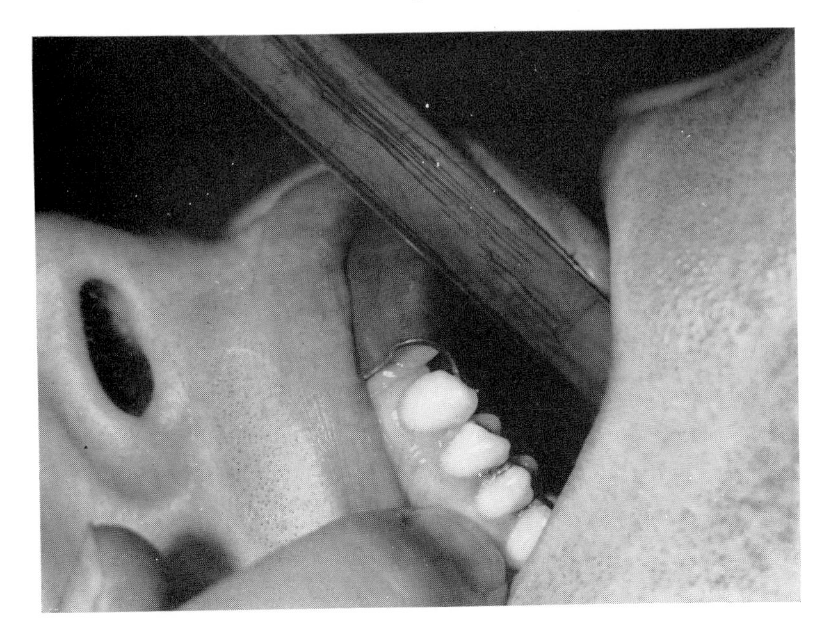

Fig. 15-8. Upper anterior teeth protected by lead strip.

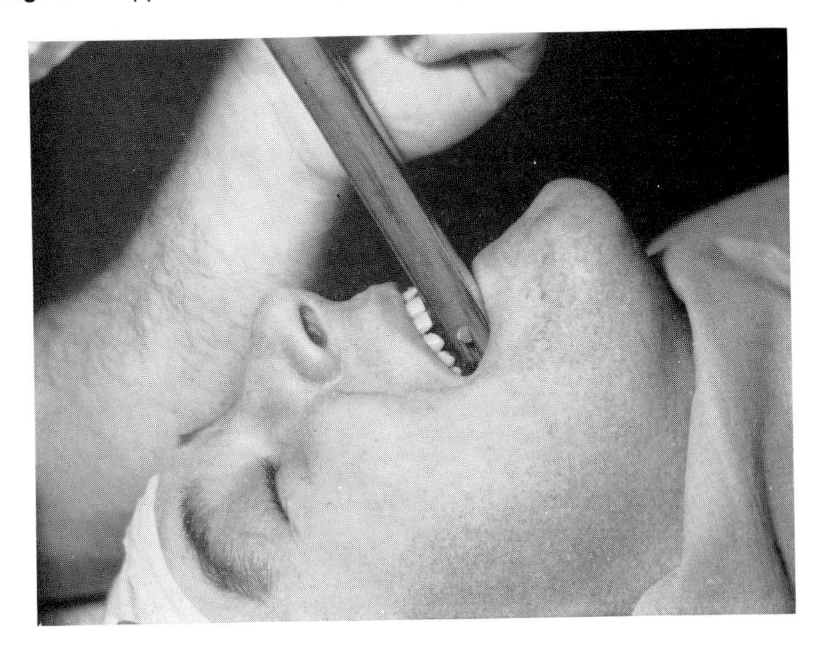

Fig. 15-9. Lower lip traumatized between lower teeth and blade of laryngoscope.

sure. The misuse of mouth props and an attempt to force the jaws apart with excessive pressure may chip, loosen, or dislodge anterior teeth.

Cuts or bruises about the lips. The lips may be severely bruised or cut if they are compressed between the upper or lower anterior teeth and the laryngoscope (Fig. 15-9) or prop. Care should be exercised to make certain that the lips are free and not impinged on by any instrument or instrumentation.

Corneal abrasions or irritation of the eyes. Corneal abrasions or irritation may occur if the eyes are not protected against injury. Eye injuries are not only painful but also can be disabling.

TECHNICAL COMPLICATIONS

Technical complications cover a variety of complications that may directly affect other systems and include a large number of unforeseen situations. However, if the equipment is scrutinized closely and the basic techniques are observed, these complications may be kept at a minimum. Technical complications include epistaxis, complications associated with intubation, complications associated with venipuncture, complications associated with overdistension of the breathing bag, and complications arising from failure of equipment.

Epistaxis. Epistaxis is likely to occur if proper care is not taken when a nasopharyngeal or nasotracheal catheter is inserted. All such catheters should be examined periodically to make certain that there are no rough areas that may irritate or injure the mucous membrane of the nasal passages. All catheters should be well lubricated and of the proper size. No attempt should be made to overcome resistance by force. In addition to nasopharyngeal and nasotracheal airways, suction catheters inserted roughly into the nasal passages, with excessive suction, may produce epistaxis.

Profuse epistaxis into the nasopharynx and laryngopharynx in an anesthetized patient can be an annoying and sometimes serious complication. It will undoubtedly interfere with respiration to varying degrees. When bleeding occurs, the head should be immediately lowered and suction applied. The patient's ozygenation should be closely observed to make certain that pulmonary ventilation is adequate. In extreme conditions it may be necessary to quickly insert a cuffed orotracheal tube to protect the tracheobronchial tree until the bleeding can be controlled. A postnasal plug may be inserted as a temporary control.

In the vast majority of patients, bleeding may not be sufficient to cause a serious complication. However, I have witnessed epistaxis in more than a few patients that caused some anxious moments. Epistaxis can occur when one is inserting a nasopharyngeal airway, as well as with nasotracheal intubation. For this reason, it is considered a separate technical complication.

Complications associated with intubation. A variety of technical complications may occur incidental to intratracheal intubation. If an attempt is made to intubate an unrelaxed patient, the pharynx may be unduly traumatized. Glottal edema, particularly in children, may result from traumatic intubation. Ulcerations of the cords have occurred secondarily to manipulation. It is also possible by exerting undue pressure to penetrate the posterior wall of the trachea and enter the mediastinum and esophagus. A not uncommon complication is due to the insertion of an unmeasured tube into the right main bronchus (Fig. 15-10). Since the right main bronchus is practically an extension of the trachea, as compared to the much more nearly horizontal left main bronchus, a tube that is too long will usually enter

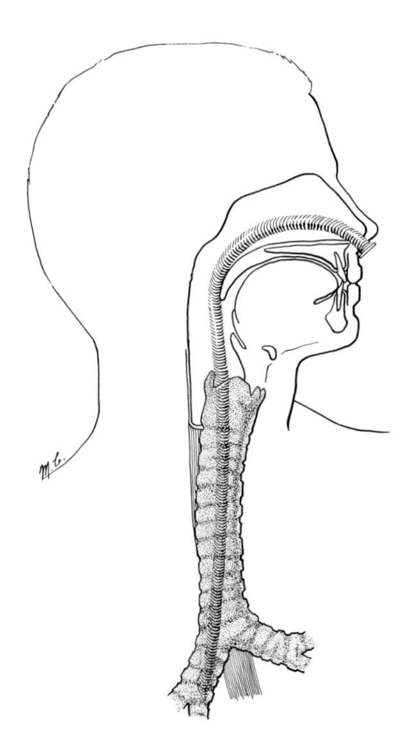

Fig. 15-10. Unmeasured nasotracheal tube extends into the right main bronchus.

the right bronchus, which eliminates the ventilation of the left lung and possibly produces atelectasis.

The inadvertent kinking of an intratracheal tube (Fig. 15-11) is a technical complication that can be readily corrected, but kinking or compression of the tube within the pharynx may occur. To avoid this difficulty, one should use intratracheal tubes of sufficient body to resist kinking or compression. Old tubes that have become soft and easily compressed should be discarded.

An unusual complication that was brought to my attention occurred when a nasotracheal tube penetrated the mucous membrane and entered the pharynx beneath the mucosa. Another unusual complication is rupturing of the inflated cuff, which may injure the trachea. Also, an overinflated cuff may produce ischemia of the tracheal endothelium.

Adapters for intratracheal tubes should be firmly affixed to the tube to minimize the danger of the tube's becoming loosened from the adapter and slipping unattached into the trachea. An adapter that fits loosely into a particular tube should not be used. It is our policy to attach the tubes to the adapter and use the two as a unit until the tube is discarded. The adapter then may be forcibly removed and attached to another tube.

Undoubtedly there are a wide variety of technical complications

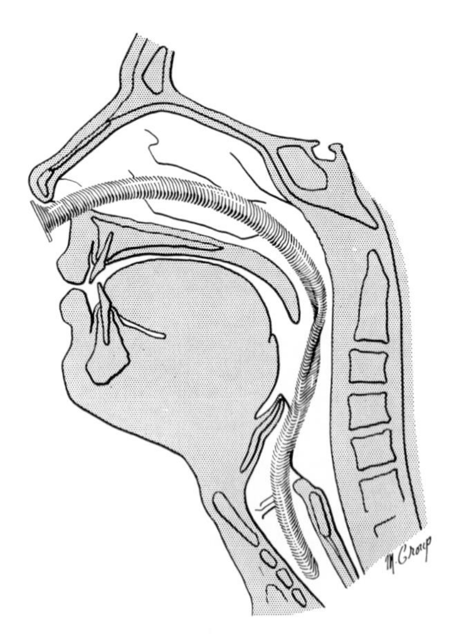

Fig. 15-11. Inadvertent kinking of the intratracheal tube.

that may be associated with intratracheal intubation. To discuss them all would be difficult and time-consuming. It should suffice to state that all necessary precautions should be taken to prevent the occurrence of these annoying difficulties.

Venipuncture. Since venipuncture is an essential part of intravenous anesthesia, the complications secondary to this maneuver should be discussed. These complications will be considered technical difficulties because they are associated with the technique of venipuncture. The most frequent ones are hematoma, tissue extravasation, intra-arterial injection, infection, and thrombosis; in addition, if a plugged needle is used in a venipuncture, distressing complications do arise.

Hematoma. A hematoma may occur as the result of an inept or difficult venipuncture that lacerates the vessel wall and permits blood from the vein to extravasate into the surrounding tissues. It is probably the most frequent complication associated with venipuncture. It may be caused by dull needles that rupture the vessel, the needle penetrating through the vein instead of into it, or by the removal of the needle while the tourniquet is in place.

Once a hematoma has occurred, the tourniquet should be removed, if it is in place, and pressure should be applied at the site of the needle insertion to reduce the internal hemorrhage.

Tissue extravasation. A faulty venipuncture may permit the extravasation of fluid into the tissues. The venipuncture should be checked and the needle stabilized. As a rule the extravasation of small amounts of fluid into the tissues will cause no harm, but larger volumes may become painful or even produce slough. Small amounts of Pentothal or other barbiturates in strong concentration (4% or more) may produce severe irritation or slough.

All venipunctures should be observed closely for the possibility of extravasation. If it does occur, hot moist compresses can be applied. Medical consultation should be sought for extreme conditions.

Intra-arterial injection. An intra-arterial injection of an intravenous anesthetic can be a serious complication. It is not very common, and it may be difficult at times to determine that the needle has penetrated an artery. Serious complications are less likely to occur with dilute solutions and small volumes.

Before a venipuncture is made, the vein should be palpated for the absence of pulsations. Immediately after the puncture has been completed, the color of the blood and the force of its return into the observation tube should be observed. If there is any doubt whatsoever, it is advisable to withdraw the needle and make a second venipuncture in another area.

Because intra-arterial injections, particularly with concentrated solutions (4% or more), may produce serious complications, the best treatment is prevention. If the complication does occur, weak concentrations of procaine should be injected in small volumes, but it is advisable to immediately seek competent medical advice as to the possibility of a sympathetic block.

Infection. Strangely enough, infections following venipunctures are not a frequent complication, and, as a matter of fact, they should not occur if basic fundamentals are adhered to. Only sterile needles (Fig. 15-12) should be used, and care should be exercised that they are not contaminated during preparation for the venipuncture. The puncture site should be thoroughly cleansed and painted with an antiseptic solution. If these basic principles are followed, infections following venipunctures will be uncommon.

The site of venipunctures should be checked during postoperative rounds or when the patient returns for the first postoperative visit if he is ambulatory. Any inflammation in the area is probably due to a low-grade infection. If it appears to be of any consequence, medical consultation should be sought.

Thrombosis. Thrombosis following intravenous anesthesia is comparatively uncommon, and I have witnessed very few such cases dur-

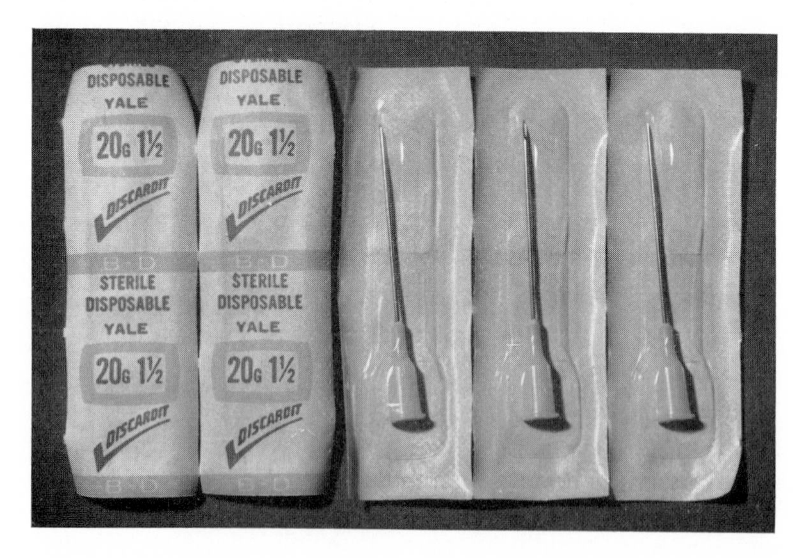

Fig. 15-12. Sterile disposable needles prevent infection that is caused by contaminated needles.

ing the past twenty years. This may be due to the fact that a demonstrable thrombosis may not appear until a week or so after the original venipuncture and injection and therefore may be missed.

If this condition is to be avoided, it is important that the tourniquet not be allowed to remain in position so that it may obstruct venous return, which allows the intravenous agent to remain in the veins. It is equally important that nothing be permitted to interfere with the circulation and venous return.

Plugged needles. The unfortunate condition that results when a plugged needle is used can be listed as a complication of venipuncture. It can be most distressing to complete a venipuncture in a sensi-

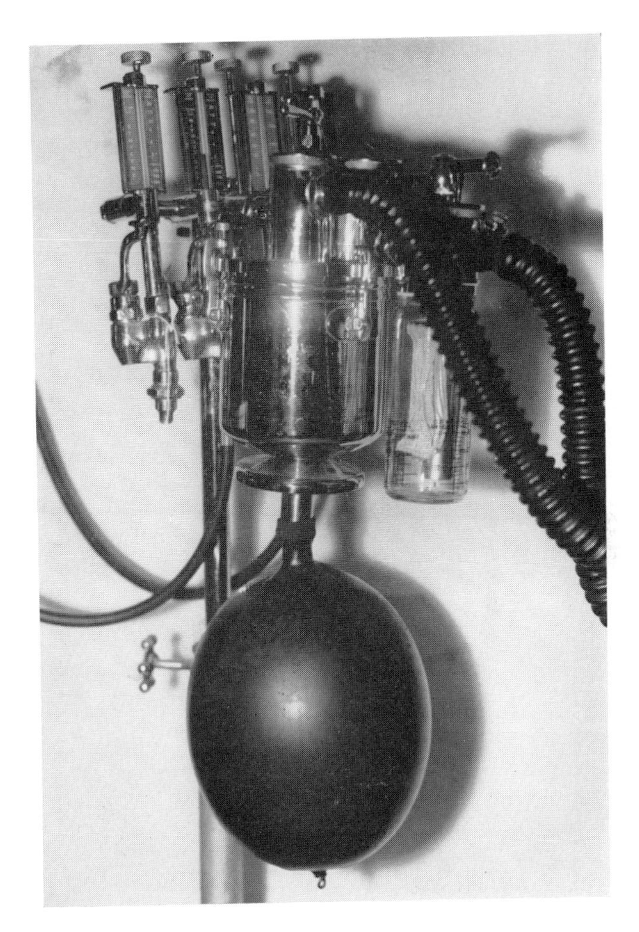

Fig. 15-13. Overdistended breathing bag.

tive patient or to enter a difficult vein and then learn that a plugged needle has been used. The needle must be removed and another venipuncture must be made.

All needles should be checked before use to make certain that they are patent. Also, after an unsuccessful venipuncture, the needle should be rechecked before it is reinserted.

Complications associated with overdistended breathing bag. An overdistended breathing bag (Fig. 15-13) may eventually interfere with both respiration and circulation. If this situation continues over a period of time, the increased pressure may produce pulmonary edema. Also, expirations against the increased pressure may interfere with pulmonary ventilation and permit a buildup of carbon dioxide.

The increased carbon dioxide retention can have a deleterious effect upon cardiac function and circulation. Also, the increased pulmonic pressure may result in compression of the large thoracic veins (vena cava) and the right side of the heart, both of which are thin walled. This compression may interfere with venous return and eventually cardiac output.

Complications resulting from failure of equipment. Many anesthetic complications are the result of faulty equipment. To list all the equipment and discuss each apparatus individually would be

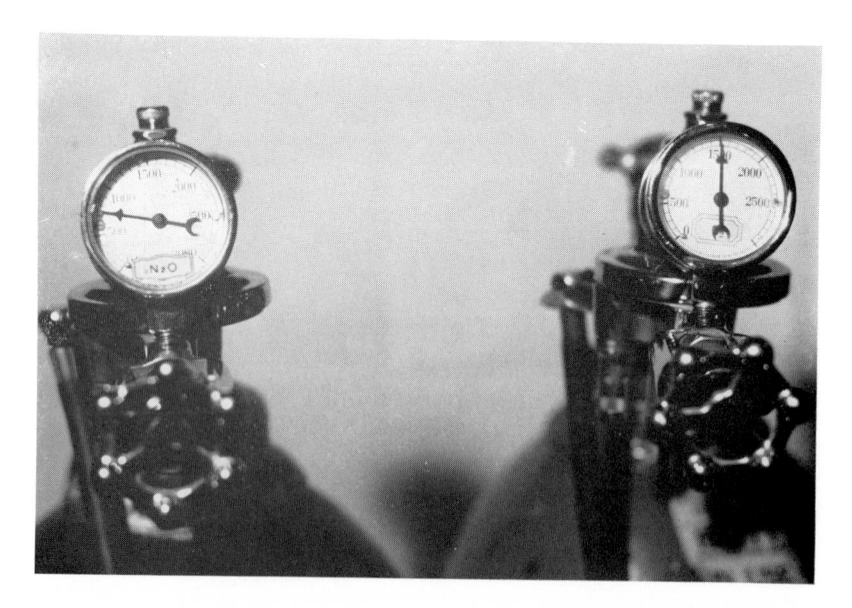

Fig. 15-14. Gauges showing adequate supply of gases for immediate use.

superfluous. It is sufficient to state that all equipment should be thoroughly checked and maintained in near-perfect condition. It is particularly important that all necessary equipment be on hand before induction is begun. To find a necessary piece of equipment missing when it is needed most is a distressing situation and may permit a primary, mild, and transitory complication to become a primary, severe, and perhaps permanent one.

Tanks should be inspected to see that adequate volumes of gases are available (Figs. 15-14 and 15-15). Oil and dust should be kept away from oxygen gauges. The care of cylinders, regulators, breathing bags, and so forth is discussed in Chapter 19.

The treatment and, better still, the prevention of complications are important aspects of anesthesia. However, to discuss every complication that might occur is practically impossible since there is no limit to the different complications that may occur. Nevertheless, any dentist administering dental anesthesia should take every precaution to prevent complications and should be prepared to treat them when

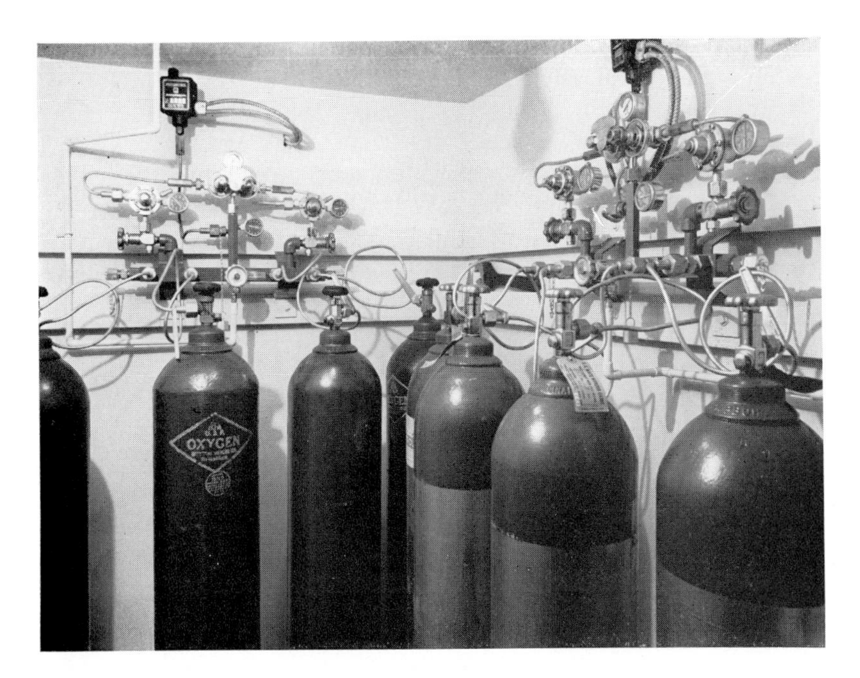

Fig. 15-15. Central gas supply with automatic cut-in measures assures an adequate supply of gases. (Courtesy National Cylinder Gas Division of Chemetron Corporation, Chicago, Ill.)

they do occur. Major complications can be very distressing and minor ones very annoying.

RESUSCITATION

Even though all precautions to prevent complications are taken, an occasional situation may arise in which resuscitation is necessary. Resuscitation is defined as "the restoration of life or consciousness of one apparently dead." It is unfortunate that resuscitation is not fully appreciated until an emergency demands its use. When a sudden need arises, there is no time to seek other professional help or to peruse the literature for necessary information. A responsible person should make certain that all needed equipment is readily available and in good working order. It is advisable for the anesthetist to check the available emergency drugs (Fig. 15-16) frequently and to refresh his memory as to their indicated uses.

Most unsuccessful attempts at resuscitation are due to unnecessary delay in ventilating the patient. Since the majority of emergencies requiring resuscitation are respiratory in origin, the establishment of adequate ventilation will be all that is necessary. It should be remembered, however, that in order for a patient to be ventilated adequately, a patent airway must be established. It will be of no avail

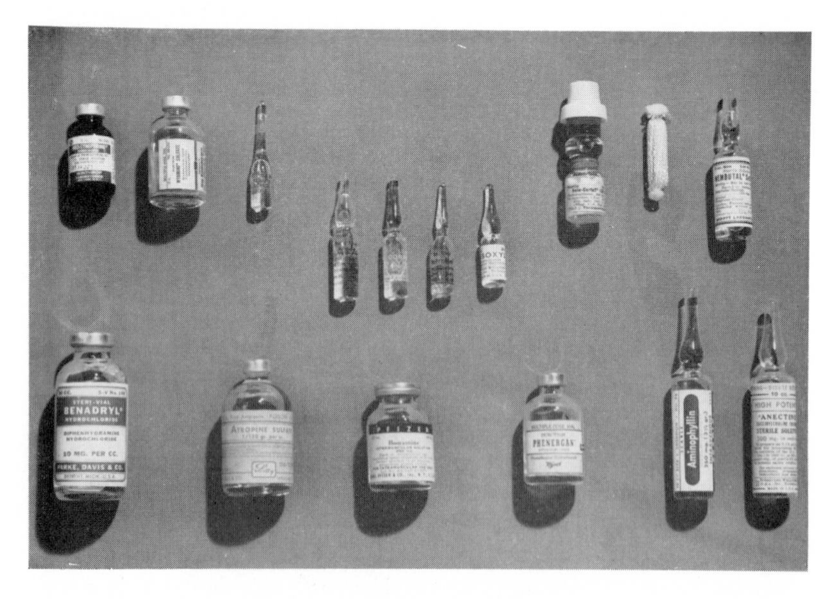

Fig. 15-16. Emergency drugs available for immediate use.

to apply positive-pressure oxygen or a positive-negative resuscitator to a patient whose airway is completely obstructed.

Various respiratory stimulants (analeptics) should not be used in lieu of artificial ventilation. Analeptics may be employed as an adjunct to oxygenation, but not to replace it.

Since the vast majority of emergencies requiring resuscitation are respiratory in origin, they can be managed by adequate oxygenation of the patient, using controlled positive-pressure ventilation. There may be occasions, however, when cardiac or circulatory resuscitation is necessary. There have been case reports of the use of an artificial external electric pacemaker. It will be interesting to observe the future of this apparatus and its possible place in the oral surgeon's office. The procedures to use in case of cardiac arrest are discussed on pp. 275 to 280.

Chapter 16

Anesthesia for dental procedures in the pediatric patient

Joseph H. Marcy, M.D.

Controversy continues to exist among dentists, physicians, and parents as to the necessity and wisdom of general anesthesia for dental procedures for children. Some persons, chiefly physicians, are very strongly opposed to its use except in extraordinary situations. Others advocate its liberal use. The latter argue that the child should not be exposed to fear or pain, that dental anesthesia is minor in contrast to that used in general surgery, and that the risk in recent years has been greatly reduced by newer drugs and techniques.

Both of these extreme points of view fail to come to grips with the issue at hand—weighing the necessity against the risk. It should be remembered that any anesthetic, anywhere, at any time, constitutes an abnormal state and carries with it a tangible risk. No patient —child or adult—should be subjected to that risk without sufficient cause. General anesthesia should be considered only in those situations where it is unlikely or where it has proved impossible that the work at hand can be accomplished with the child awake. General anesthesia should never be used as a substitute for skill or patience.

CRITERIA FOR GENERAL ANESTHESIA

It is difficult to be dogmatic in setting down indications or contraindications for general anesthesia because they will not necessarily be the same for all patients, all dentists, all offices, or all hospitals.

However, the following five points (the five P's) should be considered before general anesthesia is elected:

1. *The patient.* Is there any physical handicap or behavior problem of sufficient magnitude to prevent the child from being cooperative?
2. *The procedure.* Is the work to be done of sufficient magnitude that the child cannot or will not be able to cooperate?
3. *The place.* If general anesthesia is elected, are there satisfactory equipment, emergency drugs, means of resuscitation, and adequate postanesthetic recovery facilities available? If the patient has a medical problem requiring special medical care, can he be safely treated in the office or will he be better off as a hospital patient?
4. *The personnel.* Is the dentist or other person who will administer the anesthetic experienced in treating children and familiar with the peculiarities of pediatric anesthesia?
5. *The preparation.* Has the child been prepared emotionally by the parents to have a general anesthetic? Have an adequate history, a physical examination, and laboratory studies been done? Will the child receive adequate preanesthetic medication?

PREANESTHETIC MANAGEMENT OF PEDIATRIC INPATIENTS

The psychological effect of hospitalization on the child varies considerably from patient to patient. Much depends on the personality and family background of the individual child. It is difficult, then, to know how best to prepare the child for a trip to the hospital. In general, it is best to be frank, to tell him what he may expect, to answer all his questions but without going into too many details. Tricks and deceit to lure the child to the hospital should be avoided.

Once admitted, most children adjust remarkably quickly to hospital routine. The tears of separation from parents are quickly dried when the child sees other children in the same circumstances.

Experience has shown that children who are placed in wards in close association with other children do far better, require less sedation, and undergo induction of anesthesia more calmly then those who come from private rooms where they tend to be isolated from other children. This should be explained to the parents, since many mothers, in their anxiety to provide the best care for their children, will opt for a private room over the apparently less desirable ward accommodations. If the parent insists on a private room, it should be one that permits the mother to stay with the child.

Ideally, children should be admitted to the hospital 24 hours before operation so that the child has time to adjust to his new surroundings. This practice also provides a period in which upper respiratory or other infections not noticed before admission may become manifest. Furthermore it allows sufficient time for a complete history, physical examination, and the necessary routine laboratory work.

Any abnormal findings in the work-up should be evaluated before anesthesia is undertaken. Temperature elevations of over 100° F. or hemoglobin values of less than 10 grams are generally sufficient cause to postpone elective procedures. There seems to be little risk, however, in proceeding with anesthesia for a child who has mild nasal discharge but no fever or other signs of upper respiratory infection.

Restriction of food and fluids

It is important for the safe conduct of anesthesia in children that the stomach be empty at the time of induction of anesthesia. It is equally important, however, that children not be allowed to go for excessively long periods without food or, more important, fluids. Solid food, *including milk and fruit juices,* should be withheld 6 to 8 hours preoperatively, but clear fluids such as water, soft drinks, and the like should be encouraged to within 3 or 4 hours of the time of operation.

It is sometimes difficult or impossible to impress the child (and occasionally his parents) with the importance of abstaining from solid food before anesthesia. One must emphasize *nothing at all by mouth,* because food and candy not eaten as part of a regular meal sometimes are not considered "eating" by some lay people. The parent may allow the child to eat fruit or candy "just to tide him over" the period of enforced fasting. Children may also hide candy or chewing gum among their personal effects, to be consumed when no one is looking. Therefore, every child's mouth should be inspected before anesthesia is induced.

Patients with certain medical problems require special preparation that may require several days or more. It is essential that the physician be notified and the child admitted to the hospital sufficiently far in advance for such preparation to be carried out.

A history of congenital heart disease should be carefully evaluated before anesthesia and operation are undertaken. All such patients should be "covered" with antibiotics before and for several days after the dental procedure. Children should receive 600,000 units of both crystalline penicillin and a long-acting penicillin at least 1 hour before surgery. This medication should be followed by 250 mg. of an oral penicillin preparation four times a day for at least 2 days after surgery. Some physicians feel that oral penicillin should also be given for at least 2 days before the operation.

Diabetic children must be stabilized by way of diet and insulin dosage and be ketone-free at the time of the operation. It is essential that the child receive adequate insulin and caloric content on the day of operation. This is generally accomplished by using multiple small doses of regular insulin and by starting an infusion of 5% dextrose in water some hours before the operation. The time of day of the operation will have considerable bearing on the details of management. Frequent reductions of urine will be necessary during the immediate preoperative and postoperative periods.

Children who have received steroids within the past two years probably should receive steroid therapy before and during major surgical procedures. This does not seem necessary, however, for very short dental procedures.

PREPARATION OF PEDIATRIC OUTPATIENTS

In principle there is no difference between the preparation for anesthesia of children who are outpatients and that of hospitalized patients. However, the degree of medical work-up will depend to a large extent on the type of procedure done in the office and the results of a careful history and physical inspection.

Even if the anesthesia is limited to the minimal case, the work-up must consist of at least a detailed medical history and physical inspection and a hemoglobin determination. The history should particularly seek out past or present respiratory or cardiac disease as manifested by cough, nasal discharge, shortness of breath, limitation of exercise tolerance, cyanosis, clubbed fingers, murmurs, and the like. Previous illnesses, any history of allergy or drug sensitivity, significant drug therapy, abnormal development, unusual weight gain or loss—all should be carefully noted. Any positive findings, including an elevation of temperature above 100° F. or a hemoglobin value below 10 grams, should be reported to a physician for evaluation before anesthesia is undertaken.

Any dental procedure, other than a minimal one, for which anesthesia is administered on an outpatient basis, should be preceded by a physical examination by a physician. Except in special circumstances, a procedure that is more than minimal is more safely carried out in the hospital than in the office, particularly if the patient has, in addition, a medical problem.

The restrictions on intake of food and fluids are the same for outpatients as described above for inpatients, but it is even more difficult to control the ingestion of food when the patient is not in the hospital environment.

PREANESTHETIC MEDICATION

Preanesthetic medication plays a much greater role in anesthesia for children than in that for adults. The following are some of the reasons why this is so:

1. The child needs and is entitled to sufficient sedation to avoid fear and anxiety.
2. Because of the nature of the procedure and the type of general anesthesia used, preanesthetic medication is often an important part of the anesthetic. The success of many pediatric anesthetic techniques for children presupposes moderately heavy sedation.
3. Children tend to salivate more than do adults; it is important to control these secretions in order to be able to maintain a patent airway.
4. Heart action as reflected in pulse and blood pressure is relatively labile in children and is readily affected by drugs and reflex stimuli. Halothane, succinylcholine, and cyclopropane exert significant vagal effects, with resultant bradycardia and hypotension. These effects may be minimized or completely prevented with adequate doses of belladonna derivatives.

It is important, therefore, that premedication not be treated perfunctorily and that one be familiar with the commonly used drugs, their actions, their doses, and their dangers.

Drugs

The belladonna derivatives. For the reasons just mentioned, the child who is about to have major anesthesia should receive atropine, scopolamine, or similar drugs before anesthesia. There is no contraindication to the use of scopolamine for children; in fact, in most situations it is preferable to atropine because of its better drying effect and because it tends to produce amnesia. In an occasional patient scopolamine may lead to some disorientation and confusion. For this reason it probably should not be used for outpatients. Either drug may cause tachycardia, flushing of the skin, anhidrosis, and hyperpyrexia in excessive doses. Doses are given in Table 16-1.

The barbiturates. Secobarbital (Seconal), pentobarbital (Nembutal), and other similar short-acting barbiturates are widely used for children. By varying the dose almost any effect from slight quiescence through drowsiness to light sleep may be achieved with little danger

Table 16-1. Dosage schedule for scopolamine and atropine

Age	*Scopolamine*	*Atropine*
2-5 years	0.15 mg. (1/400 grain)	0.2 mg. (1/300 grain)
6-10 years	0.2 mg. (1/300 grain)	0.3 mg. (1/200 grain)
11 years	0.3 mg. (1/200 grain)	0.4 mg. (1/150 grain)

of depression of respiration or circulation. Barbiturates, however, do not have much analgesic effect and hence will not protect the child from the environment. External stimuli such as noise and pain tend to counteract the effect of the drug or to cause excitement and irrational behavior. Barbiturates are therefore frequently used in conjunction with narcotics.

Within reasonable limits, children tolerate barbiturates exceedingly well, and the size of the dose is not too critical. The average pediatric dose for secobarbital or pentobarbital may be estimated at 1 to 2 mg. per pound of body weight. Double this amount should be used when the rectal route is used. The barbiturates are available in capsules, as an elixir, in glycerine suppositories, and as a solution for intravenous or intramuscular use. Parenteral injection is the most effective method; the oral route is less effective. The rectal route is slow and unpredictable and should be avoided when possible.

The narcotics. The place of opiates in preanesthetic medication is controversial. It is pointed out that the primary function of an opiate is to relieve pain and that the usual preoperative patient is not in pain. Another objection, and a valid one, is that the opiates depress respiration and circulation. A third factor that might seem to militate against their use for children is that in doses that will not impair adequate ventilation they appear to have little sedative effect, although considerable analgesia may be achieved.

In spite of these objections, this group of drugs fulfills a useful place in the medication of children, particularly if more than minimal sedation is required. Their chief value is in conjunction with other drugs. For example, better sedation with less risk of hypoventilation may be achieved by using a small amount of narcotic, together with a barbiturate or similar drug, than can be achieved with relatively larger doses of either one alone. Such a scheme using morphine, secobarbital, and scopolamine is given in Table 16-2. The textbook dose of morphine (for pain) is given as 0.1 mg. per pound of body weight. For premedication of children, this dose must be reduced by about one half for use with other drugs (Table 16-2). Meperidine (Demerol)

Table 16-2. Suggested preoperative sedation

	Atropine or scopolamine		*Secobarbital pentobarbital*	*Morphine OR Meperidine*		*Chlorpromazine*
Outpatient, minimal	See Table 16-1		2 mg./kg. (1 mg./lb.) (by mouth)			
Outpatient, heavy	See Table 16-1		2 mg./kg. (1 mg./lb.) (i. m.)	0.1 mg./kg. (0.05 mg./lb.) (i. m.)	1 mg./kg. (0.5 mg./lb.) (i. m.)	
	N.B. Child will remain drowsy for several hours.					
Inpatient, minimal		See Table 16-1	2 mg./kg. (1 mg./lb.) (i. m.)			
Inpatient, moderate		See Table 16-1	2 mg./kg. (1 mg./lb.) (i. m.)	0.1 mg./kg. (0.05 mg./lb.) (i. m.)	1 mg./kg. (0.5 mg./lb.) (i. m.)	
Inpatient, heavy I		See Table 16-1	4 mg./kg. (2 mg./lb.) (i. m.)	0.1 mg./kg. (0.05 mg./lb.) (i. m.)	1 mg./kg. (0.5 mg./lb.) (i. m.)	
Inpatient, heavy II		See Table 16-1	4 mg./kg. (2 mg./lb.) (i. m.)	0.2 mg./kg. (0.1 mg./lb.) (i. m.)	2 mg./kg. (1 mg./lb.) (i. m.)	
Inpatient, maximal		See Table 16-1	4 mg./kg. (2 mg./lb.) (i. m.)	0.2 mg./kg. (0.1 mg./lb.) (i. m.)	2 mg./kg. (1 mg./lb.) (i. m.)	1 mg./kg. (0.5 mg./lb.) (i. m.)

N.B. This combination will provide intense sedation and should be used only with local or minimal general anesthesia.

1. Atropine alone may be given 15 minutes before anesthesia.
2. Barbiturate-narcotic-scopolamine combinations should be given 45 to 60 minutes before anesthesia.
3. Chlorpromazine should be given 60 to 90 minutes before anesthesia.
4. Atropine or scopolamine may be given in the same syringe with the narcotic. Barbiturates must be given separately.

may be used instead of morphine at a dose of 0.75 to 1 mg. per pound of body weight.

These drugs are most frequently given by the intramuscular or subcutaneous route. Intravenous administration may be used, but the dose must be well diluted and injected slowly.

Codeine is of little use for premedication in spite of its known value for pain. Its use should be restricted to this latter purpose.

Other drugs. Chloral hydrate is a safe but relatively mild and slow-acting agent that can be substituted for the barbiturates. The dose is 10 mg. per pound of body weight. Chloral hydrate is available in a relatively palatable orange-flavored syrup for children.

Chlorpromazine (Thorazine) is a useful adjunct to other drugs when more intense sedation is required. It is best administered (0.5 mg. per pound of body weight) intramuscularly ½ to 1 hour before the regular medication is given.

The choice and modification of premedication

The previous section has listed the drugs commonly used for premedication, and a standard dose has been given for each. However, if medication for the child is to be adequate and at the same time safe, one cannot blindly follow a standard formula. The choice of the drug and dose must be adapted to the particular patient and situation. The following are some additional considerations beyond the size, weight, and age of the child.

Status of the patient. A hospital patient who sleeps or remains drowsy for some time after operation does not usually present any problem in care. However, an outpatient in the same state is in a precarious situation unless recovery facilities are available. Outpatients, therefore, should receive only minimal amounts of sedation if they must be discharged immediately following the operation. *No patient should be allowed to walk or even stand unassisted, nor should he be left unattended for a moment if he has received more than the slightest sedation.* The danger of syncope in a patient in the upright position, particularly when narcotics are used, is a real one. Moreover, there is the risk of fracture and other injuries as a result of fainting. stumbling, or falling. This last point may have medicolegal significance.

The physiological makeup of the patient. The apprehensive child will invariably require heavier sedation. It is wise also to observe carefully the apprehensiveness of the parents, because their anxiety is frequently transmitted to the child. Major behavior problems occasionally present a formidable challenge. In most situations, a firm but understanding approach, along with moderately heavy sedation, will provide a manageable patient. In some cases, psychiatric help is indicated before any procedure is undertaken.

Previous anesthetics. Children who have had previous anesthetics generally require larger doses for premedication. It is not clear whether this is wholly a psychological problem or an increased tolerance to the drugs themselves.

The type of anesthetic. When a combination of nitrous oxide and oxygen is to be the basis of general anesthesia, heavy medication will facilitate induction and minimize the need for supplementation with other agents. On the other hand, if the open drop technique is used (for example, with ether or divinyl ether), medication should be light, and opiates should not be used, since no means of assisting ventilation is available.

Miscellaneous factors. Careful inquiry should be made for possible idiosyncrasies or specific allergies to drugs. Depressant drugs and particularly opiates should be used with extreme caution in patients with impaired pulmonary function—e.g., kyphoscoliosis or deformities of the chest.

Timing of medication

In order for any drug to be effective, sufficient time must be allowed for it to reach its full effect. Not all the drugs mentioned reach their peak effect at the same time, nor do they have the same duration of action. The narcotics and barbiturates reach their peak effect after intramuscular injection in 30 to 40 minutes. Atropine, on the other hand, is effective after 15 minutes and has little vagolytic effect after 30 minutes.

Because it is seldom possible or practical to give several drugs at different times, multiple drugs should ideally be given 45 minutes to 1 hour before induction. If atropine has been used, it may be necessary to repeat the dose either intravenously or intramuscularly just before induction or to add it to the succinylcholine injection.

ANESTHETIC AGENTS

Nitrous oxide. The numerous advantages of nitrous oxide, particularly its nonflammability, make it the agent of choice for children as well as adults. The effect of nitrous oxide on the child is much the same as that on the adult. However, because it is a relatively weak anesthetic in safe concentrations and because the child's metabolism is generally higher than the adult's there is greater need for supplementation with other drugs, either as premedication or as additional anesthesia.

In order that nitrous oxide may be used as effectively as possible, the following points in its administration are emphasized:

1. Induction with tight full face mask to exclude ambient air
2. Induction over a sufficient period of time to allow denitrogenation and tissue saturation (3 to 5 minutes)
3. Use of concentrations as close to 80% as possible
4. Use of large flows
5. Assistance of respirations to facilitate oxygenation and uptake of nitrous oxide
6. Rapid transfer at end of induction to nasal inhaler or other maintenance technique

For any but the shortest procedures nitrous oxide–oxygen alone may not be sufficient. It is usually supplemented with other anesthetic agents or with drugs. Trichloroethylene and halothane are the most frequently used anesthetic agents. Ether and divinyl ether may be used, but they introduce an explosion hazard. Barbiturates or narcotics may be given intravenously in combination with nitrous oxide. Any of these intravenously administered drugs should be used with extreme conservatism in children. They should always be given as supplements for nitrous oxide and never as primary agents supplemented by nitrous oxide. The ultrashort-acting barbiturates, Pentothal and Surital, are most frequently used. Nembutal and Seconal may also be used, although the onset of action is slower and the effects more prolonged.

Demerol injected intravenously in small fractional doses makes an excellent supplement to nitrous oxide. Demerol must be well diluted (for example, 5 mg. per milliliter) and injected slowly until the desired effect is achieved. An alternate method is to use a very dilute intravenous drip (100 mg. in 250 ml. of 5% glucose and water). The onset of action is not as rapid, and sufficient time must be allowed for the desired effect to be achieved. Otherwise, there is a danger of overdose, with the possibility of respiratory or circulatory depression. The total dose of Demerol should not exceed 0.5 mg. per pound of body weight.

Succinylcholine or other muscle relaxants, although not anesthetic agents, frequently are used to facilitate anesthesia. As always, a patent airway and means of assisting ventilation are essentials when these drugs are used.

Other agents. Any of the commonly used agents—ether, divinyl ether, cyclopropane, or ethylene—technically may be used for dental procedures. In fact, most of them would be superior to nitrous oxide if the drug were the only consideration. But all these drugs are flammable. The consideration of the safety of the patient and others, together with the medicolegal implications of anesthetic fire or explosion, is sufficient deterrent to the use of flammable agents, regardless of their pharmacological or practical virtues.

TECHNIQUES

There are many approaches to the administration of general anesthesia, and no attempt will be made here to recommend one over another. Only a few points of general importance will be emphasized.

Induction

In general, the child fears the "stick" of the needle more than the application of a face mask. Therefore, inductions are generally accomplished by a mask. If, however, an infusion has already been started, there is no contraindication at any age to a "sleep dose" of an intravenous barbiturate. Some anesthetists are extremely skillful at venipuncture with small needles. When venipuncture can be done, it makes an ideal induction for the child. Ordinarily, however, if an intravenous injection or infusion is to be used, it is best accomplished

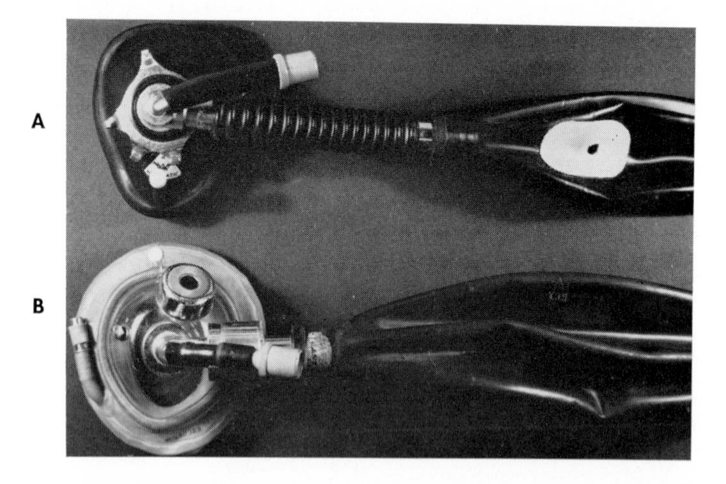

Fig. 16-1. Two types of bag-mask units for induction. **A,** Jackson Rees principle. Gases are introduced at the elbow and exhausted through thumbhole in the bag. Large gas flows are required to prevent rebreathing. Thumbhole is occluded during manual compression of the bag. **B,** Stephen nonrebreathing mask, modified with finger part on exhalation valve to facilitate occlusion during manual compression of the bag.

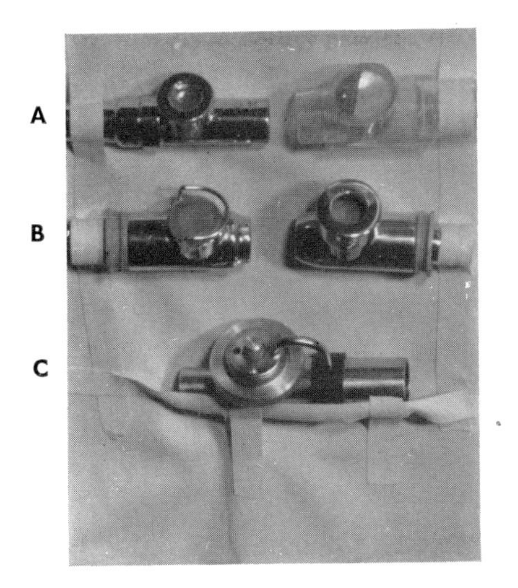

Fig. 16-2. Nonrebreathing valves. **A,** Digby-Leigh valve. **B,** Stephen-Slater valve. **C,** Fink valve. (From Marcy, J. H.: Anesthesia. In Kiesewetter, W. B., editor: Pre and postoperative care in the pediatric surgical patient, Chicago, 1956, Year Book Medical Publishers, Inc.)

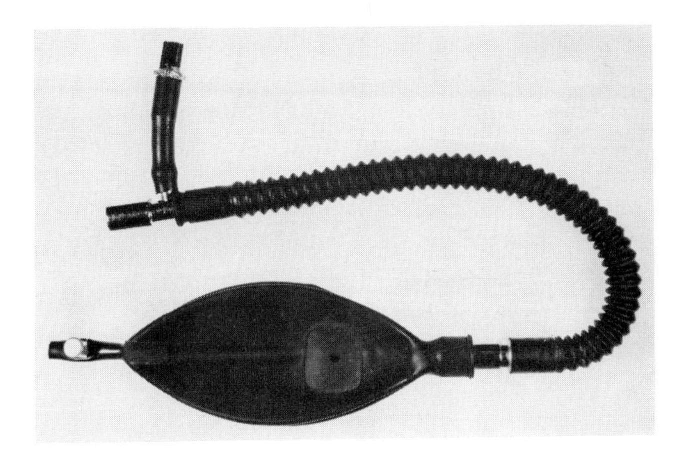

Fig. 16-3. Ayre's T-piece as modified by Jackson Rees with tailpiece and bag. The large gas flow escapes through thumbhole, which is occluded when bag is compressed for assisted ventilation.

after anesthesia has been induced. This reversal of the usual procedure prevents considerable anxiety on the part of the patient and the anesthetist alike.

The anesthetic mask, with high flows of gases running, should be brought into position by holding it low over the chest where the child cannot readily see it, and then slowly fixing it in place, first at the chin and finally tightly over the nose and mouth but only after some degree of anesthesia has been achieved. Once the mask is in place it should be held tightly to prevent leaks and dilution of the anesthetic. It should not be removed, nor should any leak be permitted until induction is completed. The induction should be "pushed" by adding the inhalation agents as rapidly as the larynx will tolerate them and by assisting the ventilation by manual compression of the bag.

Children seldom require the insertion of pharyngeal airways, and their use should be avoided if at all possible. Every effort should be made to maintain the airway by extending the head and supporting the mandible. In the time required to insert the airway, the nitrous oxide mixture may become diluted, and the smoothness of the induction may thus be lost. Furthermore, stimulus of the pharynx by a rigid airway at a light plane of anesthesia frequently induces laryngospasm or vomiting.

Once the induction is completed, the changeover to a nasal inhaler or some form of endotracheal technique is made as quickly as possible to prevent the complications that may occur with a lightening plane of anesthesia.

Maintenance of anesthesia

If the procedure is a very short one, the mask is simply removed and the procedure accomplished. For longer procedures one must decide whether anesthesia can be maintained with a nasal inhaler or whether it must be continued by means of an endotracheal tube.

Endotracheal intubation. The use of endotracheal anesthesia with the assurance of an open airway has undoubtedly widened the scope and increased the safety of general anesthesia in all fields of surgery. This statement is particularly true for children. However, in many situations in operative dentistry, maintenance of anesthesia with a nasal inhaler or a nasopharyngeal airway will be perfectly adequate.

The decision to perform endotracheal intubation depends ultimately upon the particular conditions of each case. Intubation is indicated under the following conditions: (1) if maintenance of the airway may be difficult because of malformations, congenital anomalies, cerebral palsy, etc.; (2) if respiration must be assisted or controlled or if high oxygen concentrations are essential, as in the case of poor-risk patients with heart or lung disease; (3) if it may be difficult to keep blood, pus, or other foreign matter out of the larynx and trachea; and (4) if a long or difficult procedure is anticipated.

Extubation. The larynx of the child is quite irritable. Extreme caution must be exercised, therefore, when the tube is removed. Toilet of the pharynx and larynx should be done before the tube is removed. *The tube should never be removed while the suction catheter is in the endotracheal tube.* Since hypoxia will increase the irritability of the larynx, it is wise to hyperventilate the patient with 100% oxygen while the tube is in place and again after it is removed. This maneuver will prevent laryngospasm in many patients and is well worth the few additional minutes it requires.

Possible complications of intubation and their prevention and treatment. Tracheal intubation for the child is not without risk. The possibility of causing trauma to the teeth and soft tissues is probably greater in the child than in the adult.

Nasal intubation deserves special comment. Children characteristically have a large adenoid bed. The passage of a large endotracheal tube through this bed may cause profuse bleeding, and there is the danger, theoretical at least, of carrying a piece of adenoid tissue into the trachea or bronchus. For this reason, some anesthetists try to avoid nasal intubation in children whenever possible.

The greatest danger in this age group is laryngeal edema. Since the child's larynx is smaller than the adult's in an absolute sense, any degree of mucosal edema results in occlusion of a relatively larger percentage of the cross-sectional area of the airway. Thus the margin of safety is narrower. Two factors are chiefly responsible for the formation of postintubation edema: (1) infection, which may be either already in the respiratory tract or introduced by a tube that is not sterile or at least not scrupulously clean; and (2) trauma, resulting from unskillful instrumentation or the use or attempted use of tubes of improper size.

The means of preventing the complications of intubation are apparent from their description. Elective intubation should be avoided if there is any question of upper respiratory infection. Intubation should be done only when the anesthetist is experienced and skilled in working with children, and it should not be attempted until there is adequate depth of anesthesia to provide good muscular relaxation. The equipment must be of the proper size for the individual child, and if it is not sterile, it must be surgically clean and free from pathogenic bacteria.

In the event that laryngeal edema does occur following extubation, as indicated by a brassy cough, stridor, or suprasternal retraction, the child should immediately be placed in an oxygen tent with maximum humidity. Very light sedation should be used; it should be sufficient to decrease restlessness but not to increase respiratory depression. Careful suctioning of the trachea should be performed as indicated. The use of steroids in the treatment of postintubation edema is still controversial. However, there is a strong clinical impression that they are effective, and in any case their short-term use is apparently harmless. One or two large intravenous doses are recommended (dexamethasone [Decadron], 8 to 12 mg).

The patient with laryngeal edema must be watched extremely carefully by a physician on a minute-to-minute basis until it is certain that edema is subsiding and the airway is patent. Although tracheotomy is necessary only rarely, it may be lifesaving. Preparation for tracheotomy must be made so that valuable time is not lost in the event that it is indicated.

EQUIPMENT

In order to provide suitable anesthesia for children, a considerable amount of equipment is required since the range of body size demands an equally wide range of tubes, laryngoscopes, masks, and the like.

Endotracheal tubes

A wide variety of sizes and types of endotracheal tubes are now commercially available for pediatric use. Present-day high-quality plastic tubes are preferable to rubber; they appear to be less irritating to the mucosa and are less traumatic since they become more malleable when warmed to body temperature.

Tube sizes have now been standardized throughout the industry, but unfortunately, the standard adopted has been the *lumen* rather than the outside diameter. Thus tubes are now labeled in millimeters I.D. (inside diameter). Since wall thickness is not standardized, it is impossible to know the exact external diameter without measuring each tube with a catheter guide. Anesthesiologists usually measure the outside diameter (O.D.) in millimeters or with the "French" scale (1 mm. equals 3 Fr.). Pediatric tubes are available in 0.5 mm. (I.D.) gradations—e.g., 5, 5.5, 6, etc. Although the relation between internal and external diameter is not exact for the reasons mentioned,

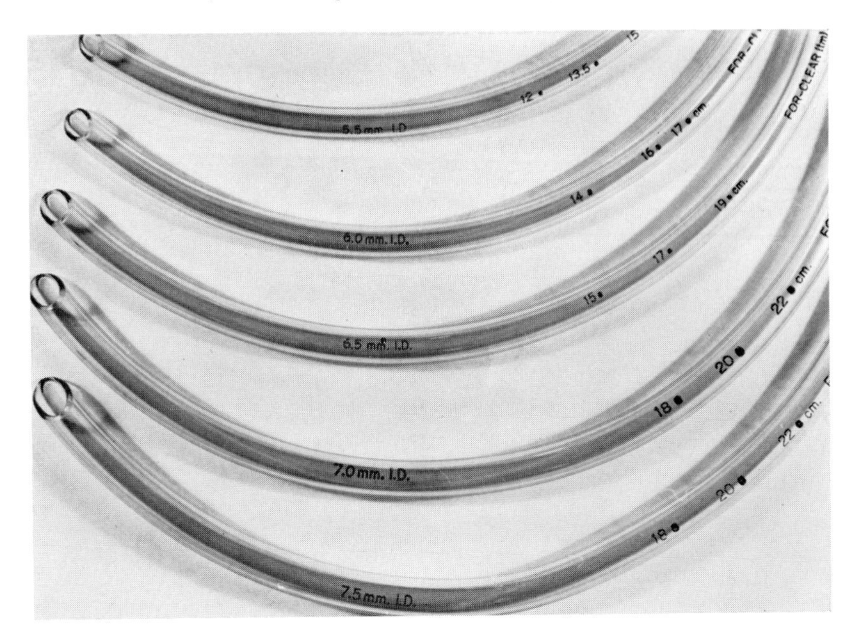

Fig. 16-4. Plastic endotracheal tubes showing markings of *internal diameter* in millimeters. An approximation of French size may be made by multiplying this number by 4.

the inside diameter multiplied by 4 will give the approximate outside "French" diameter. Thus, 5 mm. I.D. equals 20 Fr., 5.5 mm. I.D. equals 22 Fr., 6 mm. I.D. equals 24 Fr., etc.

It is important to use a tube of the proper size, i.e., the largest tube that will just pass the glottis and cricoid ring without forcing. Tubes of several sizes should be available for each patient. Experience is the best guide in selection of size; however, a rough rule of thumb is that the proper "French" size is obtained by adding 20 to the age in years. This rule is fairly reliable from 2 to 12 years of age.

Endotracheal connectors

Connectors and adapters may be curved or straight, with either slip-joint or rubber connections. The connectors should have a lumen as large as that of the tube to which it is connected in order that an added source of resistance to breathing is not introduced.

Laryngoscopes

A great many types and sizes of laryngoscopes are available for children (Fig. 16-5). The ordinary type of blade used for adults if it

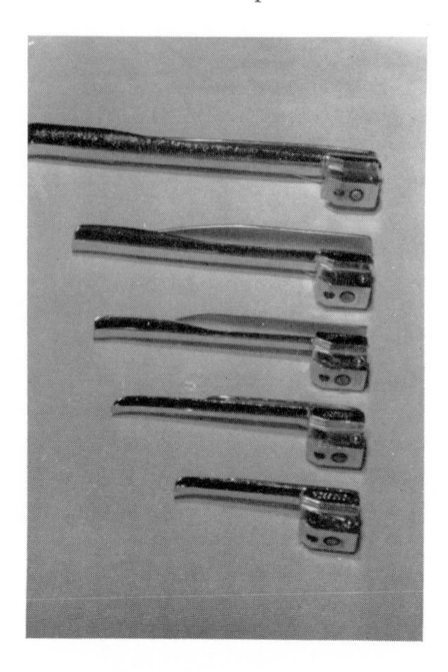

Fig. 16-5. Laryngoscope blades. Reading from top to bottom: Wis-Foregger medium adult No. 3; Flagg child No. 2; Flagg small child No. 1½; Miller infant; Miller premature infant. (From Marcy, J. H.: Anesthesia. In Kiesewetter, W. B., editor: Pre and postoperative care in the pediatric surgical patient, Chicago, 1956, Year Book Medical Publishers, Inc.)

is not too wide, will be satisfactory for children 10 years of age and over. The so-called child-size blades (approximately 10 to 15 cm. long) are suitable for patients under 10 years of age.

Catalogs of the various manufacturers of anesthesia equipment should be consulted for more details on the type of equipment available for children.

Pediatric anesthesia systems

In the past, considerable emphasis has been placed on the importance of specialized breathing devices for children. It has been argued that the standard adult circle apparatus is unsuitable for the pediatric patient because of high resistance, excessive dead space, etc. Recent work has shown that with modern types of circle absorbers, at least, these criticisms are not valid except perhaps in the very young patient. There seems, therefore, to be no contraindication to a standard absorber for children. This is not to imply, however, that there is no place for the usual pediatric "gadgets"—nonrebreathing valves, the Ayre's T-piece or its modifications, or the miniaturized circle absorber of Bloomquist. In fact, most pediatric anesthetists still prefer these devices because they are less cumbersome than the adult equipment. Since dental patients do not include the very young, and since dental procedures generally are not of very great length, the choice of anesthesia apparatus is then of relatively minor importance. Dental anesthesia machines that employ high flows of gas and some sort of nonrebreathing principle are well-suited to use with children.

Chapter 17

Fire and explosion hazards from flammable anesthetics

George J. Thomas, M.D.

Explosions from flammable anesthetics are rare, but because of their dramatic nature they receive widespread publicity. Such accidents occur once in about 150,000 anesthesias. While rare indeed, even one such incident is too many, especially if it could have been prevented.

FACTORS CONDUCIVE TO FIRES AND EXPLOSIONS

Three essential factors are required for the development of fire or explosion: combustible gases or vapors, oxygen, and a source of ignition.

Combustible gases or vapors. In ordinary anesthesia practice, the gases or vapors employed are ethylene, cyclopropane, diethyl ether, and divinyl ether, or a combination of these. We must not exclude the mixtures of nitrous oxide, oxygen, and ether because they, too, are flammable.

Oxygen. Oxygen is essential to all ordinary combustion and for life. In anesthesia, oxygen is supplied in the pure state, dilute in air, or in chemical combination with nitrogen in nitrous oxide.

Ignition source. The explosion of flammable mixtures requires an ignition source. Ignition sources may be small flames, incandescent surfaces, local combustion initiated by catalysts, or electric sparks.

Of the factors mentioned, the first two are essential to practical anesthesia. Factor three, the ignition source, is not essential and should be controlled or eliminated.

Open-flame. Open flames, such as those provided by alcohol lamps, Bunsen burners, matches, and smoking, should be rigidly excluded from rooms in which anesthetics are being administered or stored.

No incandescent or high-frequency *cautery* or *coagulator* must ever be used within 2 feet of the mouth of a patient receiving a flammable anesthetic unless a rubber sheet and wet drapes are properly applied to isolate the surgical field.

Electrical equipment. All electrical equipment should be inspected frequently to detect faulty operation, broken switches and plugs, frayed cords, and open sparks. Unless the equipment is explosion-proof, it should not be used where concentrations of flammable anesthetic gases may be present.

Roentgen ray apparatus. Roentgen ray apparatus is often brought into the room during the administration of an esthetic. Modern shock-proof equipment decreases the hazard of fire and explosion but does eliminate it entirely.

Static electricity. Static electricity is the cause of a high percentage of explosions that occur with the use of flammable anesthetic vapors. It is usually produced on nonconductors, but it can be transferred and retained on insulated conductors. Friction between dissimilar, non-

Table 17-1. Limits of flammability of anesthetics*

Anesthetic agents	*Density of air taken as 1*	*Limits of flammability*					
		In air		*In oxygen*		*In nitrous oxide*	
		Lower	*Upper*	*Lower*	*Upper*	*Lower*	*Upper*
Ethylene	0.97	3.05	28.6	2.90	79.9	1.90	40.2
Propylene	1.45	2.00†	11.1	2.10	52.8	1.45	28.8
Cyclopropane	1.45	2.40	10.3	2.48	60.0	1.60	30.3
Ethyl chloride	2.23	4.00	14.8	4.05	67.2	2.10	32.8
Ether divinyl	2.42	1.70†	27.0†	1.85	85.5	1.40	24.8
Ether diethyl	2.56	1.85†	36.5†	2.10	82.0	1.50	24.2
Nitrous oxide	1.52	Not flammable		Not flammable		Not flammable	
Chloroform	4.12	Not flammable		Not flammable		Not flammable	

*From Jones, G. W., Kennedy, R. E., and Thomas, G. J.: Technical paper 653, United States Bureau of Mines, 1943.

†Tests made in 8 liter, cylindrical, closed steel bomb.

conductive materials produces static charges—for example, the shuffling of feet across a rug on a dry day, running a comb through the hair, rubbing a glass rod with a silk or synthetic fabric, and the separating of woolen garments. Static charges can also accumulate by inductive processes on articles that are near electrically charged objects.

Most materials permit electricity to pass through them, but some are such poor conductors that they are considered insulators. Metals and carbon are good conductors; acids, salt solutions, plants, and animals are poor conductors. Various oils, dry wood, silk, rubber, plastic, glass, and air are considered insulators.

Of all the sources of ignition, static electricity is probably the most difficult to control. There is so much activity in a surgical area that frictional contact with one of the many nonconductive materials present in the room can frequently generate charges. Paths should be provided for electrostatic charges to flow away as fast as they are generated in order to prevent accumulation of static charges. In general, the use of conductive floors and efficient conductive contact thereto is helpful. All movable conductive objects and all personnel should have proper electrical contact with the floor.

On rare occasions, explosions from peroxides have occurred, due to the effect of sunlight on ether. Ether should always be stored in original cans or dark glass bottles. Unless amber glass jars are supplied by the manufacturers, all ether remaining in the anesthesia machine should be removed and properly stored at the end of the day's work.

PRECAUTIONARY MEASURES

Grounding. Grounding as it applies to hazards in the operating room must be understood in a special, limited sense—namely, the interlinking of all sources of static electricity to one large object of great capacitance, such as the building itself. It does not imply that such objects are linked to the earth via water pipes or other low-resistance conductors. The following methods of grounding may be used.

Conductive casters. Hard rubber casters impregnated with acetylene or carbon black have proved to be satisfactory for grounding, provided that they are not covered with a film of powder, lint, dirt, etc. These contaminants insulate the equipment and therefore must be removed.

Grounding chains. Grounding chains are useful for removing static electricity from operating room equipment, but only if the following conditions are observed.

1. Floors must be conductive or have metal dividing strips closely spaced.

2. Chains should make long-line contact with the floor if the floor is conductive or with at least two metal strips if it is not. To ensure greatest benefit, two diagonal chains should be used on each piece of equipment.
3. Chains should be cleaned frequently to remove foreign substances that may accumulate between the links and cause high resistance. For cleaning, use a stiff brush and a greaseless detergent.
4. Chains with open links are preferable to those of the ball, or beaded, type. The latter consists of balls connected by means of loose-fitting, double-headed pins that permit dirt to accumulate on the inside. The dirt raises the resistance of the chain; since the contaminated area is inaccessible for cleaning, the chain loses its property of conductivity.
5. Chains should be of rustproof metal that does not give off abrasive sparks when dragged over concrete or other hard surfaces; No. 45 or 50 bronze or brass chain is recommended for this purpose.

Conductive floors. Floors of rubber, linoleum, porcelain tile, or marble are very poor electrical conductors. Charges neutralize slowly through such floors, and a dangerous spark may occur before neutralization is complete. Satisfactory homogeneous conductive floors of reasonable cost, durability, and good appearance are now available.

Humidity. Good ventilation or air conditioning is desirable for comfort. A fair degree of humidification (not less than 50%) in operating suites also contributes to the electrical conductivity of materials, particularly cotton. However, high relative humidity is not the only solution or the most satisfactory one to the problem of preventing static charges; it is better to eliminate any material that has the property of electrification with static electricity.

EQUIPMENT

Electrical equipment. The electrical wiring in all new constructions should conform to the latest approved regulations of the National Fire Protection Association and the National Electrical Code.

Explosion-proof electrical receptacles and attachment plugs must be used for all cord connectors for line voltage in anesthetizing areas if they are placed within 5 feet of the floor. All electrical circuit devices for line voltage that are not explosion-proof must be limited to regions above the 5-foot level.

Illuminating instruments that are to be brought into the immediate proximity of the patient should operate at 8 volts or less. All receptacles and attachments for low-voltage circuits must not be interchanged with those of higher voltage.

It is very important that all electrical equipment used in the presence of flammable anesthetics have explosion-proof motors and switches. Likewise, variable-speed controls, rheostats, foot-pedal switches, etc. must be explosion-proof.

The use of approved electrical equipment, careful routine inspection, and proper maintenance are prime requisites in eliminating hazards of fire and explosions from flammable anesthetics.

Anesthesia equipment. The following precautions should be taken when anesthesia is being used:

1. Gas machines should be equipped with conductive rubber breathing tubes, masks, and bags.
2. Each end of the conductive rubber breathing tubes should have only conductive connectors.
3. Conductive rubber casters should be used on gas machines in place of the high-resistance type of caster.
4. Caution should be practiced when the connection is altered or changed during the course of anesthesia. It is much safer to move the patient with the gas machine completely disconnected; then, after the proper grounding has been accomplished, reconnect it and continue with the anesthetic.

Operating room equipment. Operating room equipment may be adjudged safe if the following precautions are taken:

1. Mattresses, pads, pillows, and stretcher carriers should be covered with conductive rubber.
2. Operating tables, anesthesia stands, stools, and instrument tables should be equipped with conductive material at the points at which they contact the floor.
3. Wool blankets, plastic sheets, and most of the synthetic fabrics should not be used on patients or equipment in the anesthetizing area.
4. Endoscopic instruments that operate on 6 or 8 volts do not constitute a hazard.

PERSONNEL

1. Uniforms of cotton are preferable; they retain satisfactory conductivity at fairly low humidities and do not produce or acquire electrostatic charges by frictional contact.
2. Shoes with conductive soles are desirable. Persons wearing rubber- or synthetic-soled shoes may be static carriers, regardless of the type of floor used.

The anesthetist can also minimize explosion and fire hazards from static electricity by maintaining contact with the patient and the anesthesia apparatus.

OTHER IMPORTANT POINTS

1. Keep visitors away from the anesthetist and his equipment when he is using a flammable anesthetic agent.
2. Remove paper wrappings before placing gas cylinders in service so that the cylinder label may be clearly visible.
3. Open cylinder valves fully when the cylinder is in use.
4. Keep cylinder valves closed at all times when the cylinder is not in use.
5. Never allow oxygen to enter the regulator suddenly. Open the cylinder valve slowly, keeping the face of the regulator gauge away from the operator and other personnel.
6. Do not use oxygen fittings, valves, regulators, or gauges for any service except oxygen.
7. Never let personnel mix or add gases to any cylinder.
8. Never lubricate any part of the cylinders or fittings, regulators, and gauges with oil or any other combustible material.
9. Do not use defective regulators or cylinders with improperly functioning valves. Permit only properly trained and qualified personnel to make repairs on medical gas equipment.
10. Use block anesthesia, spinal analgesia, or nonvolatile agents rather than flammable gases and vapors whenever the former are suitable. If a patient already anesthetized with a flammable mixture requires electrocauterization in the vicinity of the neck or face, the following procedures are recommended:
    a. Discontinue administration of the flammable agent, turn off the ether and all gases at the machine and cylinders, and move the anesthesia equipment at least 5 feet away from the patient.
    b. Allow the patient to breathe room air for not less than 3 minutes.
    c. Insert a 10 ml. syringe halfway into the oral cavity and take a sample of exhaled gas from the patient (Fig. 17-1).
    d. Without moving the plunger, take the syringe containing the sample of exhaled gas to a nearby room where it is safe to light an alcohol lamp.
    e. After the lamp has been lighted by an assistant, remove the plunger of the syringe and bring the mouth of the barrel into contact with the flame (Fig. 17-2). If any flammable gas is present in the barrel, it will be ignited and a puff of flame will be seen. Electrocauterization should not be attempted

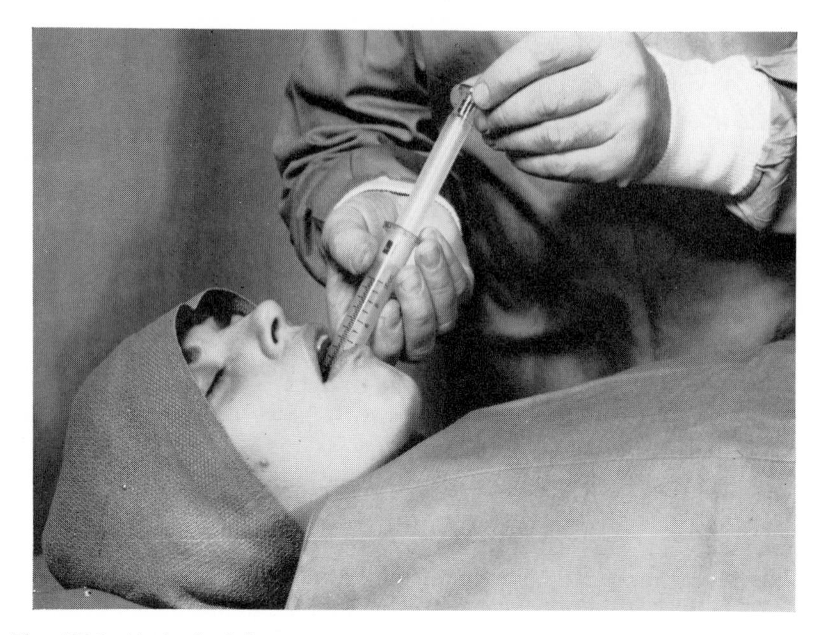

Fig. 17-1. Method of drawing a sample of exhaled gas and air.

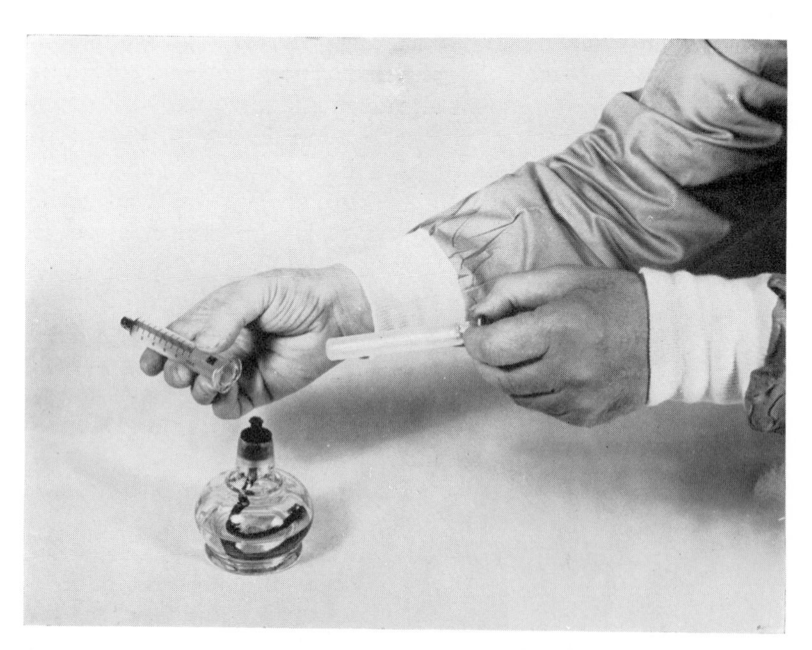

Fig. 17-2. Plunger is removed and mouth of syringe barrel is applied to flame of alcohol lamp.

until a sample of the exhaled gas gives a negative reaction.

11. Use carbon dioxide absorption technique in the administration of inhalation agents. The anesthetist should observe the following routine carefully to avoid causing static charges:
    a. Run water through the mask and breathing tubing and wet the hands immediately before starting inhalation anesthesia.
    b. Bring the mask into contact with the face after it has been connected to the apparatus.
    c. Touch the patient and the gas machine before releasing vapors or gases.
    d. Allow only a nonflammable mixture to flow until all contacts are made.
    e. Use deliberation in all movements. Break and remake connections of the mask with the patient or of parts of the breathing apparatus only when each part is in the anesthetist's hands and when gas is not flowing.
12. Always be on the alert against that silent, unseen hazard, static or frictional electricity. A spark that can scarcely be seen or felt can prove disastrous.

CONCLUSIONS

Some of the fire and explosion hazards with the use of flammable anesthetic agents have been described, and procedures and precautions necessary to provide a safe environment for the employment of these flammable gases and vapors have been discussed. In dental offices today, it is not necessary to use flammable anesthetics; with proper facilities, patients can be given a combination of intravenous barbiturates and nitrous oxide–oxygen anesthesia for almost any type of oral surgery. Should all intravenous barbiturate be contraindicated, the patient may receive a combination of nitrous oxide–oxygen with fluothane or with a less expensive agent, such as trichloroethylene. However, the anesthetist must be well acquainted with these techniques and well trained to meet the various emergencies that may arise during the administration of these valuable but potent agents. Research has done much to define the problems and point the way to a solution, but only the constant vigilance of an experienced and well-informed staff can ensure the safety and well-being of the lives entrusted to our care. Research at the many medical teaching centers continue to find better solutions to these problems. Accidents from fire or explosion can be prevented if the dentist and oral surgeon, as well as the anesthetist, keep well informed of the latest safety procedures.

Chapter 18

Legal aspects of general anesthesia

Neal A. Harper, D.D.S., LL.B., M.S.

Just as fear of pain has long been a factor of disproportionately great influence in the attitude of patients toward dental treatment, there has been a generally unreasonable association of risk and general anesthesia. Statistics do not support this premise. While there are occasional injuries incident to the administration of general anesthetics, death is relatively rare.

> The main factors which determine this risk are the type of anesthesia, the nature of the operation, and the physical condition of the patient. When a suitable form of anesthetic is competently administered; when the operation is not of undue severity or duration; when the operation is performed by a skillful surgeon; and when the preoperative physical condition of the patient is good, the risk to life is minimal. There may be a serious risk to the life of a patient, however, when an unsuitable form of anesthetic is administered; where operative shock is marked; when an operation is unskillfully performed; or when the general condition of the patient is poor before the operation.*

It is well to approach this subject with mention of who may administer general anesthetics. Qualification under the laws of licensure bestows upon the dentist, as well as upon the physician, the privilege of using general anesthetics as an integral part of the practice of his profession.

---

*Gordon, I., Turner, R., and Price, T. W.: Medical jurisprudence, ed. 3, Edinburgh and London, 1953, E. & S. Livingstone, Ltd., p. 510.

> In some jurisdictions the statutes regulate the administration of anesthetics, at least to the extent of limiting the persons by whom they may be administered. . . . One statute permits registered nurses who have qualified themselves by a special course of study of the subject to administer anesthetics under the direction and in the presence of licensed physicians or surgeons. . . . And it has held that a dentist whose right to administer general anesthetics by statute is a surgeon within the meaning of such a statute.*

And it is well settled that "the rules governing the duty and liability of physicians and surgeons in the performance of professional services are applicable to practitioners of the kindred branches of the healing art, such as dentists."†

While the law recognizes the right of the dental licensee to employ general anesthetics, it also holds him to account for competence in their use. The general rule is that he shall use the skill and care prevailing among the dental practitioners of the community. The law not only holds him responsible for this degree of performance but also regards the selection of one who is to administer the anesthetic as of such importance that if the dentist is incompetent to give it himself, he must exercise due care in choosing one capable of doing so, Likewise, the dentist's use of a "less safe method" of anesthetization, rather than other well-known ones that may be more safe in the circumstances, may be held to be actionable negligence. This is true even though the dentist lacks the equipment for using a safer method, and even though in all probability no injury would result from the use of the method he employs.‡ It is important legally that the proper physical equipment be on hand, together with such instruments, resuscitants, and medicaments as the reasonably careful and skillful practitioner of the locality would have available when administering general anesthetics. This armamentarium takes on added significance in dealing with emergencies that may arise.

Consent, express or implied, is always an important part of the relationship of the dentist and his patient, especially with regard to the employment of general anesthesia, not only as to the administration of the anesthetic, but also as to the operations accomplished under its effects. "Generally, a dentist who is instructed by his patient to do certain work only cannot go beyond his instructions and do other

---

*State v. Borah, 51 Ariz. 318, 115 Am. Law Rep. 254.

†21 Rule, Case Law 386.

‡Vigneault v. Dr. Hewson Dental Co., 15 N. E. (2d) 185.

work without first obtaining his patient's consent,"* but "where the patient relies entirely upon the dentist's judgment, the latter is not negligent in performing properly what he considered the right thing to do."† While the dentist anesthetizes and operates at his peril without proper consent, most courts allow leeway in emergency cases. "In one jurisdiction, at least, it has been held that the employment of anesthesia has extended the power and authority of an operating surgeon in this respect, during the period of unconsciousness resulting from the anesthetic, where the patient has not appointed a representative to act for him."‡

Accidents and emergencies occur in the administration of general anesthetics as they do in other activities of dental practice. The law regards them leniently if they are unavoidable, but it assures itself that there are no factors constituting negligence. The yardstick of appraisal generally is that of control. Did the dentist have complete control over the physical conditions from which the accident arose? Was he entirely in command of the situation causing the accident? Was he careless in his responsibility to the patient? The answers to these questions are those the courts determine in arriving at decisions relating to suits wherein a plaintiff patient, or his proper representative, alleges injury due proximately to the negligence of the dentist and a resulting avoidable accident.

A case illustrating the degree of case follows.

A dentist administered nitrous oxide–oxygen for the extraction of three teeth. The patient was strapped to the chair. Despite this precaution and the limitation of movement, the patient, during the excitement stage of anesthesia, clutched the dentist's testicles with a very painful grip, requiring great force to release. After recovery from the anesthetic, the patient complained of pain in the right little finger. The following day an x-ray picture showed a fracture of the second phalanx. In the suit that ensued the court adopted the holding of another court as its decision in this case:

> There was nothing hurtful in the anesthetic administered to the patient, and the fact that he was put under its influence is material only in determining the amount of care which the defendants were called upon to exercise. They knew that the plaintiff, while under the influence of the anesthetic, had no control of his faculties; that they were powerless to act, and that he was unable to exert the slightest effort to protect himself from any of the probable or possible consequences of the opera-

---

*Moscicki v. Shor, 107 Pa. Supreme Court 192.
†69 Am. Law Rep. 1145; 129 Am. Law Rep. 107.
‡26 Am. Law Rep. 1037; 53 Am. Law Rep. 1056.

> tion which they had undertaken to perform. He was in their charge and under their control to such an extent that they were required to exercise the highest professional skill and diligence to avoid every possible danger, for the law imposes duties upon men according to the circumstances in which they are called to act. In this case skill and diligence must be considered as indissolubly associated. The professional man, no matter how skillful, who leaves an essential link wanting or a danger unguarded in the continuous chain of treatment is guilty of negligence, and if the omission results in injury to the patient, the practitioner is answerable.*

The trial court, in another instance, found similarly and under circumstances more difficult, from the dentist's point of view, to reconcile with his responsibilities. Suit was instituted by a patient alleging injuries to her foot sustained through the carelessness of the dentist engaged in the extraction of a tooth. She was anesthetized by inhalation of nitrous oxide gas administered by a trained nurse in the defendant's office. The whole time the plaintiff was in the dentist's chair did not exceed five minutes, and the period of complete unconsciousness, during which the tooth was extracted, did not exceed forty seconds. The plaintiff did not claim that anything was wrong with the administration of the anesthetic or with the operation, only that her foot was injured at that time. She testified that she was in a perfect condition of health before the treatment; that immediately afterward she felt a sharp pain in her left foot, and cried out; that the defendant said, "Your foot is all right. Get up and walk"; that she walked into an adjoining room, where she rested a few minutes on a couch and then left the dentist's office, suffering great pain. During the afternoon duties of her employment the foot was very painful, and on arriving home in the evening she found a bruise about the size of a half dollar on the instep. She called a physician, who treated her. She claimed that she was unable to work at her job as a schoolteacher for six weeks.

The defendant and his assistant testified that nothing happened while the patient was in the chair that could have caused the injury. The plaintiff's attorney argued:

> We do not, I contend, have to go further than to show that this accident happened at that place. It happened in her helpless condition. It was something that would not ordinarily happen in a dentist's chair, and that is all we have to show; it is all we can show and it is all you or anybody else can show under the same circumstances.*

The appellate court, in reversing the judgment and awarding $300 to the plaintiff, gave its opinion in the following language:

---

*Wolfe v. Feldman, 158 Misc. 656, 286 N.Y. Supp. 118.

> Where a dentist gives an anesthetic to his patient for the purpose of extracting a tooth, the dentist is not an insurer against all possible injuries or accidents, and a presumption of negligence on the part of the dentist does not arise from proof of the mere fact that the plaintiff without her fault sustained an injury of unusual character while she was in the care and control of the dentist . . . The doctrine of *res ipsa loquitur* can only be properly invoked where there is some evidence tending to prove that an injury complained of was caused by something under the defendant's control . . . The injury might have been caused by pure accident or by something not at all within the control of the dentist, the cause of the injury being a question of fact and one of the main issues in the case.*

Further, with regard to accidents in which general anesthesia is involved, the following opinion is held generally:

> The risks arising from anesthetics will differ markedly as they are incurred by an individual who is (1) in normal health, except for the accident; (2) in abnormal state of health, or disabled in some manner which interferes with the taking of anesthetics. . . . In actual practice it is sometimes impossible to separate the two risks or to determine accurately, in a fatal case, to what extent the result was due to operation and to what extent to the inhalation of an aneshetic. . . . The risks of anesthesia may be regarded, broadly speaking, as slight. In fact, when it is a question of an operation which is not in itself dangerous from extent, severity, or loss of blood, when the anesthetic is in skilled hands, and when the subject is in average health, it may fairly be said that the risk is negligible. This holds true whatever anesthetic may be chosen. Given, however, chloroform as the selected anesthetic, and an inexperienced administrator to give it, the risk is so greatly increased that no comparison can be made between the two sets of circumstances.†

Even those accidents resulting in the death of the patient may be held unavoidable if it is clearly found that reasonable care, ability, and prudence were demonstrated in the service rendered.

In accidents creating emergencies of a serious nature it is often necessary to proceed with quick and bold treatment to preserve life or health. The courts take the circumstances into consideration when hearing suits alleging injury or death resulting proximately from unauthorized treatment or the dentist's having exceeded the scope of his abilities. They generally view with leniency the lack of consent, particularly if the patient is unconscious and/or time is essential to dealing successfully with the situation. The courts insist that a true emergency be proved, that it was not due to the negligence of the

---

*Dawson v. Allen, 191 Ill. Appellate Court 399.

†Knocker, D.: Accidents in their medicao-legal aspect, London, 1910, Butterworth & Co., Ltd., and Baillière, Tindall & Cox, Ltd., p. 74.

dentist, that due care and skill were employed in dealing with the emergency, that the dentist procured able assistance if indicated, and that he did not abandon the patient. They also hold that even an emergency does not warrant overtreatment, that the services rendered must be those necessary for the immediate physical welfare or life of the patient, that insofar as possible the accepted methods of treatment must be used, and that no experimentation must be tried. All reasonable efforts to meet the emergency will be upheld—revival from fainting, the treatment of shock, heroic measures in complications or impending death from reactions to anesthetics, sudden and serious injury or illness, or other conditions in which prompt action is imperative. Courts may even regard these efforts as a duty owed to the patient, irrespective of results.

Negligence in the administration of general anesthetics, like that pertaining to other kinds of dental service, is a serious dereliction of duty. Negligence is the basis of suits in malpractice. While the dentist is held only to that degree of care and skill obtaining in his locality, the law insists that he meet those standards. The negligence may be due to commission or omission; if injury ensues, there is a legal cause of action. Mistakes in judgment do not establish liability if prudence has been exercised. The dentist is not an ensurer of his diagnosis or of the treatment he provides unless he has been unwise enough to bind himself by contract guaranteeing the success of his services. "The surgeon is charged with the duty of acting on his best bona fide judgment, and is not liable for injuries or death resulting without negligence, from honest errors of judgment."* However, the following has been said:

> [The surgeon] is liable if his mistake of judgment is so gross as to constitute negligence. . . . He may be liable, also, if he fails to observe plain physical laws or physical facts which are governed by ordinary principles of intelligence, and it has been held that if a surgeon persists in the use of an anesthetic after a warning which would impel one of reasonable prudence to desist, he should be answerable for the consequences. . . . It has been held negligence for a surgeon to administer a certain anesthetic without first advising himself by an examination as to the condition of the patient.†

Because of the many kinds of anesthetics, the administration of them is becoming increasingly more of a specialty. If the services of a specialist in anesthesia are procured, he is held at law for the following.

---

*Loudon v. Scott, 58 Mont. 645, 194 P. 488; 12 Am. Law Rep. 1487.

†12 Am. Law Rep. 1494, 1495.

> To bring to the discharge of his professional duties that degree of skill, care and learning ordinarily possessed by specialists of a similar class, having regard to the existing state of knowledge in medicine and surgery, that is, a higher degree of skill, care and learning than that of the average practitioner.*

"Authorities are to be found, however, in which no higher standards of skill and care have been imposed upon specialists than upon general practitioners."†

The general interpretation is expressed well in the language of a court in which the question was one at issue:

> The question whether a physician or surgeon is a specialist, while one of fact, is primarily for his own determination, and if he holds himself out as such, he must bring to his patients that degree of skill which a specialist assumes to possess.‡

As has been noted in the findings of one case, "Specialists in dentistry or any of its branches fall within the general rule."§

Usually the specialist administering the anesthetic is not held liable for any of the operative procedures of the physician or dentist. In a case involving fracture of the jaw and other injury in the course of extracting an impacted tooth, the court held the following:

> Where a physician recommended the extraction of a tooth by a certain dentist and was employed by the patient to administer the anesthetic and watch over her interest, the evidence was held not to raise the issue of joint employment for extraction of the tooth on which to base liability of the physician for negligence of the dentist. . . . Mere recommendation of one doctor by another does not make the latter liable for malpractice of the former. . . . Generally, the physician administering the anesthetic is not liable for negligence of the operating surgeon.‖

Under a statute that establishes that death under general anesthesia is not by natural cause, the following is observed:

> Although other factors are often responsible for a death under anesthesia, the terms of this statutory provision are such that there is a tendency at inquest proceedings to place the entire responsibility for such death upon the anesthetist. Actually, few deaths are due to the administration of anesthetics in operative procedures.¶

---

*41 Am. Juris. 208, sec. 90.

†59 Am. Law Rep. 1074.

‡Coleman v. Wilson, 85 N.J.L. 203.

§Turner v. Sanders, 247 Ky. 90, 56 S.W. (2d) 718.

‖Nelson v. Sandell, 202 Iowa 109, N.W. 440

¶Gordon, I., Turner, R., and Price, T. W.: Medical Jurisprudence, ed. 3, Edinburgh and London, 1953, E. & S. Livingstone, Ltd., chap. 18, pp. 513, 515.

The authorities just quoted, writing with regard to deaths that are the direct result of the administration of general anesthetics, note as causes the explosion and fires that may occur through the ignition by an electric spark of flammable vapor caused by a mixture of air or oxygen with anesthetic gas, that the most dangerous mixtures are cyclopropane-oxygen and ether-oxygen, and that the necessary ignition may come from a faulty electric appliance, x-ray apparatus, or static electricity. They observe further that deaths due to respiratory failure may be due to depression of the respiratory center or to obstruction of the respiratory tract. Legal inquiry takes into consideration the fact that serious anoxia may develop if the anesthetist fails to keep the patient under constant observation. It is also interested in ascertaining whether or not respiratory failure may have been due to overdose of the anesthetic or overpremedication, to the administration of relaxant drugs, such as curare, that may paralyze the intercostal muscles and diaphragm, to functional obstructions, or to acute cardiovascular failure.

The law relies upon evidence for the determination of its findings and decisions. Where the care and skill of the dentist are involved, lay opinion on this question is not admissible. Neither is reputation for care or skill.* And evidence cannot be based on conjecture or speculation.† The testimony of expert witnesses, qualified by their greater training and skill, is the usual means of proof. This testimony is held to be an exception to the rule of direct evidence; the expert may give opinions and conclusions.

Courts, it appears, now often permit cases to go to the jury without expert testimony or allow less of it. In one involving fracture the State Supreme Court of Michigan stated:

> It is claimed lay witnesses were erroneously permitted to testify to the plaintiff's physical condition. One does not have to be an expert to testify to what he sees and knows. There is no rule which can prevent ordinary witnesses from describing what they see, or from testifying concerning the kind of injury or sickness of others whom they have had occasion to consort with, unless it is something out of the common course of general information and experience, or unless the question presented involves medical knowledge beyond that of ordinary unprofessional persons. It would be ridiculous to shut out testimony of what any juryman would understand well enough for all the exigencies of the case before him, simply because no physician had seen or examined the party. It would lead to a denial of justice in all cases of bodily injuries and

*48 Corpus Juris. 1145, sec. 155; 41 Am. Juris. 238, sec. 128.
†Mayer v. Hipke, 183 Wisc. 382, 197 N.W. 333.

sickness which did not occur within range of medical help, and which were not regarded as so difficult of treatment as to demand it.*

Some jurisdictions enforce strictly the expert witness rule. As stated by a Connecticut court: "Ordinarily, where the exercise of proper professional skill or care on the part of a physician, surgeon, dentist, or other similar practitioner is an issue, expert testimony tending to establish want of such skill or care is essential to a recovery."† This legal view is the one usually held.

Evidence may be submitted by a defendant dentist that the plaintiff patient was guilty of contributory negligence, by acts of commission or omission. If sustained, this usually has the effect of defeating the liability of the defendant. However, some states, including New York, Oklahoma, Oregon, Utah, and Wisconsin, hold that contributory negligence does not bar recovery but merely mitigates damages.

Of great importance, too, is the general holding that the doctrine of *res ipsa loquitur,* "the thing speaks for itself," is not applicable to an action against a dentist charged with "causing the death of a patient through use of an anesthetic."‡ In fact, *res ipsa loquitur* generally should have no place in malpractice suits.

"Admission against interest" may be received in evidence. Such statements by the dentist as "I've made a mistake," "That regulator valve went bad again," and so forth, may be used against him with great weight. Presumptions and inferences, on the other hand, ordinarily do not apply to cases of the type discussed. An adverse result creates "no presumption of negligence."§ Nor, as has been pointed out, "can negligence be inferred from the fact alone that the patient died under anesthesia . . . or from the fact that the patient was in an alcoholic condition and that it is dangerous to administer the anesthetic to one in that condition, since there is an element of danger in every instance where a patient is anesthetized."‖ Further, in most states, textbooks cannot be read in the presence of the jury, and cannot be used in the cross-examination of expert witnesses, except when the witness has testified that he bases his opinion on the knowledge acquired from reading such textbooks. The important reason for this is that the author is not under oath and cannot be cross-examined.

The proper keeping of records is essential in the office of the prac-

---

*De Groot v. Winter, 265 Mich. 274, 251 N.W. 425.

†Chubb v. Holmes, 111 Conn. 482.

‡Dolan v. O'Rourke, 56 N.D. 416, 217 N.W. 666.

§Donoho v. Rawleigh, 230 Ky. 11, 18 S.W. (2d) 311.

‖Loudon v. Scott, 58 Mont. 645, 194, P. 488; 12 Am. Law Rep. 1487.

titioner. They should contain the medical history of the patient, x-ray pictures, dates and nature of services rendered, and other pertinent information. While not considered "best evidence" because they could contain self-serving or afterthought entries by the dentist, they are admitted in court to "refresh the memory." They should be simple and understandable to be of the greatest value. If they are neat, accurate, orderly, and concise, they may well mean the difference between success and defeat in the case at court. An eminent authority has stated:

> Juries are disposed to conclude, and perhaps justifiably so, that a doctor who has been slack in his records is very likely to have been slack in other aspects of his conduct of the case. The greatest protection available to the individual doctor against a malpractice suit is the taking and preserving of a complete, written medical case record.*

In conclusion, and for emphasis, it should be repeated that the law recognizes the right of the licensed dentist to administer general anesthetics, holding him liable only for injury or death to his patient through negligence or the lack of care and skill employed by his fellow practitioners in the community. It expects him to receive proper consent before performing his services but is lenient when unconsciousness or other real emergency prevents its being given or refused. It does not hold him liable for unavoidable accidents or treatment or for using any reasonable means to save life or to preserve health in an emergency. It recognizes the specialist and generally holds him to the bestowal of higher-than-average skill in the services he performs for his patients. Evidence that establishes, by preponderance, the proof of facts must form the basis of legal determination of the issues of a case, and the dentist's office records may play an important part in that evidence.

While these rules have general application to all departments and endeavors in dentistry, they apply with special weight to the field of general anesthesia. The very nature of that service, so important to the progress of dentistry, demands thoroughness of training, the employment of care, skill, and prudence commensurate with the risks involved, and the ability to deal with anesthetic emergencies. It is due essentially to the observance of that need for preparation and care that injury or death from the administration of general anesthetics is rare. It is gratifying to realize, however, that in the few cases that occur, the law and the courts that interpret and apply it are as zealous

---

*Regan, L. J.: The doctor and patient and the law, ed. 2, St. Louis, 1949, The C. V. Mosby Co., p. 386.

in the protection of the dentist as in that of his patient. The courts should hold no terror for the dentist or the anesthetist who has followed the rules, professionally, ethically, and legally, to the reasonable best of his ability. In promoting further security in the administration of general anesthetics, the dentist should do all within his power to assist his insurers, in the event of suit, by supplying witnesses and making available the facts, circumstances, records, and other pertinent information.

Chapter 19

Armamentarium

In very few fields is the armamentarium as important as in anesthesia. During the administration of an anesthetic, we depend constantly upon anesthesia machines, gauges, tanks, airways, laryngoscopes, syringes, stopcocks, needles, and so forth. While it is not necessary for the anesthetist to be a mechanical genius, he should at least understand the basic workings and functions of the various devices of his armamentarium.

GAS MACHINES

The gas machine is basically an apparatus for administering inhalation anesthetics (gaseous and volatile) to the patient under controlled conditions. It is composed of storage tanks for compressed gases (oxygen, nitrous oxide, etc.), regulators that reduce the pressure of the gases as they leave the tank or cylinder, flow meters to control the volume of gas administered to the patient, rebreathing bag, vaporizers for administering volatile anesthetics, carbon dioxide absorbers for removing excess carbon dioxide from rebreathed mixtures, breathing tubes for carrying gases to the patient, and full face masks or nasal inhalers to facilitate ventilation of the patient with the gases and vapors. In essence, the gas machine is an artificial atmosphere wherein the anesthetist controls the percentages and volumes of gases that the patient is breathing.

GAS CYLINDERS

Cylinders made of steel are used to transport and store compressed gases. Compressed gases are classified by the Interstate Commerce Commission, and therefore their transportation is regulated by the United States Government. Any gas with a pressure exceeding 25 pounds per square inch at 25° C. is classified as a compressed gas and is subject to these regulations. These specifications require that the steel used in cylinders must meet certain chemical and physical requirements and that cylinders must pass a hydrostatic pressure test.

Because of the tendency of any gas in a closed container to increase in pressure with rising temperature, the possibility always exists that a cylinder charged with gas at a safe pressure at normal temperatures will reach a dangerously high pressure at elevated temperatures. This is equally true whether the contents of the cylinder are in the gaseous or the liquid state. In the latter case, the liquid may expand to such a degree that excess hydrostatic pressure develops within the cylinder.

Table 19-1. Approximate dimensions and contents of cylinders

Cylinder	*Quantity*	*Oxygen*	*Nitrous oxide*	*Ethylene*	*Cyclopropane*
A	gal.	20	50	40	40
(3″ o. d. × 7″)	lb.–oz.	0–3.75	0–12.5	0–6.25	0–9.4
B	gal.	40	100	100	100
(3½″ o. d. × 13″)	lb.–oz.	0–7.25	1–9.0	0–15.75	1–7.5
C	No longer commonly used				
D	gal.	95	250	200	230
(4½″ o. d. × 17″)	lb.–oz.	1–1.0	3–14.5	1–15.5	3–5.5
E	gal.	165	420	330	
(4½″ o. d. × 26″)	lb.–oz.	1–13.25	6–9.0	3–4.0	
F	gal.	550	1280	1100	
(5½″ o. d. × 51″)	lb.–oz.	6–2.0	20–0.0	10–12.0	
M	gal.	800	2000	1640	
(7⅛″ o. d. × 43″)	lb.–oz.	8–14.0	31–4	2800	
G and H	gal.	1400	3200	2800	
(8½″ o. d. × 51″)	lb.–oz.	15–8.5	50–0.0	27–8.0	

To prevent these conditions from occurring with normal usage, the Interstate Commerce Commission has drawn up regulations that limit the amount of gas that may be charged into a cylinder.

The Interstate Commerce Commission prescribes definite markings for each type of cylinder, and these markings must not be changed except as specifically provided in the regulations of the Interstate Commerce Commission.

A color code to aid in the identification of medical gas cylinders has been adopted by the Medical Gas Industry, The American Society of Anesthesiologists, and the American Hospital Association. These colors are as follows:

Oxygen	Green
Carbon dioxide	Gray
Nitrous oxide	Light blue
Cyclopropane	Orange
Helium	Brown
Ethylene	Red
Carbon dioxide and oxygen	Gray and green
Helium and oxygen	Brown and green

Medical gases are supplied in standard cylinders (Fig. 19-1) designated by the letters A, B, D, E, F, G, H, M, and HH. All medical gases are not supplied in each cylinder size, but are limited to the most advantageous quantity. Table 19-1 shows the approximate dimensions and contents of the cylinders.

G and H cylinders are identical in size and contents. The type of valve denotes the difference. The G cylinder has a flat type of outlet face and requires a washer. The H cylinder has a ground connection and requires no washer. The HH cylinder is a manifold type of cylinder containing 300 cubic feet, as compared to 244 cubic feet for the G and H cylinders.

Recommended safe practices for handling and using medical gases. Following are recommended safety procedures for the handling and use of medical gases:

1. Never permit oil, grease, or other readily combustible substance to come in contact with cylinders, valves, regulators, gauges, hoses and fittings. Oil and certain gases such as oxygen or nitrous oxide may combine with explosive violence.
2. Never lubricate valves, regulators, gauges or fittings with oil or any other combustible substance.
3. Do not handle cylinders or apparatus with oily hands or gloves.
4. Prevent sparks or flame from any source from coming in contact with cylinders and equipment.
5. Never interchange regulators or other appliances used with one gas with similar equipment intended for use with other gases.

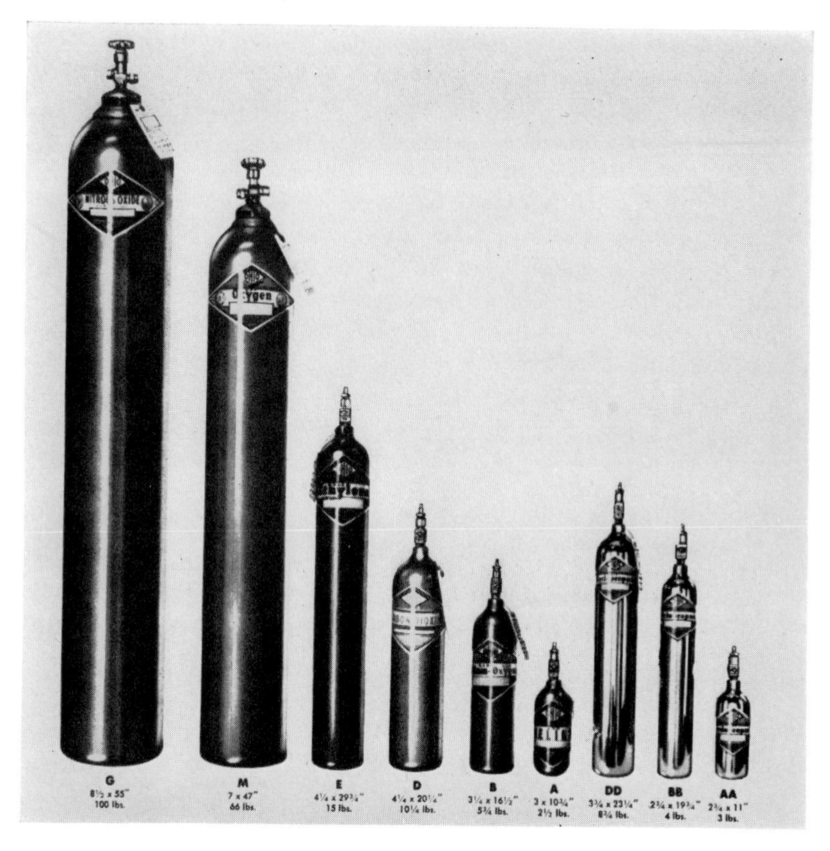

Fig. 19-1. Standard cylinders. Approximate dimensions and weight of empty cylinders, including valve. (Courtesy Ohio Chemical & Surgical Equipment Co., Madison, Wis.)

6. Fully open the cylinder valve when the cylinder is in use.
7. Never attempt to mix gases in cylinders. (Mixtures should be obtained already prepared, from recognized suppliers.)
8. Before placing cylinders in service any paper wrappings should be removed so that the cylinder label is clearly visible.
9. Do not deface or remove any markings which are used for identification of contents of cylinder. This applies to labels, decals, tags, stenciled marks, and upper half of shipping tag. Cylinders should not be refilled using label of previous filling.
10. No part of any cylinder containing a compressed gas should ever be subjected to a temperature above 125° F. A direct flame should never be permitted to come in contact with any part of a compressed gas cylinder.

11. Never tamper with the safety devices in valves or cylinders.
12. Never attempt to repair or to alter cylinders.
13. Never use cylinders for any purpose other than to contain gas.
14. Cylinder valves should be closed at all times except when gas is actually being used.
15. Notify supplier of cylinder if any condition has occurred which might permit any foreign substance to enter cylinder or valve, giving details and cylinder number.
16. Cylinders should be repainted only by the supplier.

Moving cylinders

1. Where caps are provided for valve protection, such caps should be kept on cylinders when cylinders are moved.
2. Never drop cylinders nor permit them to strike each other violently.
3. Avoid dragging or sliding cylinders. It is safer to move large cylinders even short distances by using a suitable truck, making sure that the cylinder retaining chain or strap is fastened in place.

Storing cylinders

1. Cylinders should be stored in a definitely assigned location.
2. Full and empty cylinders should be stored separately, with the storage layout so planned that cylinders comprising old stock can be removed first with a minimum of handling of other cylinders.
3. Storage rooms should be dry, cool and well ventilated. Where practical, storage rooms should be fireproof. Storage in subsurface locations should be avoided. Storage conditions should comply with local and state regulations.
4. Cylinders should be protected against excessive rise of temperature. Do not store cylinders near radiators or other sources of radiant heat. Do not store cylinders near highly flammable substances such as oil, gasoline, waste, etc. Keep sparks and flame away from cylinders.
5. Do not store reserve stocks of cylinders containing flammable gases in the same room with those containing oxygen or nitrous oxide. (It is good practice to include cylinders containing carbon dioxide in the storage room with those containing flammable gases, since carbon dioxide gas is in itself a fire extinguisher.)
6. Large cylinders should be placed against a wall to offer some protection against being knocked over. They should not be placed along an aisle used for trucking traffic. The best practice is to provide means for a chain fastening of large cylinders to the wall.
7. Cylinders may be stored in the open but in such cases should be protected against extremes of weather and from the ground beneath to prevent rusting. During winter, cylinders stored in the open should be protected against accumulations of ice or snow. In summer, cylinders stored in the open should be screened against continuous direct rays of sun.
8. Cylinders should not be exposed to continuous dampness and should not be stored near corrosive chemicals or fumes. Rusting will damage the cylinders and may cause the valve protection caps to stick.
9. Never store cylinders where oil, grease or other readily combustible

substance may come in contact with them. Oil and certain gases such as oxygen or nitrous oxide may combine with explosive violence.
10. Cylinders should be protected against tampering by unauthorized individuals.
11. Valves should be kept closed on empty cylinders at all times.

Withdrawing cylinder contents

1. Never attempt to use contents of a cylinder without a suitable pressure regulating device. Pressure regulators are preferred for reducing pressure from cylinders. If needle valves are used, particular attention shall be given to preventing excessive pressure from building up beyond the needle valve.
2. After removing valve protection cap, slightly open valve an instant to clear opening of possible dust and dirt.
3. When opening valve, point the outlet away from you. Never use wrenches or tools except those provided or approved by the gas supplier. Never hammer the valve wheel in attempting to open or to close the valve.
4. Regulators, pressure gages and manifolds provided for use with a particular gas or group of gases must not be used with cylinders containing other gases.
5. It is important to make sure that the threads or regulators or other auxiliary equipment are the same as those on cylinder valve outlets. Never force connections that do not fit.
6. Never permit gas to enter the regulating device suddenly. Open the cylinder valve slowly.
7. Before regulating device is removed from a cylinder, close the cylinder valve and release all pressure from the device.
8. Always close valves in empty cylinders*

The Compressed Gas Association strongly urges that smaller tanks not be refilled from larger cylinders and that all cylinders be returned to charging plants for refilling.

To eliminate the possibility of wrong gases being used or wrong cylinders being inadvertently substituted for correct cylinders, the Compressed Gas Association, in cooperation with the American Society of Anesthesiologists and the American Hospital Association, has devised a Pin-index safety system (Fig. 19-2). This system is based on the matching of pins with holes and is aimed at the prevention of the erroneous interchange of medical gas cylinders equipped with flush valves. There is only one combination of pins and holes for each gas. Unless the right cylinder valve is connected, the holes and pins will not match, and the two parts will not fit together. The Pin-index safety system does not replace any of the means of identification now

---

*From Safe handling of compressed gases, a pamphlet prepared by the Compressed Gas Association.

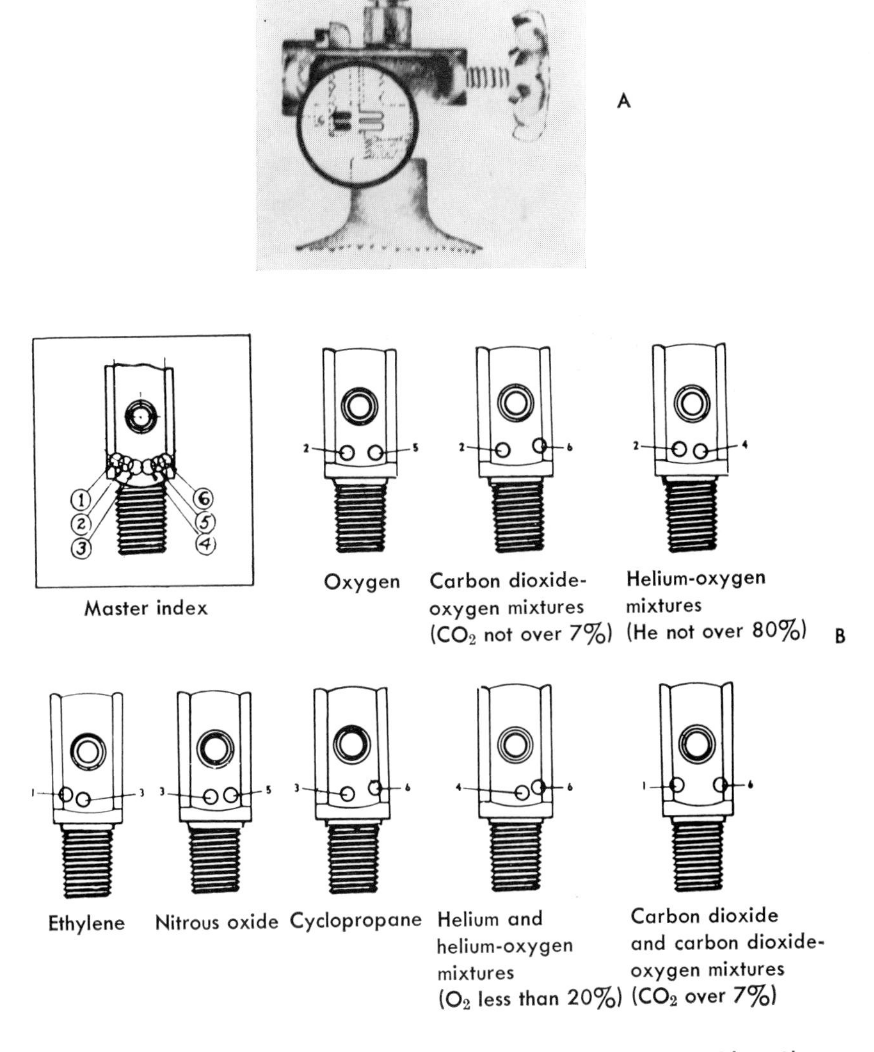

Fig. 19-2. Pin-index safety system for gas cylinders. (Courtesy Ohio Chemical & Surgical Equipment Co., Madison, Wis.)

in use for medical gases, such as labels and markings. It provides an additional and positive safeguard.

Regulators

The purpose of the regulator is to reduce the pressure of the gas as it leaves the cylinder to a safe, usable pressure, which is usually 60 pounds of pressure. The reduction of cylinder pressure to a safe working pressure can be accomplished in one or two stages. The one-stage regulator will reduce the pressure from the high pressure within the cylinder to 60 pounds in one step. If a two-stage regulator is used, the pressure will be reduced first to an intermediate pressure and then, in the second stage, to a working pressure of 60 pounds. The flow of gases from regulators may usually be adjusted to suit the individual situation. In most cases, gauges are attached to the regulator. One gauge may register the reduced or working pressure, usually in

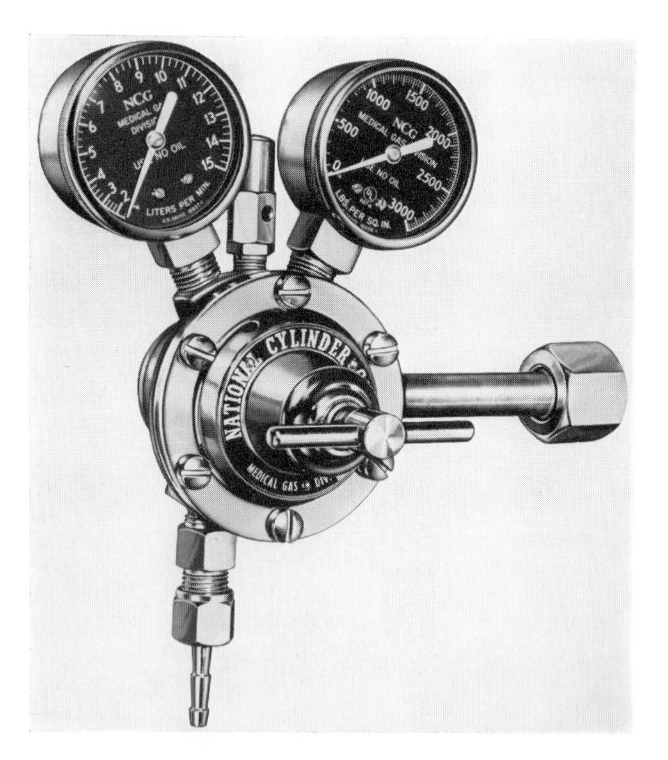

Fig. 19-3. Gauge on right measures pressure of gas in cylinder in pounds per square inch; gauge on left measures flow in liters per minute. (Courtesy National Cylinder Gas Division of Chemetron Corporation, Chicago, Ill.)

pounds per square inch, while the other gauge may measure the pressure of the gas in the cylinder (Fig. 19-3), also in pounds per square inch.

In cylinders containing liquefied compressed gas and vapor in equilibrium, the pressure in the container is determined almost solely by the vapor pressure of the liquid at the existing temperature and bears no relation to the amount of liquid that remains in the cylinder. At a given temperature, the pressure in the cylinder containing a liquefied compressed gas, such as nitrous oxide, cyclopropane, or carbon dioxide, will remain approximately constant until all of the liquid has been withdrawn, at which time the pressure drops in relation to the rate at which the remaining gas is withdrawn. As long as liquid remains in the cylinder, the true contents can be determined only by weight.

In cylinders charged with a nonliquefied compressed gas, the pressure in the container is related to both the temperature and the amount of gas in the container. For such gases as oxygen, ethylene,

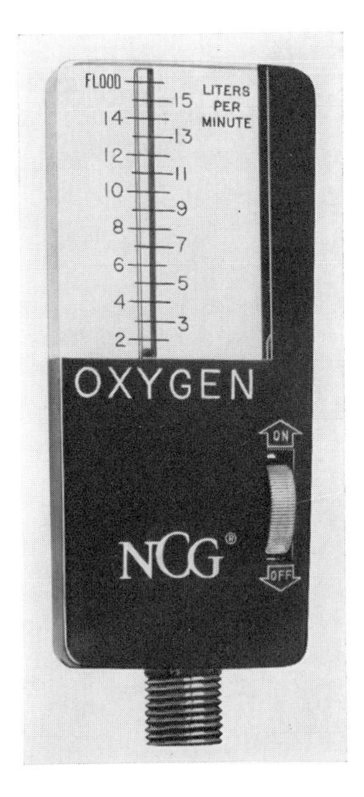

Fig. 19-4. Float type of flow meter. (Courtesy National Cylinder Gas Division of Chemetron Corporation, Chicago, Ill.)

and helium and oxygen mixtures, cylinder content may be determined by pressure; for example, at a given temperature when the pressure is reduced to half the original pressure, the cylinder will be approximately half full.

Flow meters

The flow meter (Figs. 19-4 and 19-5), in contrast to the pressure gauge (Fig. 19-3), records actual flow and not merely pressure, and therefore, when the flow is interrupted, the flow meter will register zero. The operating principle of the flow meter is comparatively simple. A float (ball or rod) of proper weight and accurate diameter is placed so that it will rise and fall within a slightly tapered and

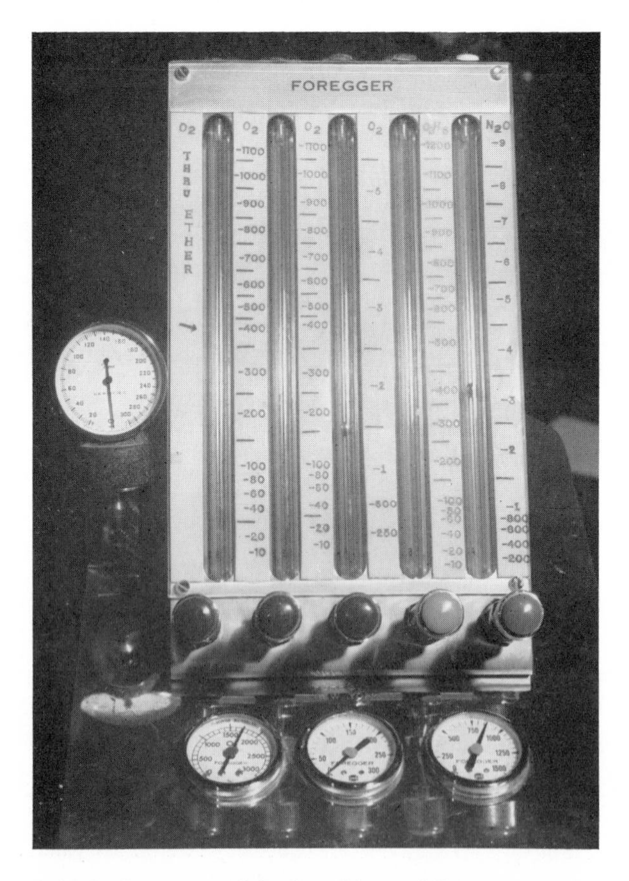

Fig. 19-5. Multiple float type of finely calibrated flow meter.

transparent tube, depending upon the quantity of gas that forces itself between the tube and the float. When the pressure rises and the volume flow increases, the float is made to rise within the transparent tube. The flow meter may be provided with an outlet valve to increase or decrease the diameter of the outlet orifice. This may not be done when a flow gauge is used because a change in outlet orifice merely registers a rising or a falling delivery pressure, regardless of the volume of flow.

Rebreathing bags

Rebreathing bags are rubber bags that vary in size from 1 to 5 liters. They are connected within the breathing circle (Fig. 19-6), and when the gases within the rebreathing bag are compressed, it is possible to augment or control respirations. If the oxygen is compressed rhythmically within the rebreathing bag, it may be used as a very efficient respiratory resuscitator.

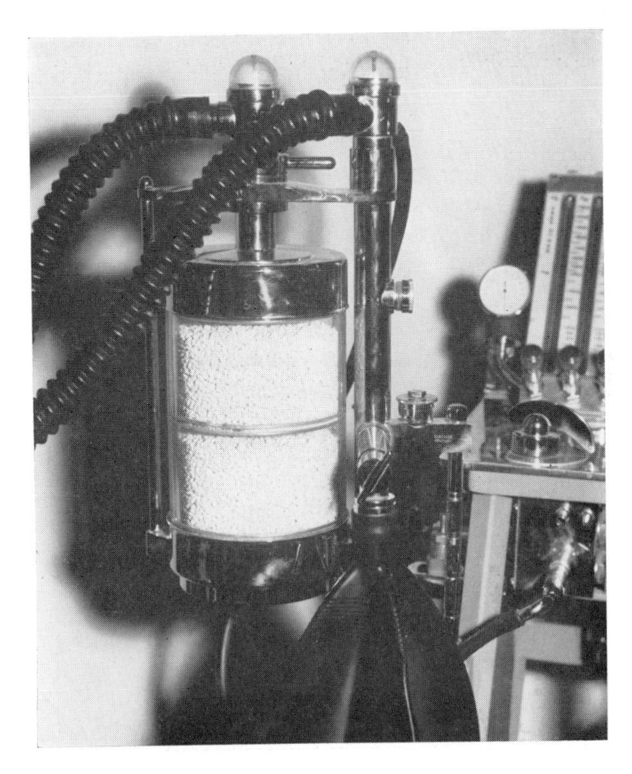

Fig. 19-6. Rebreathing bag.

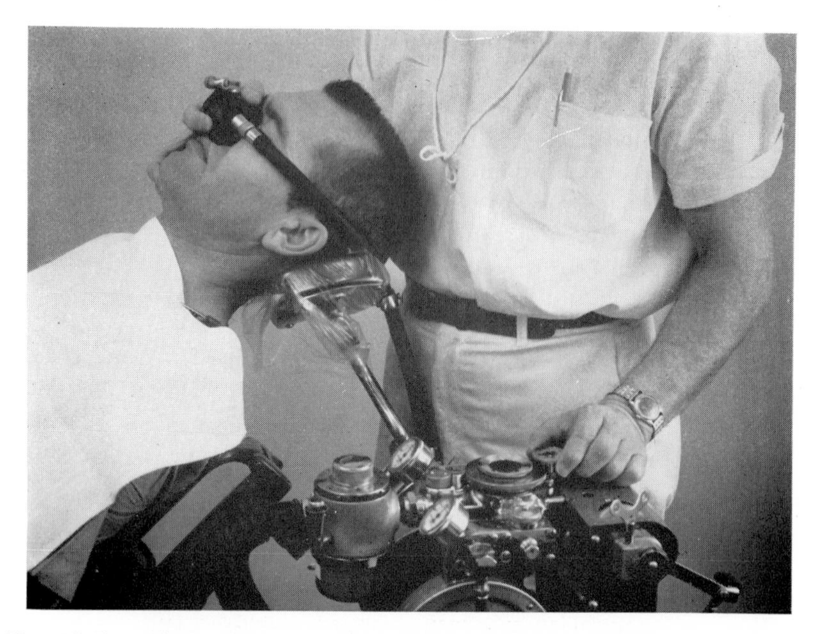

Fig. 19-7. Trichloroethylene and Vinethene cylinders attached to McKesson machine.

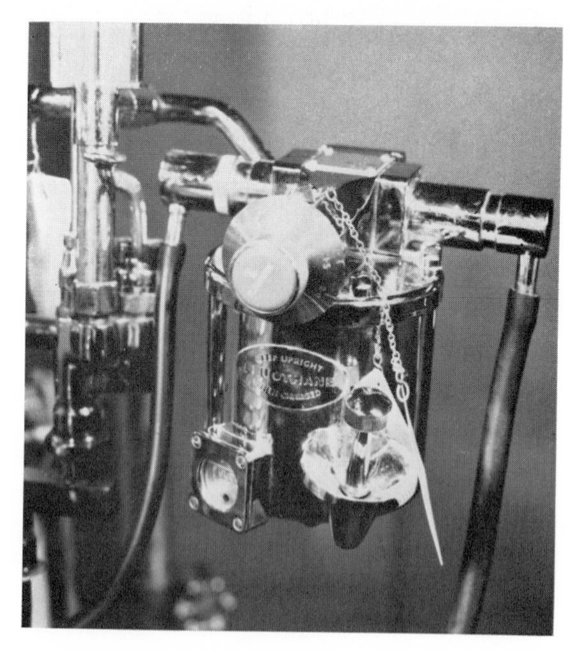

Fig. 19-8. Fluotic vaporizer for halothane.

Vaporizers

Vaporizers are reservoirs for volatile anesthetic agents (ether, divinyl ether, trichloroethylene, and fluothane). If the gaseous agents (oxygen, nitrous oxide, ethylene, and cyclopropane) are passed through the reservoir or vaporizer, varying amounts of the volatile agent are carried to the patient, depending upon the amount of the flow.

Ether vaporizers are usually effectively calibrated to contain 4 ounces of ether, with an adequate area for vaporization. A wick may or may not be used in conjunction with an ether vaporizer. Vaporizers for trichloroethylene and Vinethene are smaller, usually one-half the size of ether vaporizers (Fig. 19-7), and a wick is not necessary.

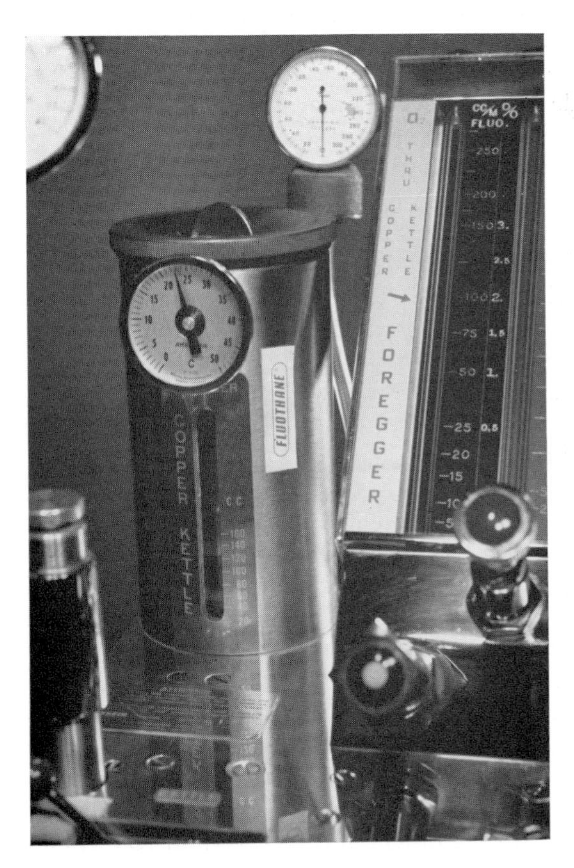

Fig. 19-9. Copper kettle vaporizer for halothane or ether.

Dropper-type vaporizers may be employed for Vinethene, trichlorothylene, or ether.

Vaporizers for fluothane (Figs. 19-8 and 19-9) must be specially calibrated for the use of this agent. It is hazardous to use fluothane in any vaporizer not specially calibrated and designated for it.

Vaporizers should be thoroughly cleansed after each use. It has been our policy not to allow volatile agents to remain in vaporizers from day to day.

Carbon dioxide absorbers

An anesthetic gas machine will operate effectively without a carbon dioxide absorber. However, if the machine is to be used for any thing other than anesthesia of short duration by the semiclosed technique, an absorber is necessary. The carbon dioxide absorber is a canister containing soda lime (Fig. 6-6) and affixed within the breathing circle for the purpose of removing carbon dioxide from the rebreathed or recirculated gases. There are a variety of designs for carbon dioxide absorbers. They may contain one or two chambers and be constructed of opaque metal or transparent plastic material.

Breathing tubes

Breathing tubes are made of corrugated rubber, which, preferably, is conductive. They may be of varying lengths, usually from 8 to 32 inches. Their purpose is to transport gases from the anesthetic apparatus to and from the patient. If the breathing valves on the machine are functioning properly, the breathing tubes will present a negligible amount of dead space.

Breathing masks

Breathing masks may be either full face masks or nasal inhalers. There are a variety of full face masks (Fig. 19-10), all anatomically designed to fit the face as snugly as possible to prevent the escape of anesthetic gases. Full face masks are available in a variety of sizes.

The nasal inhalers (Fig. 19-11) are used primarily in dentistry because they enable the patient to continue the respiratory circle through the nasal passages with the mouth open.

The American-made gas machines (McKesson, Heidbrink, and Foregger) available at the present time are all efficient, capable machines for dental anesthesia and contain most of the previously discussed essentials. It would be very difficult to judge any one machine to be superior to the others; however, certain features do make some machines more desirable for outpatient anesthesia than others. In order

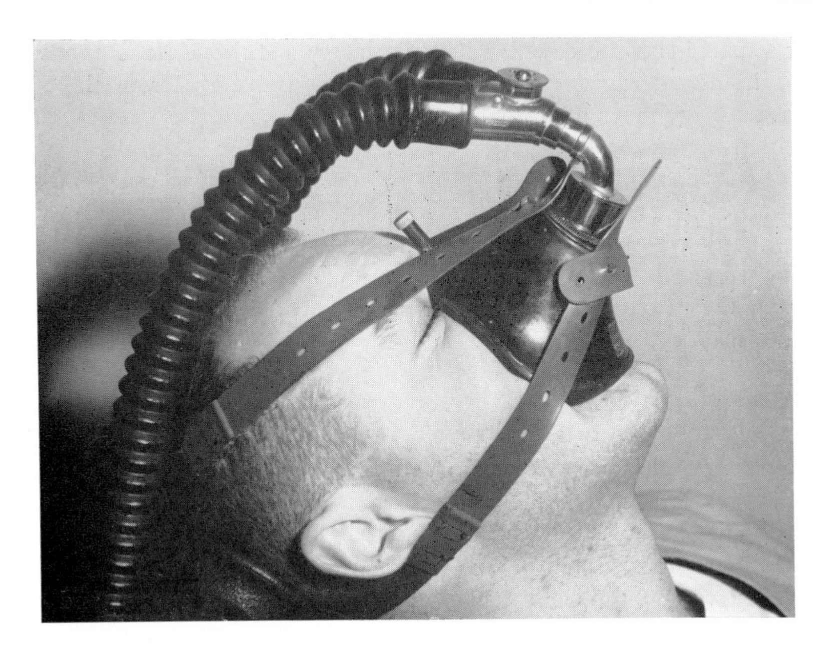

Fig. 19-10. Full face mask.

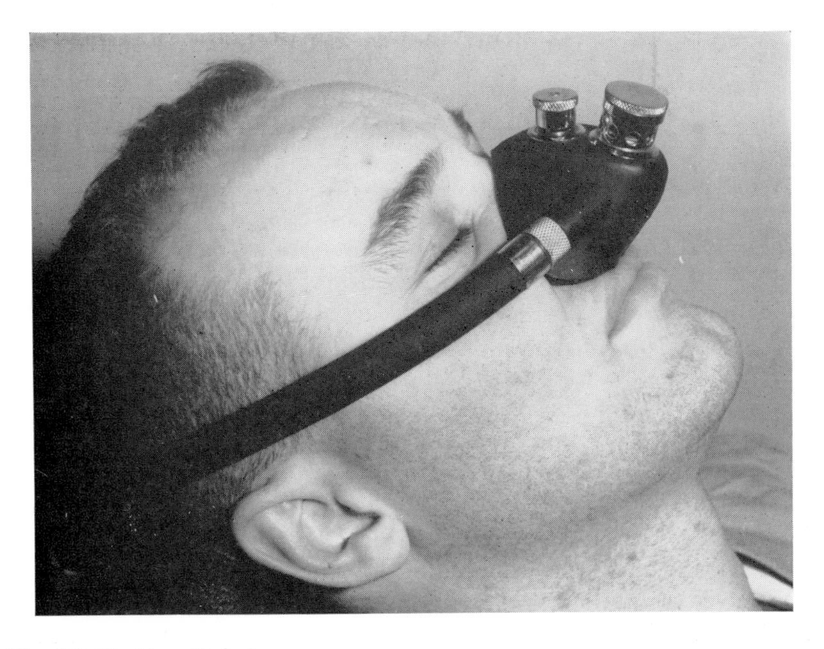

Fig. 19-11. Nasal inhaler.

for a machine to be effective in ambulatory anesthesia, it is essential that its design permit a rapid and smooth transition from the full face mask to the nasal inhaler. However, it should be stressed that regulators, gauges, flow meters, and so forth are not infallible. Therefore, regardless of the readings on the machine, during the administration of all anesthetics, the patient should be observed closely, and the anesthetist should use the manifest signs as a true guide to the patient's condition. For example, if the patient shows signs of hypoxia, these signs should be readily accepted, no matter what the readings on the machine indicate.

MECHANICAL AIRWAYS

Airways are a very important and necessary part of the anesthesia armamentarium. Various types, such as oropharyngeal airways, nasopharyngeal airways, and intratracheal airways (nasotracheal, orotracheal, and tracheotomy adapters), are available.

Oropharyngeal airways. Oropharyngeal airways are tubelike structures curved anatomically to fit over the base of the tongue and extend into the pharynx. Their prime purpose is to prevent the tongue from relaxing posteriorly and obstructing the respiratory airway. The oropharyngeal airways are designed in a variety of sizes and are made of metal (solid or ribbed), hard rubber, or plastic (see Fig. 10-1). In my experience, hard rubber has proved most adaptable and less injurious to the dentition.

Nasopharyngeal airways. The nasopharyngeal airways are rubber tube-shaped structures of appropriate diameter and length for insertion through the nasal passage and nasopharynx (see Fig. 10-5). The nasopharyngeal airway should also prevent the tongue from relaxing posteriorly and obstructing respirations.

The diameter of the nasopharyngeal tube should be such that the tube can slip through the nasal passages without undue resistance or damage to the mucous membrane. The tube should be long enough to offer support to the tongue without extending sufficiently into the laryngopharynx to become a mechanical irritant to the cords. The length of the tube should be predetermined by measuring from the tip of the nose to the meatus of the ear. The nasopharyngeal airway should have a flange or some other device to prevent it from slipping into the nares and pharynx.

Intratracheal airways. The intratracheal airway is the most positive method of maintaining a patent airway. The intratracheal airway is a tube of varying diameter and length, made of rubber, plastic, woven silk, metal, or combinations of these materials (Fig. 19-12).

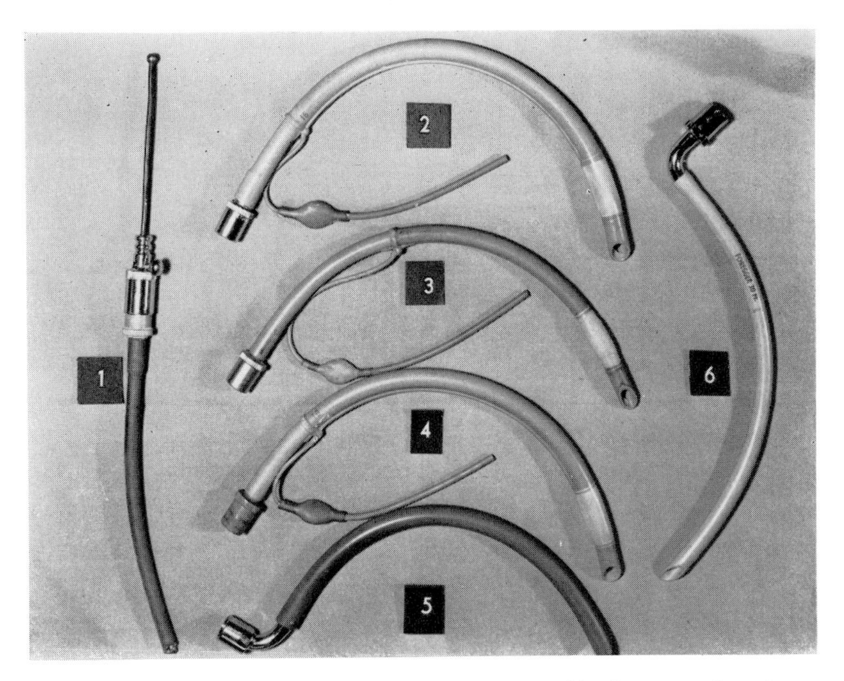

Fig. 19-12. Intratracheal tubes. **1,** Flexible metal ribbed type with stylet inserted; **2,** orotracheal tube with inflatable cuff (36 gauge); **3,** orotracheal tube with inflatable cuff (32 gauge); **4,** orotracheal tube with inflatable cuff (34 gauge); **5,** orotracheal tube, plain with curved adapter (36 gauge); **6,** nasotracheal tube, plain with curved adapter (30 gauge).

Nasotracheal airway. Nasotracheal tubes are made of rubber or plastic material and should be of sufficient diameter to ensure an efficient airway without injury to the nasal passages. Nasotracheal tubes should maintain an anatomical curvature to facilitate their passage by way of the nares, nasopharynx, and laryngopharynx and through the glottal opening into the trachea. The length of the nasotracheal airway should be predetermined by resting the tube along the side of the face and neck from the nares to the lower border of the cricoid cartilage (see Fig. 10-14). When the nasotracheal tube without a cuff is used, a pharyngeal pack around the tube (Fig. 19-13) is necessary to prevent gases from leaking around the outside of the tube between the tube and the wall of the trachea. The packing will also prevent blood and mucus from gaining entrance into the tracheobronchial tree along the outside of the tube.

Orotracheal airway. Orotracheal tubes may be made of rubber, plastic, metal, silk, and so forth and need not be curved, as are the

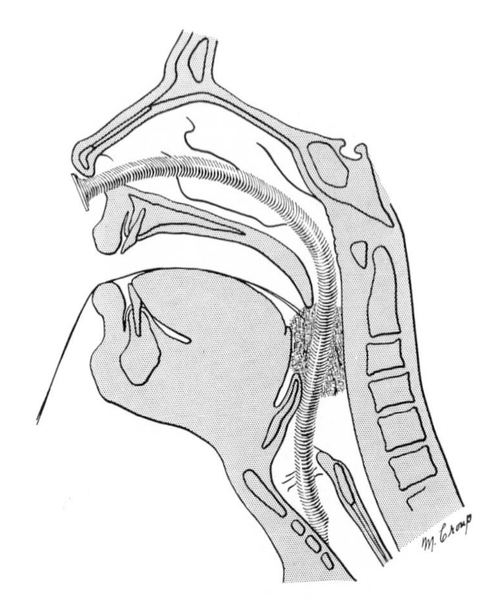

Fig. 19-13. Throat pack around plain nasotracheal tube.

Table 19-2. Scale used to classify intratracheal tubes

English	*French*	*English*	*French*
0	12	6	29
1	15	7	31
2	19	8	35
3	23	9	37
4	25	10	41
5	27		

nasotracheal airways. As a rule, they have a larger diameter. The length is usually measured from the incisor teeth to the lower border of the cricoid cartilage. When the orotracheal tube is used, an inflatable cuff (Fig. 19-14) may be employed to form a seal around the outside of the tube and the tracheal wall. In selected patients a pharyngeal pack may be used, but it is always more advantageous to use an inflatable cuff. When the oropharyngeal tube is flexible, a stylet for insertion will be necessary.

The internal diameter of intratracheal tubes varies; Table 19-2 shows the scale used to classify intratracheal tubes.

Tracheotomy adapters. If by chance the patient has had a pre-

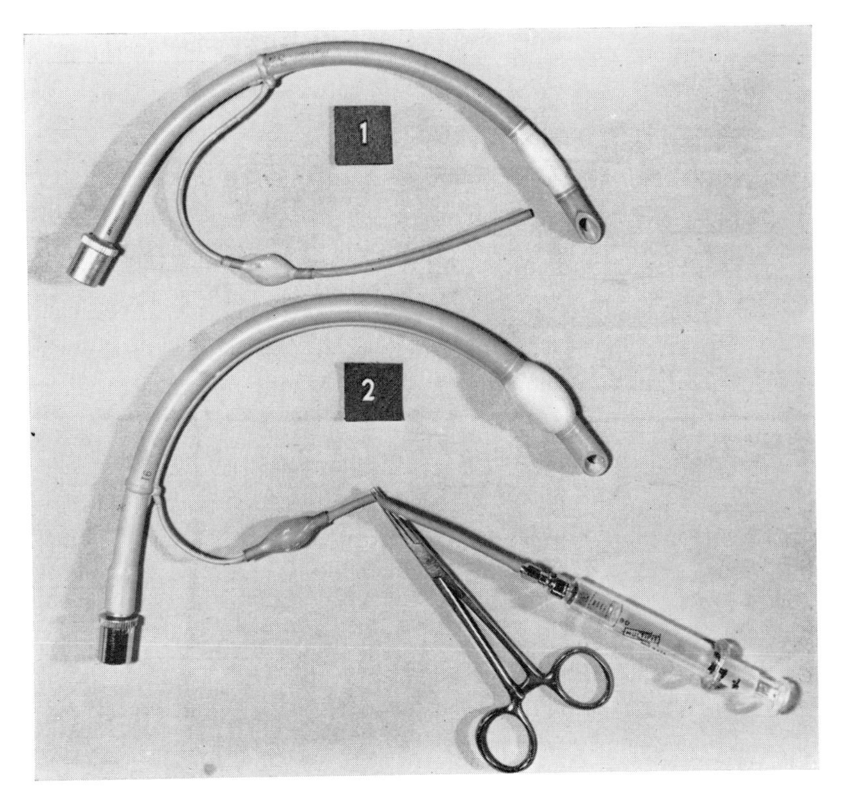

Fig. 19-14. Orotracheal tube with inflatable cuff. **1,** Cuff deflated; **2,** cuff inflated and clamped.

vious tracheotomy, it will be necessary to use an adapter that will fit into the tracheostomy tube in order to ensure an airtight connection. In this manner respirations may be augmented or controlled, as necessary. The adapters are supplied in a variety of sizes to fit standard tracheostomy tubes.

Special adapters. Special adapters are necessary when the anesthetic is administered with a nasotracheal or orotracheal tube in place. The adapters are essential because access to the oral cavity cannot be maintained when a full face mask is used. It is also more advantageous to use adapters in place of nasal inhalers in order to interfere as little as possible with the operating field.

These adapters may be curved, straight, or angled (Fig. 19-15); the shape should be chosen to fit the individual situation. One end will be of a standard size, while the other may vary according to the diameter of the intratracheal tube (Fig. 19-16).

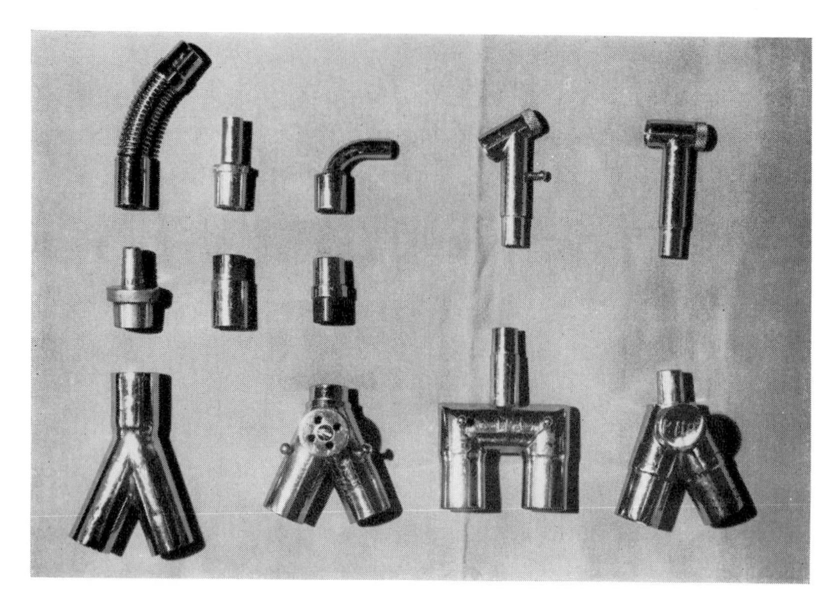

Fig. 19-15. Adapters for connecting intratracheal tubes to breathing tubes.

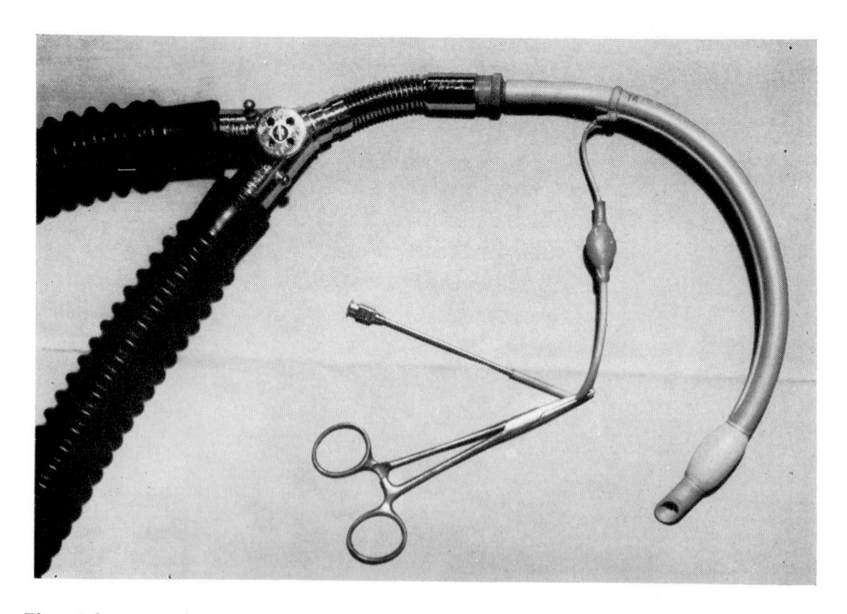

Fig. 19-16. Adapters in place connecting intratracheal tube to breathing tubes.

LARYNGOSCOPES

The laryngoscope is an instrument used to expose and view the vocal cords and larynx. Practically all the scopes used today consist of a handle and interchangeable blades (Fig. 19-17). Interchangeable blades make it possible to use the size and shape most ideally suited for an individual patient. The blades are of various lengths and have a light bulb near the tip of the blade that illuminates the structures in its path. The bulb may be on the side, top, or center of the blade. The blades may be straight or curved; there are a variety of adaptations. By experience, the anesthetist will eventually choose the type of blades that suit his individual preference. Laryngoscopes should be checked at intervals and always before they are used, because it may be embarrassing to discover at the last minute that the bulb does not light, which will make visualization of the cords impossible.

MAGILL AND ROVENSTEIN FORCEPS

The Magill (Fig. 19-18) and Rovenstein forceps are suitably curved, with flat, rounded ends to facilitate the guiding of the intratracheal tube into the trachea. They are curved to avoid obstructing the operator's vision.

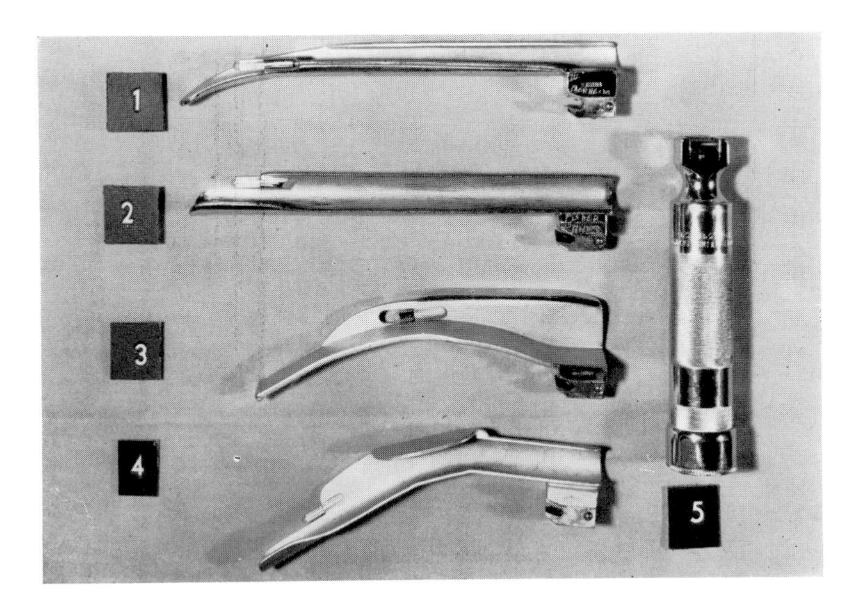

Fig. 19-17. Laryngoscopes. **1,** Miller blade No. 4; **2,** Foregger blade No. 4; **3,** Macintosh blade No. 4; **4,** Siker mirror blade; **5,** laryngoscope handle.

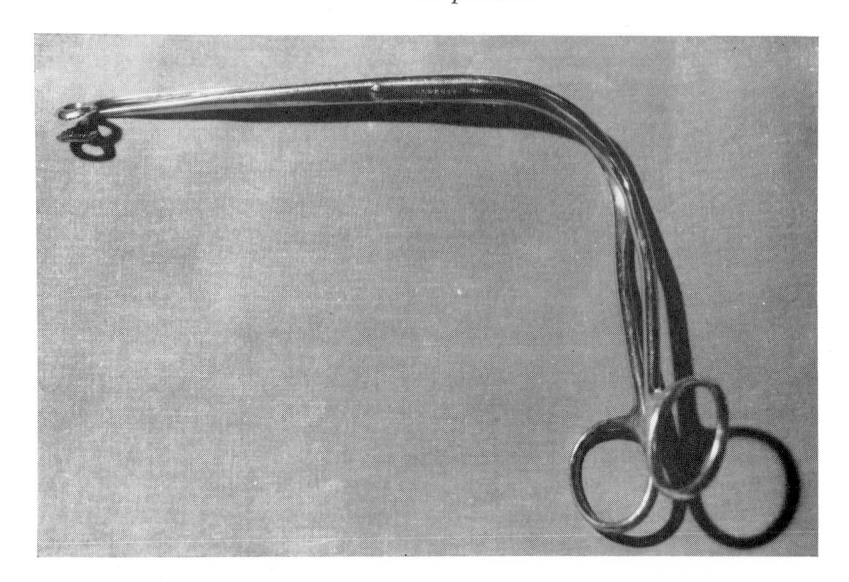

Fig. 19-18. Magill forceps.

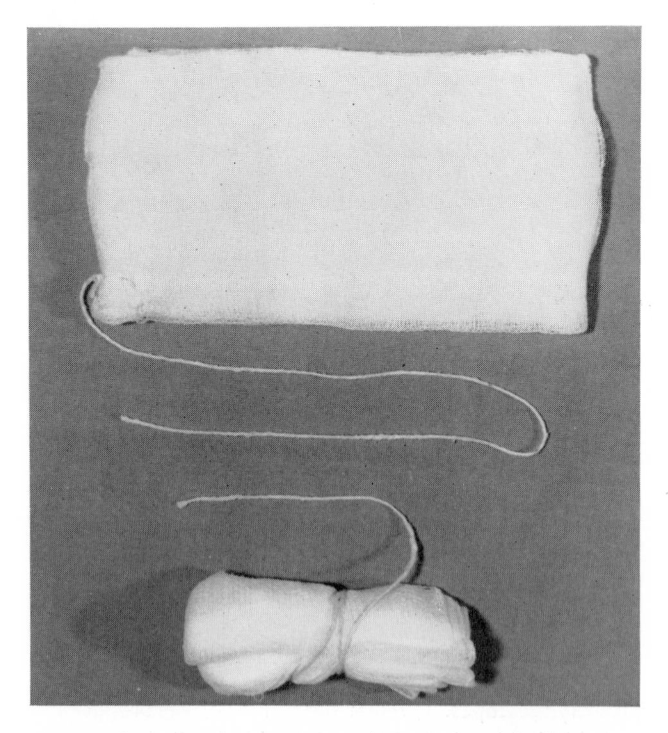

Fig. 19-19. Oropharyngeal partition with string attached.

OROPHARYNGEAL PARTITION

A properly placed oropharyngeal partition plays an important role in the administration of anesthesia for ambulatory patients. The vast majority of ambulatory patients are not intubated, which accounts for the importance of the oropharyngeal partition. Two gauze sponges, 8 × 4 inches with impregnated cotton, make an ideal oropharyngeal partition (Fig. 19-19). A piece of cord is tied through a loop in one corner of the partition so that the cord may protrude from the mouth when the partition is put into place (Fig. 19-20). This prevents the partition from slipping into the postpharynx and always presents the operator or anesthetist with a positive means of removing it. Also, the cord does not interfere with the operator. More than one partition may be used at the same time if desired. When an intratracheal tube is in place, the same partitions may be used as packs by pushing them into the pharynx around the intratracheal tube (see Fig. 19-13). It is essential that the cord attached to the gauze protrude from the oral cavity.

The oropharyngeal partition serves four important functions, which are discussed in Chapter 20.

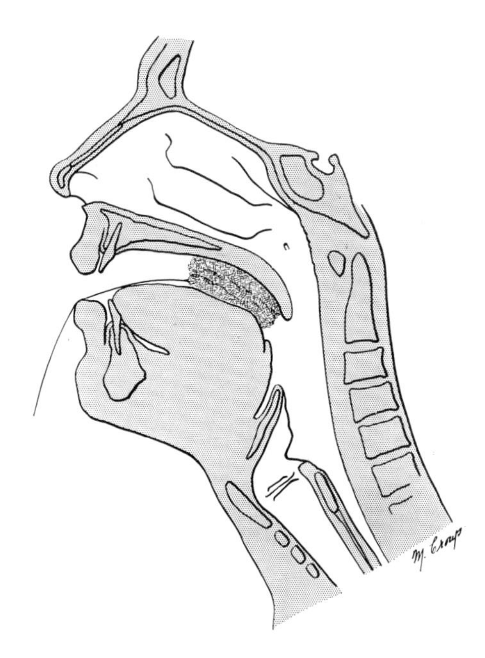

Fig. 19-20. String protruding from mouth when partition is in place.

MOUTH PROPS

Mouth props (Fig. 19-21) are instruments or devices used to facilitate opening the mandible or maintaining the mouth in an open position. A prop may be a ratchet type of instrument or a solid rubber device.

The ratchet type is designed so that its ends may be covered with rubber sleeves to protect the teeth or tissues. The ratchet permits the prop to open but prevents its closure without releasing the ratchet. This type of mouth prop has the advantage of adaptability. The solid rubber types are designed to be used with tooth-bearing or edentulous arches. The type to be used with an edentulous arch is constructed with flanges to prevent its dislodgment. Both types are made in a wedge shape to offer some adaptability to various mouth openings.

SUCTION APPARATUS AND CATHETERS

Suction apparatus and catheters are essential equipment when general anesthesia is being employed. The suction apparatus may be of the portable or wall type, but should be of sufficient force to be effective without undue injury to the tissues. Plastic or rubber suction catheters of sufficient size and length to be introduced through the

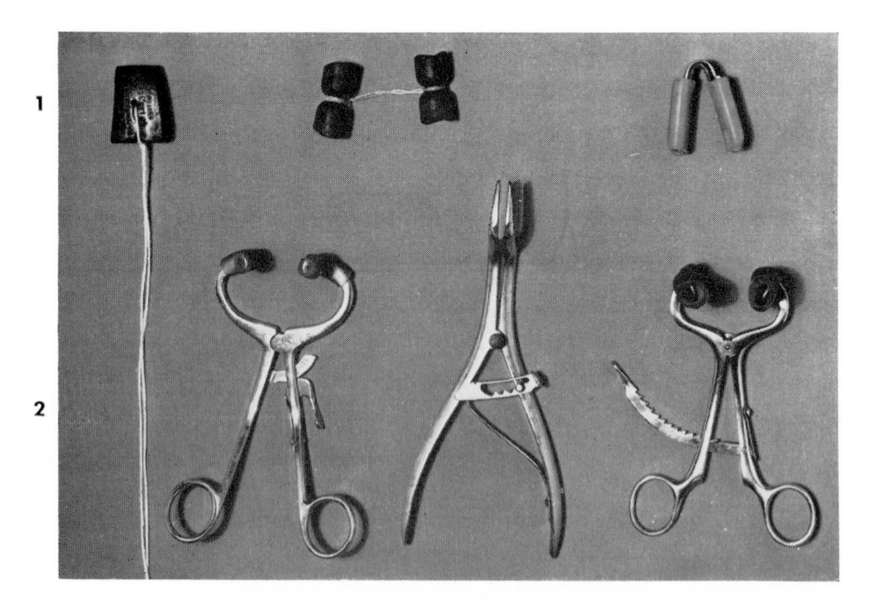

Fig. 19-21. Mouth props. **1,** Rubber; **2,** ratchet type.

intratracheal or nasopharyngeal tubes should be available. A metal tonsil suction to facilitate aspiration within the oral cavity and oropharynx should also be available. In most instances this device will be in constant use by the operator, rather than by the anesthetist.

In addition to the armamentarium just described, suitable syringes, needles, stopcocks, tourniquets, arm boards, and so forth, are necessary. Intravenous anesthetics may be administered with many different types of apparatus. For both the operating room and the office, we have found the Thomas arm board and syringe holder (Fig. 19-22) to be the most convenient.

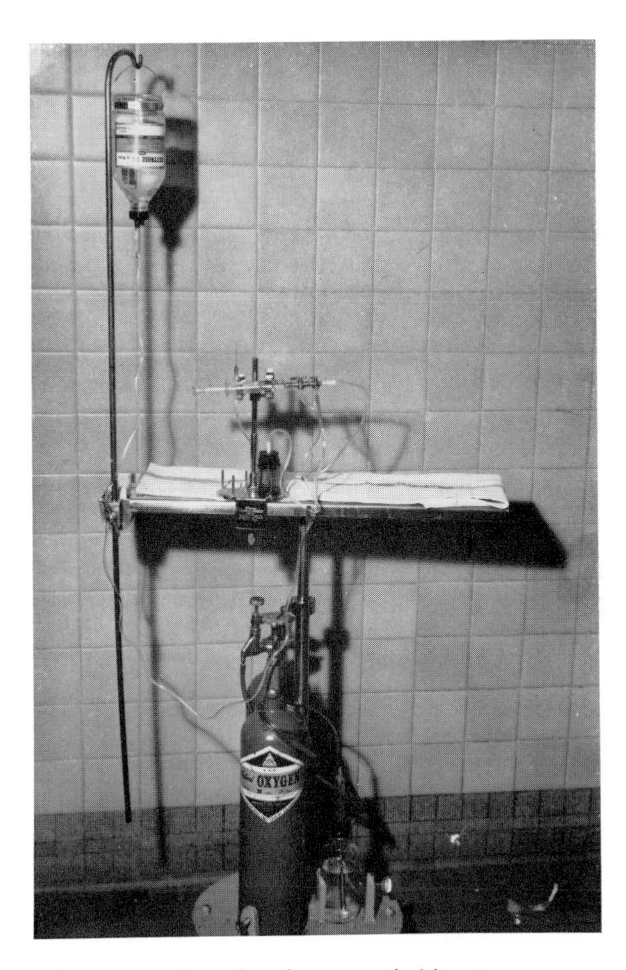

Fig. 19-22. Thomas arm board with syringe holder, intravenous stand, and oxygen tank.

A

B

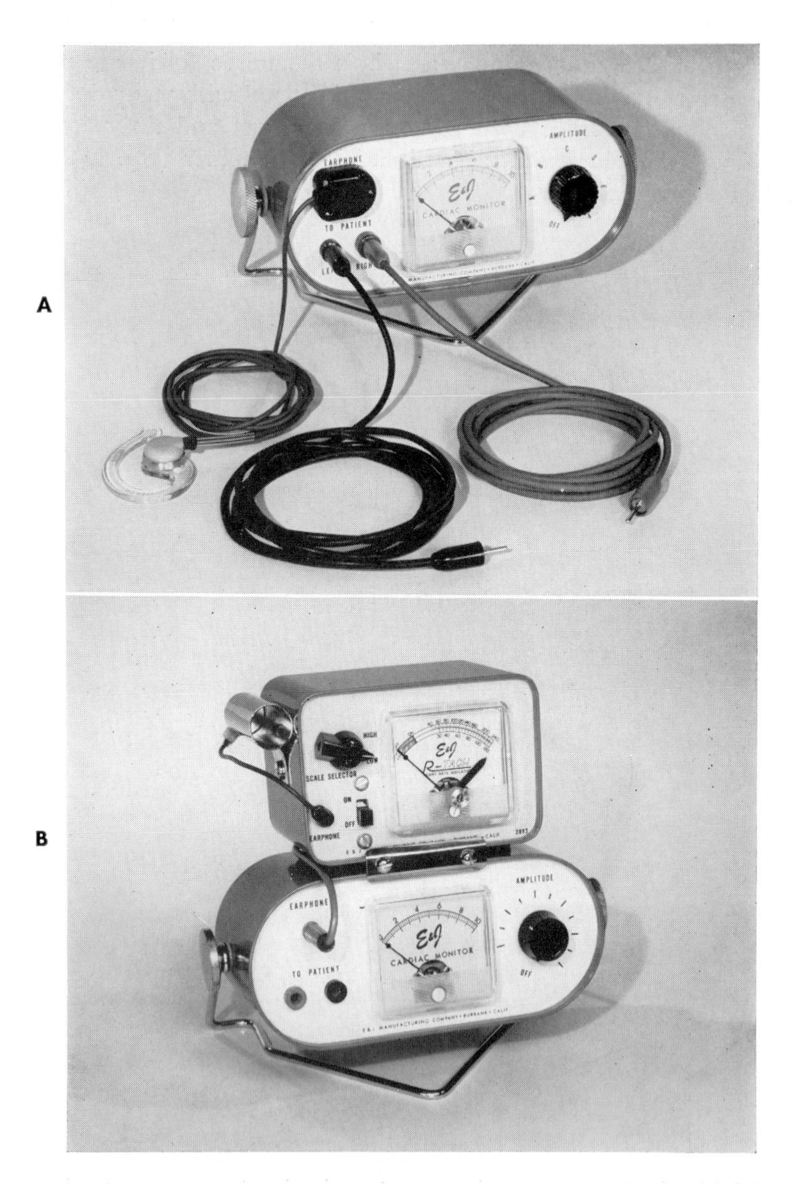

Fig. 19-23. A, Cardiac monitor. **B,** Cardiac monitor with heart rate attachment. (Courtesy E. & J. Manufacturing Co.)

MONITORING DEVICES

Monitoring devices (Fig. 19-23), both electronic and otherwise, play and will continue to play an important role in anesthesia. Electronic devices such as the electrocardioscope and cardiophone can be valuable aids in keeping the anesthetist aware of vital cardiovascular and respiratory functions. The esophageal stethoscope, which is placed in the esophagus, permits the anesthetist to monitor the respirations as well as the heartbeat, and is a valuable instrument during longer cases and when the anesthetist cannot maintain a contact with the patient (Fig. 19-24). There is no doubt that readings for pulse palpation, as well as blood pressure readings, can at times be misleading and inaccurate. However, monitoring devices will hardly replace the skill and judgment of the person administering the anesthetic.

Although it has been stated that careful preparation and preven-

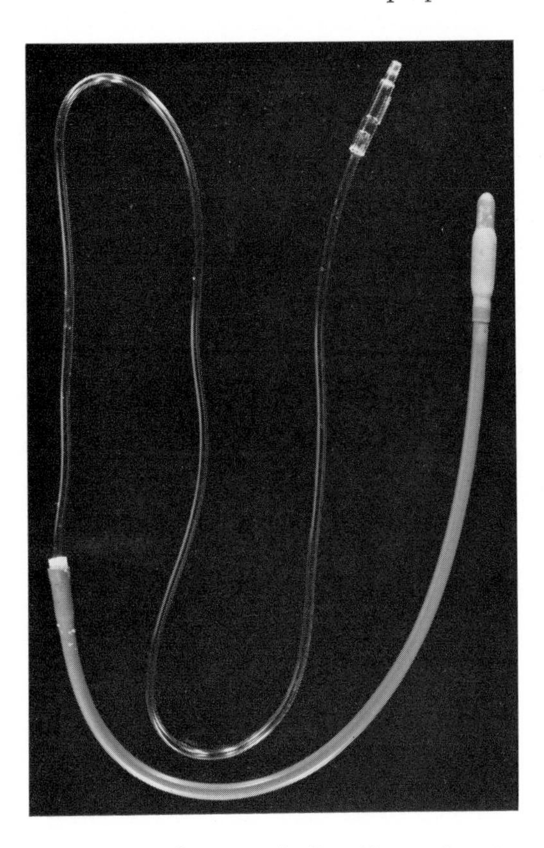

Fig. 19-24. Esophageal stethoscope—balloonlike end is inserted into the esophagus.

tion are far more important than heroic emergency efforts, it is not feasible to employ the cardioscope and other, more complex monitoring devices for ambulatory dental patients. Monitoring devices have a definite place if the procedure is to be a prolonged one. However, this may raise the question of the feasibility of prolonged anesthesia for ambulatory patients.

SUMMARY

The anesthetist should make certain that all necessary equipment is available and in good working condition. It is not only embarrassing but also hazardous to need essential equipment urgently and to find it missing. Equally distressing is the discovery that a piece of equipment, while available, is not in good working order.

Before an induction is started, the cylinders should be opened and the gauges checked. Flow meters should be briefly tested and tubing and masks examined. Suction apparatus should be used to make certain that it is functioning properly. The ready availability of syringes, needles, tourniquets, laryngoscopes, airways, and so forth should be determined. In other words, everything should be in readiness to facilitate the administration of the anesthetic and to decrease the possibility of complications.

Chapter 20

Technical aspects of anesthesia

Even though the dentist has a fundamental knowledge of the basic sciences and a satisfactory understanding of the general considerations of anesthesia, a certain degree of technical adaptability is necessary for the successful administration of a general anesthetic.

It is difficult to explain technical procedures adequately; however, the steps will be detailed, with the full understanding that there are a multitude of techniques practiced by many different individuals. It is very difficult to rate some superior to others. If anything should be stressed, it is the fact that there is no substitute for experience; within reason a person should accomplish a maneuver in the manner in which he does it best.

POSITION OF PATIENT

Most dental patients may be operated upon when they are properly positioned in a dental chair or are in the supine position on an operating table. For hospitalized patients who are to be intubated, the supine position on the table and the semireclining position in the chair are equally advantageous.

For office and ambulatory patients, we have found the reclining chair position to be most advantageous. After using the supine position for some time, we found that ambulatory patients prefer the reclining chair position. Furthermore, it offers both the anesthetist and the operator many advantages.

When placed on the operating table, the patient should be as near the head of the table as possible, with the left arm extended for the venipuncture. The right arm should rest comfortably at the patient's side and be secured there. Caution should be exercised to avoid all pressure areas and hyperextension of the left arm.

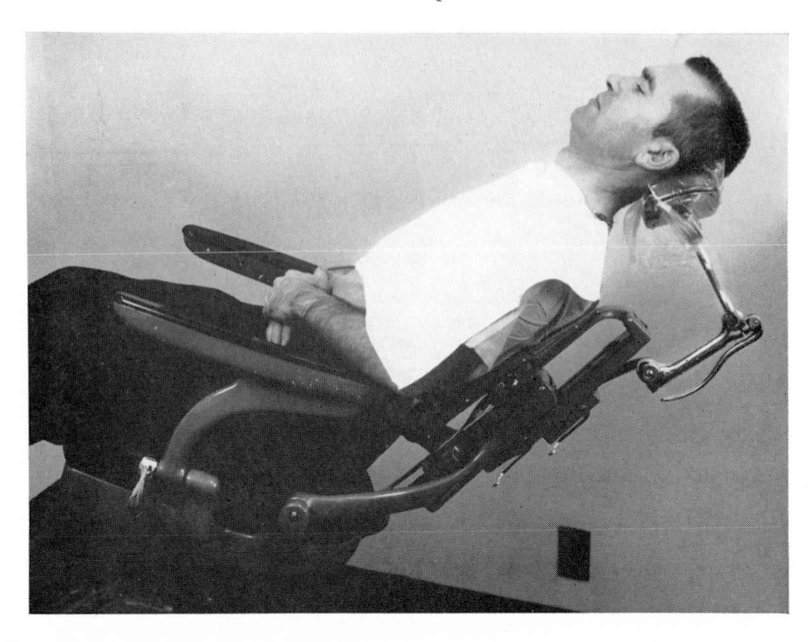

Fig. 20-1. Patient in semireclining chair position.

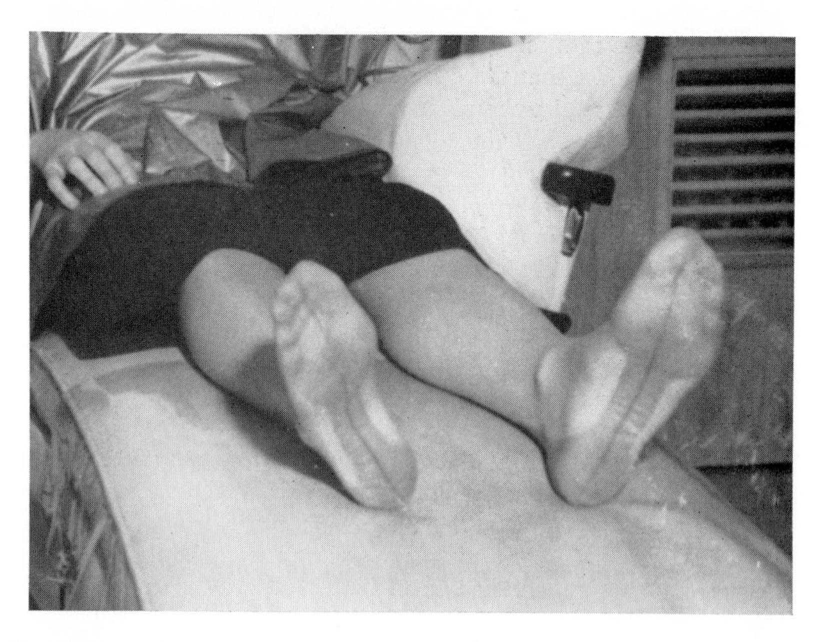

Fig. 20-2. Feet and legs are comfortably supported. Note the absence of a footrest.

When the semireclining chair position is adopted, the patient should be comfortably seated in the chair, which is then titled backward to an angle of approximately 45 degrees. (Fig. 20-1). The occipital portion of the head, the shoulders, and the hips should be in a straight line so that the center of gravity is posterior, toward the junction of the back and seat of the chair. The chin will then be elevated slightly to facilitate respirations. With the patient in this position, the abdominal viscera do not impinge upon diaphragmatic movements and thus reduce the vital capacity.

It has been some years since we have used anything but a loose restraint when a patient is in a semireclining position. As the patient relaxes, he is retained in the chair by his position. It is advantageous to have no footrest, but there should be a support for the legs and feet (Fig. 20-2). This prevents the patient from creating force by pressing his feet against the footrest.

When children are anesthetized, it may be better to use some form of light restraint. The child must not feel overly restricted but should be restrained only enough to prevent sudden, unexpected movements. It may be necessary to elevate the child in the chair if a pediatric chair is not available.

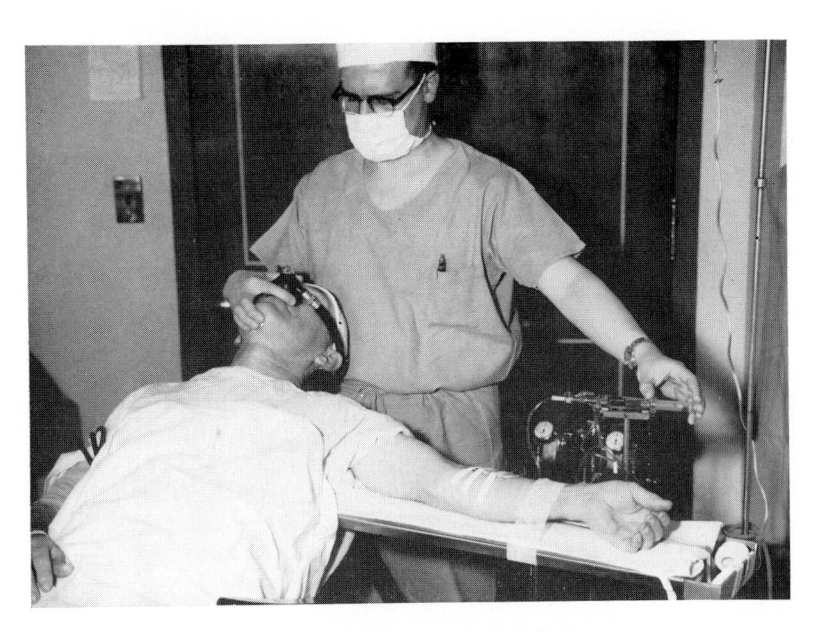

Fig. 20-3. Venipuncture in extended left arm for intravenous administration. Note oxygen being administered by nasal mask.

The venipuncture is usually made in the left arm, which may be placed on an arm board attached to the chair or on a separate stand (Fig. 20-3). We prefer a separate stand that holds the syringe and the intravenous bottle (Thomas arm board). This permits us to push the arm board and the stand out of the way when the procedure is finished. It also offers a choice of positions and permits the anesthetist better access to the arm and intravenous equipment.

The anesthetist should place himself at the head and to the rear of the patient, with the gas machine to his immediate left (Fig. 20-4). After the induction is completed and the mouth prop placed in position, the anesthetist supports the chin, mask, and mouth prop with one hand (Fig. 20-5), leaving the other hand free to augment respirations (see Fig. 20-4) or to give additional intravenous injections (see Fig. 20-3). When the operator is working on the right side of the oral cavity, the anesthetist should support the chin, prop, and nasal inhaler

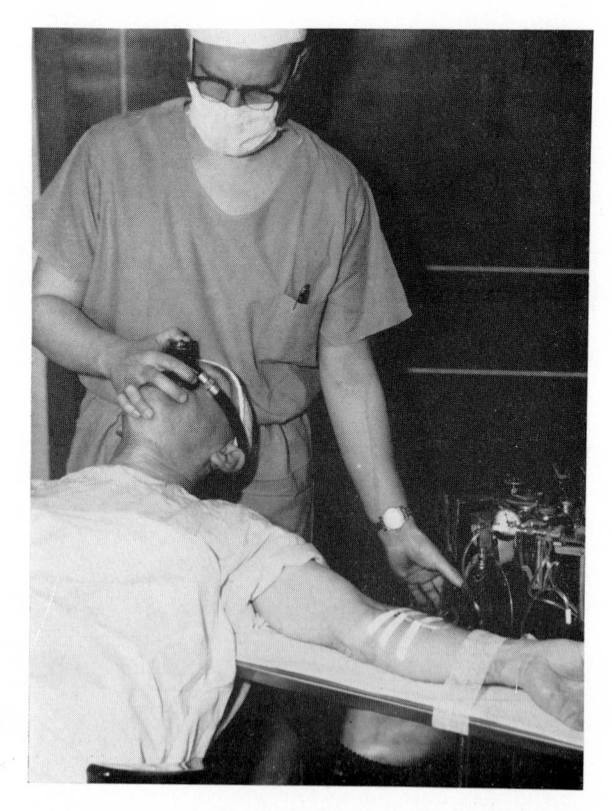

Fig. 20-4. Anesthetist at head and behind patient, augmenting respirations.

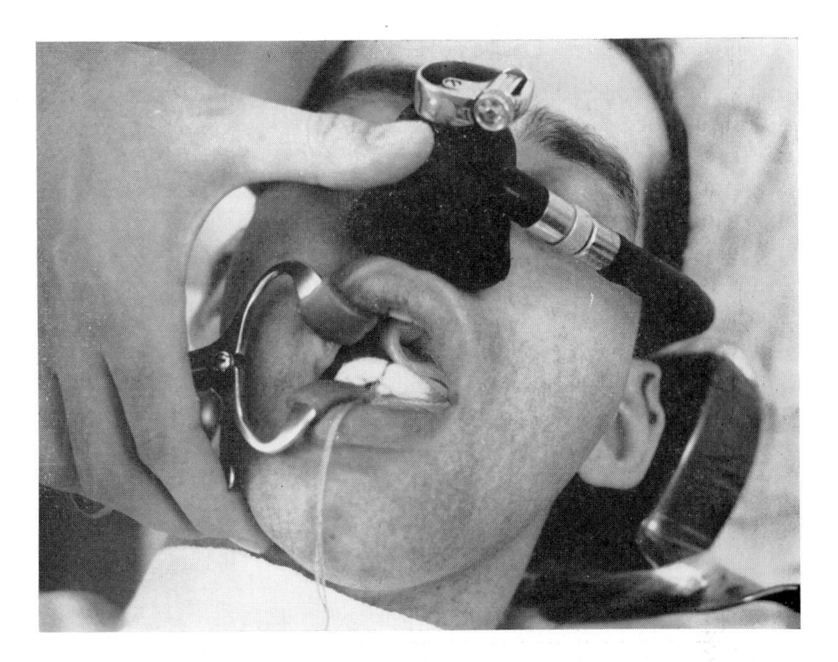

Fig. 20-5. Anesthetist supporting the patient's chin, mask, and mouth prop with the right hand.

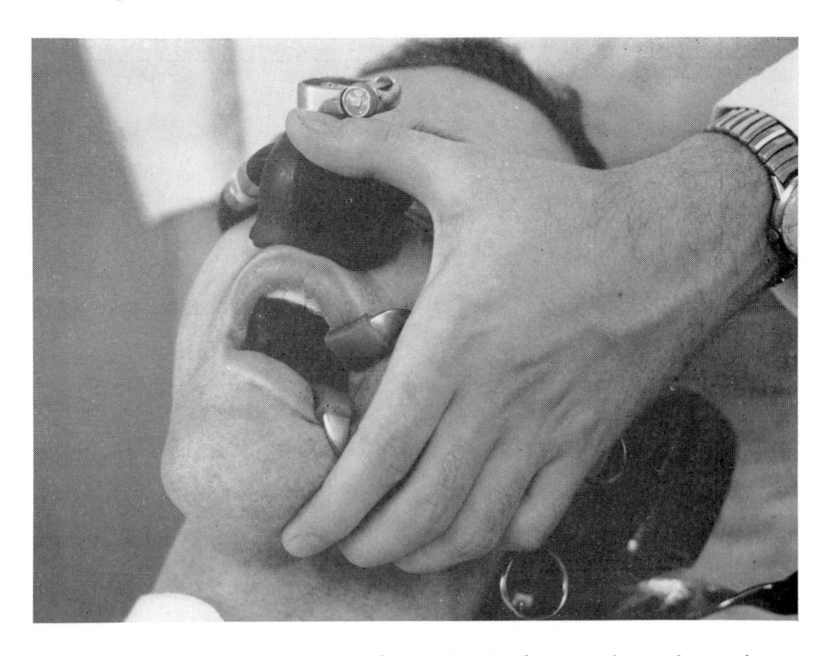

Fig. 20-6. Anesthetist supporting the patient's chin, mask, and mouth prop with the left hand.

with the left hand (Fig. 20-6) and at the same time cross the right hand underneath the left arm to augment the respirations, manipulate the intravenous syringe, or take the pulse and blood pressure. When the operator is working on the left side of the oral cavity, the anesthetist should support the chin, prop, and nasal inhaler with his right hand, leaving the left hand free to perform the duties just mentioned.

After intubation in the semireclining position has been accomplished, intratracheal adapters should be used, and the anesthetist will not be required to support the chin, mouth prop, and mask (Fig. 20-7). If the patient is in a supine position on the operating table, the left arm should be extended for the venipuncture, and the anesthetist should place himself at the head and slightly to the left of the patient. Some operators prefer the assistant to work from the left side of the table, but a few like to have him at the head of the table, in which case the anesthetist will move to the left below the extended arm.

VENIPUNCTURE

Venipuncture in itself should not be an extremely painful or unpleasant procedure. Some of the discomfort is based on emotional factors, and some is no doubt due to dull needles and poor technique.

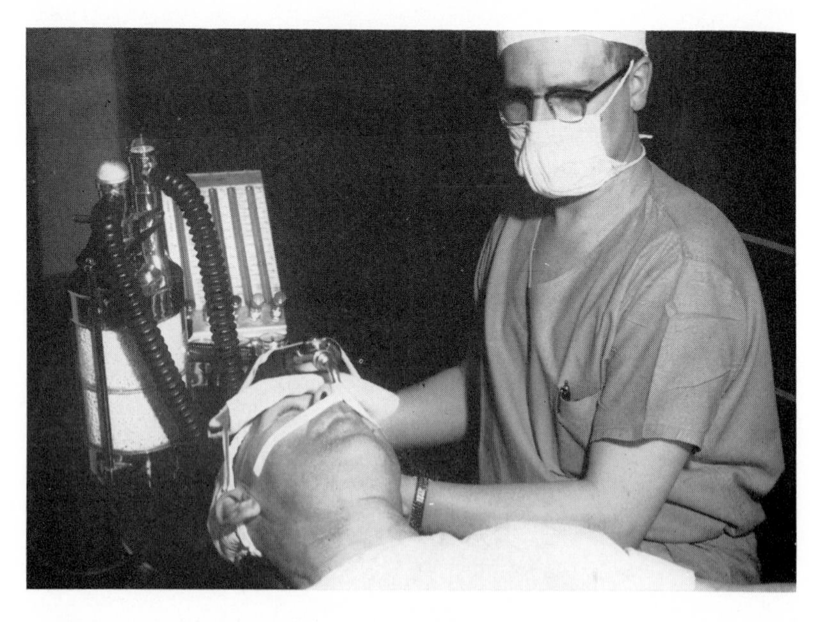

Fig. 20-7. Nasotracheal tube in place, with adapters. Anesthetist is not required to support the chin or hold the mask in place.

The patient should be reassured as to the safety and comfort of the procedure. All necessary equipment should be at hand so that the patient will not be perturbed by unnecessary delays.

The first step for successful venipuncture is selection of the proper vein. A basic knowledge of anatomy will help in locating the more prominent vessels in the antecubital fossa or the dorsum of the hand. Once a suitable vein is chosen, the tourniquet should be applied centrally to the area of insertion (Fig. 20-8). It should be kept in mind that arterial blood flows into the forearm at a pressure of approximately 120 mm. Hg. Venous blood flows away from the arm at a pressure of approximately 12 mm. Hg. The pressure of the tourniquet should not exceed 60 mm. Hg because this permits free arterial flow into the arm and maximum obstruction to the venous return. After the tourniquet is applied, 30 to 45 seconds should be allowed to elapse before venipuncture is done. This will give adequate time for venous filling, and in many cases veins that were not particularly prominent may stand out very well.

The size of the needle should be determined by the size of the vein and the purpose of the puncture. A 20-gauge, 1½-inch needle is most suitable for intravenous anesthesia. Of course, the needle should be

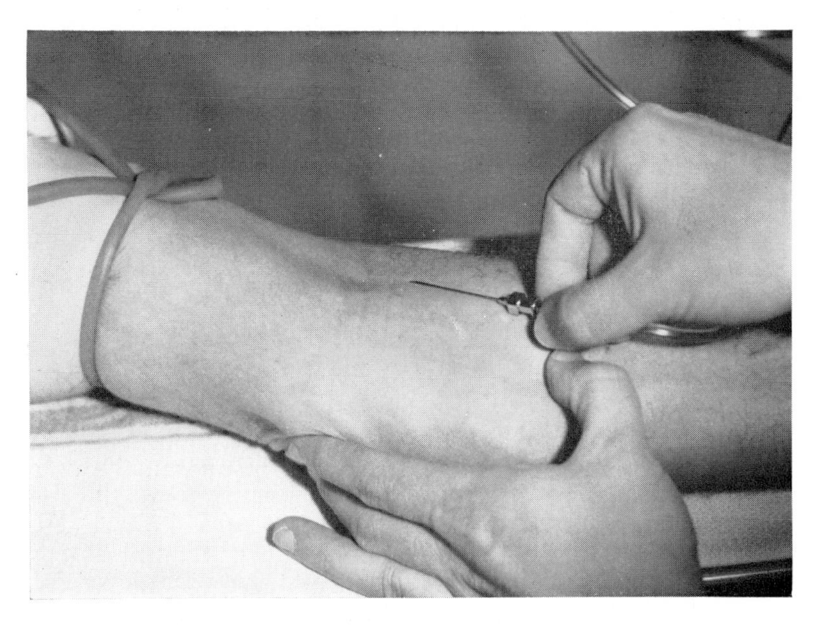

Fig. 20-8. Tourniquet is applied centrally to the area of insertion.

sterile, sharp, and patent (see Fig. 15-12). Its patency should always be tested by forcing fluid through the lumen before the puncture is started.

The patient's forearm should be extended on a comfortable arm board at a satisfactory working level. The area of penetration should be cleansed with a suitable antiseptic solution. Without contaminating the prepared area, apply pressure on the skin with the left hand (if right-handed) to counteract the thrust of the needle. The needle, with bevel up, should approach the skin at an angle of 35 to 40 degrees. Once the needle has penetrated the skin, realign it with the vein and then, with a single thrust, insert the needle into the lumen of the vessel. The needle should then be affixed to the arm (see Fig. 6-7) or the dorsum of the hand to prevent any undue movements that may dislodge the needle.

When the operation is terminated and there is no longer need for the venipuncture, a sterile piece of cotton or a gauze sponge should be held firmly in place over the site of the puncture and the needle withdrawn. The pressure should be maintained for 30 to 90 seconds, or more if necessary. If bleeding has ceased, a small sterile dressing should be applied to the area.

OROPHARYNGEAL PARTITION

The oropharyngeal partition forms a protective barrier between the oral cavity and the pharynx. It may be composed of 4 × 4 gauze sponges (see Fig. 19-19), a length of gauze dressing, or synthetic sponges. The sponge itself may consist of a variety of materials, depending on individual preference. It is mandatory in all cases that a portion of the partition or a string attached thereto protrude from the oral cavity (see Fig. 19-20). This is a precautionary measure that should never be neglected.

Regardless of the material from which the partition is made, it should serve four important functions. They are the following:

1. To prevent blood, mucus, and debris from passing into the pharynx and perhaps eventually into the trachea
2. To prevent dilution of the anesthetic mixture by mouth breathing
3. To form a sufficient seal between the pharynx and the oral cavity so that inspirations can be augmented by positive pressure when the nasal mask is used
4. To maintain the tongue in a forward position and thus prevent any possible obstruction from it

The oropharyngeal partition should be placed by the oral surgeon when the anesthetist has attained the proper plane of anesthesia and before surgery is begun. As a rule, the partition should be placed at the junction of the hard and soft palates. It thus forms an effective seal between the oral cavity and the pharynx and maintains the tongue in a forward position. The oropharyngeal partition should be of sufficient size to fulfill its purpose, without creating a respiratory obstruction by protruding into the pharynx, or interfering with the operator's vision or working area by protruding anteriorly into the oral cavity.

The partition should be changed whenever necessary. It is hazardous to allow the partition to become saturated with blood or mucus because it may then slip easily into the postpharynx and cause a respiratory obstruction. This can be avoided by changing it at frequent intervals. For the same reason a portion of the partition should protrude from the mouth, or a string should be attached to it.

THROAT PACKS

A throat pack, which is vastly different from an oropharyngeal partition and should never be confused with it, is used only when an intratracheal airway without an inflatable cuff is in place. The throat pack, composed of moistened 4 × 4 gauze sponges with a string attached, should be placed in the pharynx around the intratracheal tube to form a seal, which thus prevents the egress of air from the lungs around the tube (see Fig. 19-13). The throat pack will also prevent foreign material, blood, and mucus from passing into the tracheobronchial tree. It is impossible to seal the trachea effectively by using an intratracheal tube alone without a cuff.

It is desirable for the oral surgeon to use an oropharyngeal partition even though the patient is intubated and a throat pack is in place. Its function will be to prevent blood, mucus, and debris from gravitating into the pharynx. The throat pack should not be used as a catchall, but primarily as a seal for the intratracheal tube.

TECHNICAL ASPECTS OF ADMINISTRATION

While the fundamental technique of anesthesia is the same for ambulatory patients, outpatients, and hospitalized patients, it varies somewhat because of the special requirements of each type of patient.

Anesthesia for ambulatory patients

More anesthetics are administered for ambulatory patients in dentistry than in any other specialty requiring anesthesia. All office patients and many of those cared for in the hospital are ambulatory and, as explained in Chapter 11, are Class A patients whose surgical procedure will not consume more than 30 minutes (approximately). These patients should recover and be able to leave the office, escorted by a responsible adult, within a time approximately that required for the surgical procedure.

The ideal anesthetic agent for the ambulatory patient should meet four requirements: rapid induction, satisfactory maintenance, rapid recovery, and a high safety factor. As yet, no one agent fulfills them all to perfection. However, by combining two or more agents it is possible at times to utilize their individual advantages and to eliminate their disadvantages.

The most suitable agents presently available are nitrous oxide, trichloroethylene, divinyl ether, fluothane, ethylene, and the intravenous agents—thiopental sodium (Pentothal), thiamylal sodium (Surital), and methohexital sodium (Brevital). These agents, alone or in combination, should enable the dentist to handle efficiently practically every type of ambulatory patient. If proper and adequate premedication has been administered, they closely approach the ideal. However, it is important that each patient be considered an individual and that the anesthetic agent or combination of agents and the technique of administration be adapted to his needs.

It is no longer necessary to use hypoxic techniques with nitrous oxide and oxygen since these agents can be supplemented or complemented with other agents. On the other hand, it is not desirable to use the more potent anesthetics alone for longer procedures since they may have decided disadvantages.

Nitrous oxide and oxygen. Nitrous oxide properly used with supplemental or complemental agents is still the first choice for ambulatory patients. When properly administered, it is the safest of all general anesthetics, and if complications occur, they are usually the result of misuse. Being the weakest of the anesthetic agents presently in use, it is also the most difficult to administer and requires a considerable degree of skill and experience. Unfortunately, the technical administration of nitrous oxide has almost become a lost art. The more potent agents are too frequently used, and the full benefit of the nitrous oxide is not derived. On the other hand, nitrous oxide and oxygen should be used to their fullest advantage, and the more potent agents should be used to supplement or complement the mixture.

As for any other anesthetic, the technical administration of nitrous oxide and oxygen will differ from patient to patient, according to existing circumstances. The anesthetist should be able to vary the procedures as required to meet these conditions.

Nitrous oxide and oxygen alone may be suitable for comparatively short procedures (about 5 minutes). However, Vinethene, trichloroethylene, or fluothane should be readily available to potentiate the action of the nitrous oxide and enable the oxygen levels to be increased to safe limits. It is not unusual for a procedure that is expected to be of short duration to be protracted because of unforeseen difficulties.

It should always be assumed that prior to the administration of nitrous oxide or any other agent the patient has had an adequate preanesthetic evaluation and has been properly prepared. The patient should be positioned in the chair as previously discussed in this chapter. All necessary equipment and materials should be readily available, and an operating team of at least three people—the operator, his assistant, and the anesthetist—should be present.

The degree of cooperation that can be expected from the patient should be predetermined. If a patient appears to be extremely cooperative, the procedure and what is expected of him should be explained. On the other hand, if he is fearful and apprehensive, the dentist should attempt to calm him and gain his confidence. If this attempt does not appear to be succeeding, the patient should be well premedicated before the administration of the anesthetic. A fearful, apprehensive patient is not only more difficult to anesthetize but also may present a greater risk. Children particularly should not be denied the tremendous advantages of adequate premedication.

Induction. We usually induct the patient by using a nasal mask, with the exhaling valve as loose as possible to facilitate the blowing off of the nitrogen and at the same time to spare the patient the feeling of suffocation or resistance to expiratory efforts. The mask should be adapted gently but firmly over the patient's nose and be seated so that it does not obstruct the nares. At the same time, in a quiet, soothing voice, the anesthetist should encourage the patient to follow his instructions. (A vast majority of inductions are now accomplished by using a full face mask [Fig. 20-9].)

Whenever possible I favor comparatively slow induction (rapid induction may at times be indicated) with nitrous oxide and oxygen since it is essential that the nitrogen within the lungs and tissues be replaced with nitrous oxide to secure the maximum results with this weak anesthetic agent.

The anesthetic machine (McKesson-Nargraff) should be set at 5% oxygen and 95% nitrous oxide, with a pressure of 2 or 3 mm. Hg. This should be varied to suit the individual patient; most likely, the oxygen percentage will be increased.

The rebreather pressure key is released to facilitate unimpaired expirations. The rebreather stop lever is set according to the individual

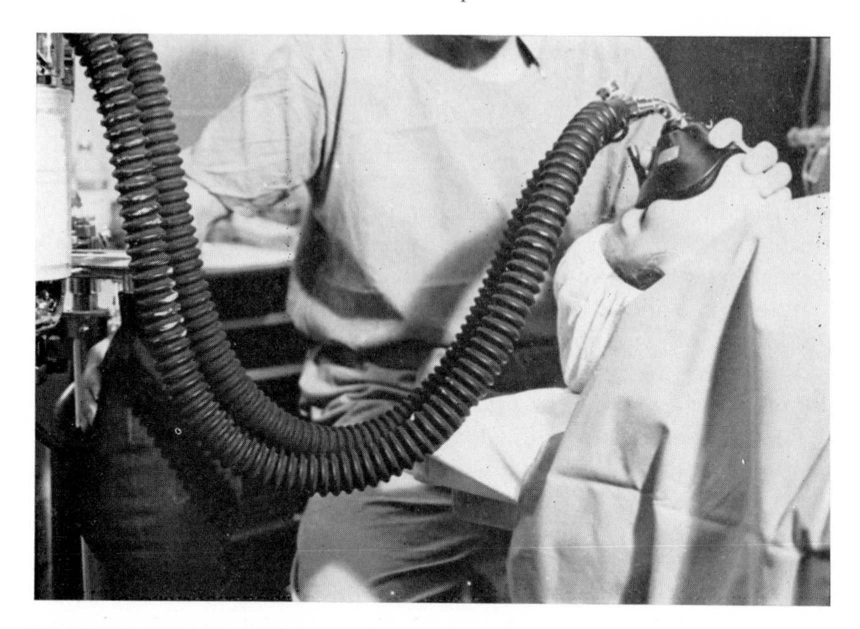

Fig. 20-9. Induction with a full face mask.

patient, with an adequate volume permitted. After the patient has taken three or four breaths, the oxygen should be gradually increased, rapidly enough to prevent any manifestations of hypoxia. In many patients this increase may be a rapid one, depending on the rate and depth of the respirations. For all patients, however, the oxygen increase should be continued, and the anesthetist should make certain that metabolic levels of oxygen are being administered. This metabolic level should be reached within a comparatively short time since in most uncomplicated procedures induction is completed in 3 to 4 minutes.

The patient should be instructed to keep the mouth closed and to breathe normally through the nose. If necessary, the mouth may be covered to facilitate nasal breathing. As the nitrous oxide begins to take effect, the patient should be told to open his mouth, and a mouth prop should be inserted in a closed position. The expiratory valve on the nasal exhaler should then be tightened so that the inspirations can be augmented by hand pressure on the rebreathing bellows to increase pulmonary ventilation. At the same time this helps prevent dilution of the anesthetic mixtures by mouth breathing.

The percentage of nitrous oxide and oxygen should be varied as necessary to secure the desired results, and one should make certain that the patient at no time exhibits the symptoms or effects of hypoxia.

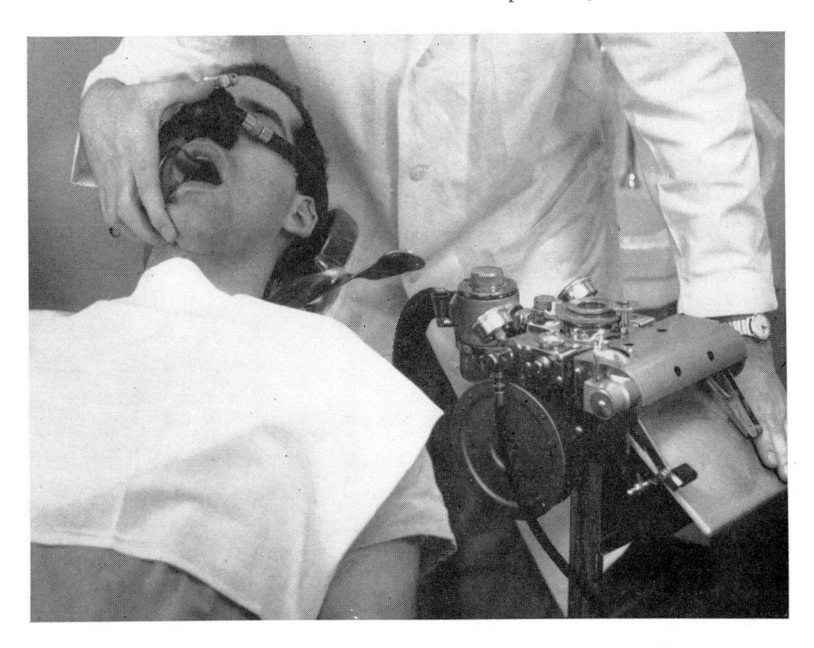

Fig. 20-10. Inspiratory phase augmented with hand pressure on rebreathing bellows.

Increasing the pulmonary ventilation by augmenting the inspiratory phase with hand pressure on the rebreathing bellows (Fig. 20-10) enhances the diffusion of nitrous oxide and oxygen and makes possible a more favorable anesthesia. No attempt should be made to control the respirations but only to augment them.

Although the patient may begin to experience a greater effect from the nitrous oxide, he will remain conscious for a short time. During this time he will be aware of external stimuli, and the operating area should be as quiet as possible, with nothing to distract the patient.

When a patient is no longer in harmony with his surroundings, he will have entered the second stage of anesthesia. This stage is characterized by its uncertainty. The patient's respiration may be regular or irregular. The lid reflex will be sluggish or absent. The pupils will probably be dilated but will react to light, and the eyeball will be active.

One feature of this stage that is characteristic of all anesthetic agents is amnesia. We have purposely stimulated patients, and they have at times reacted rather vigorously to the stimulation but upon recovery have had no memory of it. We have duplicated this procedure with other agents and noted the same results.

When the breathing becomes regular and rhythmic, the patient has entered the light surgical stage. The volume will be slightly greater than normal and the rate slightly increased. The lid reflex will be absent, but the pupils will still react to light. The eyeballs may be active. At this time the mouth prop can be opened as required and the oropharyngeal partition placed in position.

Maintenance. In order that a satisfactory level of anesthesia with nitrous oxide and oxygen be maintained, mouth breathing should be eliminated as far as possible since its diluting effect may make it impossible to maintain the proper plane of anesthesia. In order for this to be accomplished the pressure under which the gases are being administered may have to be increased, the inspirations more forcibly augmented (see Fig. 20-10), and sometimes the oxygen decreased to compensate for the mouth breathing (20% oxygen and 80% nitrogen). A well-placed oropharyngeal partition (see Fig. 19-20) will be of inestimable value in preventing or decreasing mouth breathing.

If the patient is in a proper position, the jaw is adequately supported, and the oropharyngeal partition is placed to support the tongue in a forward position, a patent airway should be assured. If a slight obstruction is evidenced, increased augmentation of the inspiratory phase (Fig. 20-10) may overcome it, or a nasopharyngeal airway (see Fig. 10-5) may be gently inserted to aid in maintaining a patent airway.

During the maintenance phase and when the surgery is in progress, the patient should be closely observed for signs of anesthesia and alterations in physical condition. As the anesthesia progresses, the oxygen should be gradually increased, perhaps 1% at a time, and care should be taken not to alter the desired level of anesthesia unduly. Many times what seems to be adequate oxygenation in the early minutes of the anesthesia proves to be inadequate as time continues. For these patients a slow increase of oxygen will be very advantageous. At times the oxygen may be increased to 20, 25, or even 30% without unduly altering the level of anesthesia.

It should be kept in mind that deep levels of anesthesia are not necessary and that, once the patient is conditioned to the stimuli, procedures can be completed in an amazingly light and safe plane.

Recovery. When the surgery is completed, 100% oxygen should be administered. Some persons disagree with the principle of switching to 100% oxygen to facilitate recovery, but I have yet to see any ill effects from this maneuver and believe that inhalation of oxygen does shorten the recovery time.

If nitrous oxide and oxygen constitute the anesthetic mixture, the patient's recovery should be complete in 2 to 3 minutes, and he will be able to proceed with help to the recovery room. He should have command of all his faculties, and within a time approximating the anesthesia time he should be able to leave the office under his own power.

Premedication. Whenever possible, it is desirable to premedicate the patient adequately before the administration of nitrous oxide and oxygen. This will produce psychic sedation and reduce the basal metabolic rate. It will also make the patient more receptive to the anesthetic and enhance the effect of the nitrous oxide. The barbiturates or narcotics have heretofore been the premedicants of choice. Recently we have been using combinations of pentobarbital (Nembutal) and promethazine (Phenergan), or meperidine (Demerol) and promethazine. These combinations have proved most effective.

When the patient has been adequately premedicated, essentially the same technique is used, with the exception that the oxygen may be started at approximately 10% and increased as indicated to 20 or 25% or more.

Supplemental agents. As previously stated, every dental anesthetic machine used to administer nitrous oxide and oxygen should be equipped with a vaporizer (see Figs. 19-8 and 19-9) for administering supplemental agents. The agents that we have used most commonly are divinyl ether (Vinethene), trichloroethylene, and fluothane.

The decision to use supplemental agents with nitrous oxide and oxygen need not be predetermined; however, the supplemental agent of choice should be available in the vaporizer on the machine for immediate use. The patient should be adequately premedicated and inducted as with nitrous oxide and oxygen, with the oxygen attaining metabolic levels. If, however, difficulty is encountered in raising the oxygen to metabolic levels without affecting the course of the anesthesia, the supplemental agent may be gradually added to the mixture to potentiate the nitrous oxide. This should then enable the oxygen level to be increased to safe limits. Under no circumstances should it be kept below metabolic limits to secure the desired results. Allowing the oxygen to fall below the metabolic level even for short periods can create serious complications because time often passes more quickly than one realizes, and what was originally intended to be a 1- or 2-minute procedure may continue for 5 minutes or more.

Divinyl ether is an excellent agent for potentiating mixtures of nitrous oxide and oxygen. In low concentrations it will adequately potentiate nitrous oxide and oxygen and stabilize the anesthetic. Like other supplemental agents, it should not replace nitrous oxide. The outstanding disadvantage of divinyl ether is that when it is added to nitrous oxide and oxygen, a flammable and explosive mixture is formed.

Trichloroethylene should be used only to potentiate mixtures of nitrous oxide and oxygen. It should be used with extreme caution in low concentrations and for comparatively short periods. When used in this conservative manner, the drug can be used in the office.

As our experience with *halothane* (fluothane) has increased, we are more and more of the opinion that this drug has many advantages for all dental patients—ambulatory, outpatient, and hospitalized. The ease and rapidity of induction, the ease of maintenance, the rapidity of recovery, and its proved safety have made it our first choice for the supplementation of nitrous oxide. So impressed have we been with halothane that we no longer attempt nitrous oxide-oxygen inductions without its potentiating effect. In fact, combination of the nitrous oxide, oxygen, and halothane has markedly reduced our use of the intravenous agents, and in many cases a venipuncture is not made until the patient is anesthetized.

All our patients are now inducted with a full face mask (see Fig. 20-9). Even when intravenous agents are used to remove patients from the realm of consciousness, the induction is completed with a full face mask and nitrous oxide, oxygen, and halothane.

Many ambulatory patients and outpatients in the office and hospital are inducted with nitrous oxide, oxygen, and halothane, a venipuncture is made, and the patient is given 40 to 60 mg. of succinylcholine chloride intravenously. A nasotracheal tube is inserted, and the patient is maintained with nitrous oxide, oxygen, and halothane. Ventilation is controlled until spontaneous breathing returns.

This technique has permitted the intubation of many more ambulatory patients and outpatients, thus assuring a patent airway and an ease of maintenance without sacrificing recovery time. In fact, when small amounts, 100 to 200 mg., of an ultrashort-acting barbiturate are used to induce unconsciousness, 40 to 60 mg. of succinylcholine chloride are used for relaxation to facilitate nasotracheal intubation, and the patient is maintained with nitrous oxide, oxygen, and halothane (0.5 to 1%), the recovery time is as fast as, if not faster than, if the patient were inducted and maintained with the intravenous drugs and nitrous oxide.

It should be realized that nitrous oxide has definite anesthetic properties, as well as considerable analgesic potency. Its inherent weakness is its principal disadvantage. However, this disadvantage in many cases can be eliminated or minimized by the judicious use of supplemental inhalation agents. When nitrous oxide and supplemental inhalation agents can be utilized for ambulatory dental patients, it is considered by many to be the method of choice.

Open drop anesthesia. The open drop method (see Figs. 6-1 and 6-2) of administering an anesthetic agent to ambulatory dental patients is limited primarily to short procedures for very young children. Divinyl ether and vinyl-ethyl ether are our agents of choice. Although many persons and some institutions have had considerable success with ethyl chloride, we have discontinued its use in favor of divinyl ether and vinyl-ethyl ether since these agents possess the advantages of ethyl chloride without its decided disadvantages. Since the introduction of halothane, the open drop techniques have been used mainly for teaching purposes.

Method of administration. Divinyl ether or vinyl-ethyl ether is administered by slowly dropping the volatile agent on a 4 × 4 gauze sponge (see Fig. 6-2) approximately six to eight layers in thickness or on a wire ether mask covered with gauze or a stockinette (see Fig. 6-1). The gauze or mask covering should be thick enough so that it vaporizes the liquid and at the same time permits an adequate intake of oxygen and an efficient elimination of carbon dioxide. We have followed the procedure of inserting an oxygen hook into the mouth and not wrapping the mask or gauze with a towel or other cover.

Whenever indicated, the child is adequately premedicated and the eyes are protected. For some patients it is best to apply the protective covering to the eyes after the induction in order not to alarm the paient unduly. Whenever possible, the child's confidence should be gained by talking to him in a reassuring voice.

The rate of drop, which is slow at first, should be gradually increased, depending on how the patient tolerates the administration.

For the majority of patients we do not insert a mouth prop prior to or during induction.

When the induction is completed and the mouth opened with a prop, an oropharyngeal partition is placed in position. A few drops of the anesthetic agent may be placed on the partition to stabilize the anesthetic. The administration is continued, and the gauze is restricted to the nasal area so that access to the oral cavity is not impaired. The anesthetic agent can then be dropped on the nasal covering or oropharyngeal partition as needed to maintain an adequate level of anesthesia.

Since this method is employed for short procedures on children, deep planes of anesthesia are not required. Even slight movements on the part of the patient should not be considered objectionable so long as they do not interfere with the procedure.

The patency of the airway must be assured since any interference, no matter how slight, will reduce pulmonary ventilation. The head should be in a proper position and the lower jaw adequately supported. When the oropharyngeal partition is in place, the tongue should be drawn forward. If necessary, a nasopharyngeal tube may be inserted to maintain the patency of the airway.

Although the open drop method does have a definite place for use on ambulatory dental patients, it should be confined to short procedures on younger children, and it should not be employed unless suction apparatus and all necessary resuscitative equipment are available.

Intravenous anesthesia. The intravenous anesthetic agents have had a tremendous influence on anesthetic procedures for ambulatory dental patients, and when properly used, they offer many advantages. Unfortunately, they have been misused and abused. Much of this abuse has been due, apparently, to the erroneous assumption that inserting a needle into a vein and pressing the plunger of a syringe to administer the anesthetic are simple procedures.

The use of the intravenous barbiturates for ambulatory dental patients has been much discussed. In my opinion, these drugs are definitely indicated for office use. It has been stated that they should not be used unless trained personnel and facilities are available, but this holds true for all the anesthetics, not just the intravenous agents.

The use of Pentothal as the sole anesthetic should be restricted to short procedures only (less than 5 minutes), and even then we believe in administering oxygen (see Fig. 20-1) during this interval. When using this technique, we employ thiopental (Pentothal), thiamylal (Surital) or methohexital sodium (Brevital). The first 3 or 4 ml. are given rather slowly, with close observation of the patient during this time and for 25 to 30 seconds following. If no untoward reactions or exaggerated effects are manifested, the induction may be completed within 45 seconds to 1 minute.

When the induction is completed, the lower jaw will be sufficiently relaxed to permit easy insertion of a mouth prop. The oropharyngeal partition should be placed very carefully, not so far posteriorly (see Fig. 15-2) that it may stimulate the phrayngeal or laryngeal reflexes, which are usually still present and active.

The proper plane of anesthesia will be attained when the lid reflex is absent and the respirations are slightly depressed. The lower jaw will be relaxed and the pupils will react to light. One of the most important signs will be the patient's reaction to painful stimuli. In my opinion it is better that an ambulatory patient react slightly to the initial stimulus than to be overdepressed in order that this slight reaction be avoided. This initial stimulation by the operator should be gentle and for the purpose of learning the patient's reaction to it. Gentle stimulation also tends to condition the patient to such an extent that lighter planes of anesthesia can be used eventually.

It is our practice to administer oxygen by a nasal mask (see Fig. 20-3) for short procedures. This not only improves oxygenation but also permits the immediate use of nitrous oxide and oxygen if the procedure becomes longer than anticipated. In addition, the benefits of the combination are advantageous.

Combined intravenous and inhalation techniques. The combined use of intravenous and inhalation agents offers many advantages in the administration of anesthesia for ambulatory patients (see Fig. 20-3). This sequence closely approaches the four requirements of the ideal anesthetic for ambulatory patients—namely, rapid induction, smooth maintenance, rapid recovery, and a high degree of safety. This combination should be judiciously employed so that the agents will complement each other, which enables one to utilize their advantages and eliminate their disadvantages.

The intravenous agents offer a rapid induction and potentiate the inhalation agent. Nitrous oxide, the inhalation agent, greatly reduces the amount of the intravenous agent required for smooth maintenance and thus permits more rapid recovery. The controllability of the inhalation agent and the smaller amounts of intravenous agent increase the safety factor.

A variety of combinations may be used. The most common are (1) intravenous ultrashort-acting barbiturate and nitrous oxide and oxygen; (2) intravenous ultrashort-acting barbiturate, nitrous oxide and oxygen, and halothane; (3) intravenous narcotic (usually Demerol), a psychosedative drug, promethazine (Phenergan), hydroxyzine (Vistaril), and nitrous oxide and oxygen; (4) intravenous narcotic (usually Demerol), psychosedative drug (Phenergan or Vistaril), an ultrashort-acting barbiturate, and nitrous oxide and oxygen; and (5) nitrous oxide and oxygen and halothane plus an intravenous narcotic (usually Demerol).

When an ultrashort-acting barbiturate has been specified, it refers to thiopental sodium (Pentothal), thiamylal sodium (Surital), or methohexital sodium (Brevital). Each may be used interchangeably without altering the technique particularly. In some few cases, very small doses of muscle relaxants may be added when specifically indicated.

Intravenous thiopental sodium and nitrous oxide and oxygen. With this combination, we routinely use atropine or scopolamine for premedication unless they are specifically contraindicated. The thiopental sodium (2%) is administered as though it were to be used alone, except that when the lid reflex is absent, nitrous oxide and oxygen are administered in mixtures of 80 to 85% nitrous oxide and 15 to 20% oxygen. By initially depressing the patient, the intravenous agent potentiates the effect of the nitrous oxide and many times permits the anesthetic to be continued with nitrous oxide and oxygen and no additional intravenous drug.

The needle, however, is left in place and its patency is maintained by a slow drip of normal saline solution or 5% glucose in water. Small amounts of the intravenous agent may be administered at intervals if necessary. The mixtures of nitrous oxide and oxygen may be varied as indicated, but the patient must be adequately oxygenated while at the same time the maximum benefits are derived from the nitrous oxide. As with nitrous oxide and oxygen when used alone, the percentage of oxygen should be gradually increased as the procedure continues; it is not unusual to use 30 to 50% or more of oxygen with a corresponding decrease in the percentage of nitrous oxide.

When this technique is employed, a mouth prop is not used until the induction is completed, after which it is inserted and the oropharyngeal partition is placed in proper position. Throughout the anesthesia the inspiration is augmented and mouth breathing eliminated or reduced to a minimum. This permits the full utilization of the nitrous oxide as well as of the intravenous agent.

The amount of intravenous agent (Pentothal, Surital, or Brevital) will necessarily vary, depending on the patient's requirements. It should be stated that the intravenous agent in this technique is a controlled premedication and basal anesthetic, although additional amounts may be added at intervals if necessary.

While the recovery time for this combination is not so rapid as that for nitrous oxide and oxygen alone, it is prolonged only slightly. As a rule, the patient can leave the chair with help within a few minutes and can depart from the office under his own power within a reasonable length of time when accompanied by a responsible adult. The amount of Pentothal (2%) used may vary from 200 to 400 mg., depending on the duration of the procedure and the individual patient.

As previously stated, the anesthesia and surgery time for our ambulatory patients usually does not exceed 30 minutes; we do not advocate prolonged procedures. These patients may or may not be intubated; however, the introduction of the muscle relaxants so facilitates intubation without an increased depth of anesthesia that it is now feasible to intubate more ambulatory patients. This does not alter the fact that for many patients a patent airway can be maintained and the patient adequately oxygenated without intubation. However, under the present setup and hospital arrangements, we prefer to hospitalize any patient who may present an anesthetic problem.

Intravenous meperidine, promethazine, and nitrous oxide and oxygen. In this technique, meperidine and promethazine in doses of 12.5 to 50 mg. of each are given slowly intravenously, and the needle is kept open by a slow infusion of normal saline solution or 5% glucose in water, After 2 or 3 minutes or when the full effect of the intravenous medication is in evidence, nitrous oxide and oxygen are administered as previously described, using the intravenous medication to potentiate the action. The analgesic and cortical-depressing effects of the intravenous meperidine and promethazine enable the anesthetist to maintain a satisfactory level of anesthesia with nitrous oxide and oxygen without reducing the oxygen to hypoxic levels. Whenever necessary, small amounts of meperidine and promethazine may be added, but as a rule this is not required.

We have modified this procedure somewhat by administering meperidine and promethazine initially, plus nitrous oxide and oxygen as previously described, with the addition of a slow, continuous drip of meperidine to aid in maintaining a satisfactory level of anesthesia.

The recovery time when this combination is used is within the range for the combination of an intravenous barbiturate and nitrous oxide. It has the added advantage of a high degree of analgesic potency, with the result that a large percentage of the patients react without pain or restlessness.

Intravenous meperidine, promethazine, thiopental sodium, and nitrous oxide and oxygen. This combination may appear to comprise an excessive number of drugs for a seemingly minor surgical procedure. However, the components blend well and each is administered for a definite purpose. The mixture of meperidine and promethazine, 12.5 to 25 mg. of each, has a high analgesic potency and a depressing effect on the cerebral cortex. The intravenous thiopental sodium is administered to complete the induction. A sufficient interval (60 to 90 seconds) should elapse between the administration of the mixtures of meperidine and promethazine and the thiopental sodium to allow the effect of the former drugs to be observed and also to prevent any contact between these drugs and the thiopental sodium, since they are incompatible and, when mixed, will produce a cloudy precipitate. The interval also permits the anesthetist to determine whether thiopental sodium will be necessary and to judge its effect if given. The nitrous oxide and oxygen is then used as previously described to maintain the proper plane of anesthesia. Small amounts of Pentothal may be administered at intervals if necessary.

It should be realized that moderate or depressed stages of anesthesia are unnecessary for ambulatory patients, and the necessary surgery can be efficiently accomplished in the light surgical plane. Even slight movements on the part of the patient are not to be frowned upon so long as they do not interfere with the surgical procedure. Therefore all that may be required of the anesthetic combinations is that one or more of the drugs possess sufficient analgesic potency to alleviate pain and that the other agents remove conscious awareness. When other undesirable reflexes can be adequately controlled, the lighter the stage of anesthesia, the safer the procedure will be.

Chemanesia and analgesia. With this thought in mind, some years ago we used various combinations to achieve this purpose. We termed the procedure chemanesia plus analgesia and gave a preliminary report in May, 1957.* Since that report and the introduction of meperidine and promethazine mixtures, we have altered our procedure. This technique has enabled us to treat ambulatory patients requiring longer and more difficult procedures than was previously advisable and also to include poor-risk patients who otherwise could not be effectively treated.

Chemanesia combined with analgesia is physiologically more normal and therefore safer for the patient than is surgical anesthesia; the advantage increases as the anesthesia time increases. Consequently, we feel that if a procedure longer than 30 minutes is contemplated and there is no definite contraindication to the drugs to be used, the patient should be offered the safety and lack of unpleasantness of this technique.

The chemanesia-analgesia technique is a highly individualized form of medication, and the dosages of the drugs will vary with the age, mental status, and physical condition of the patient and with the length of the procedure. The mental preparation of the patient is important; he should be told that he may feel pressure and hear sounds or voices but that he will be perfectly comfortable and relaxed.

---

*Peiffer, G. W., and Monheim, L. M.: Preliminary report on chemanesia combined with analgesia for the ambulatory dental patient, Oral Surg. **10**:504, 1957.

The short-acting barbiturates, pentobarbital (Nembutal) and secobarbital (Seconal), are given very slowly intravenously until a total of 50 to 100 mg. is reached, depending upon the individual patient. After the tube is clear, meperidine (Demerol) and promethazine (Phenergan) or hydroxyzine (Vistaril) in doses of 12.5 to 50 mg. each are slowly given until the patient feels "unusual" or drowsy. It is necessary to clear the tubing of the barbiturate before administering the narcotic, as the difference in pH will produce a white precipitate if the drugs or given together. After each drug is given, a short time should be allowed to elapse for the full effect to become evident. Overmedication may result if the administration is too rapid. The intravenous needle is allowed to remain in place and is kept patent by a slow drip of normal saline solution or 5% dextrose in water.

After the maximum effect of the drugs has been achieved, the nasal inhaler is placed over the nose and nitrous oxide and oxygen are administered, with the nitrous oxide kept at 50% or less.

When the desired effect of the drugs is manifested, the area to be operated on is rendered pain-free by the administration of regional analgesia (local anesthesia). The level of chemanesia may be estimated at the time of the insertion of the needle since the patient should show little or no reaction to the needle puncture. Local anesthesia is an integral part of this technique, and its effectiveness will ensure the success of the procedure.

During the procedure, the patient's reactions should be closely observed so that the mixtures of nitrous oxide and oxygen may be varied to suit his needs. In most cases it will be necessary to reduce the percentage of nitrous oxide as time elapses. It has not been unusual to use 25% nitrous oxide and 75% oxygen eventually for prolonged procedures.

It should be stressed that with this technique the patient will at no time be beyond light, second-stage anesthesia. The vast majority of patients will be able to hear and to respond sluggishly to commands but will not remember their experiences.

Anesthesia for outpatients

We arbitrarily use the classification of outpatient for patients who can be discharged the same day but not within as little time as the ambulatory patient can be discharged. These patients are cared for in the hospital as outpatients but can be admitted if the need arises. To date we have had no situation arise in which a patient had to be hospitalized.

The technique for outpatients more closely resembles that employed for hospitalized patients rather than that employed for ambulatory patients, in that the majority of patients are intubated. We do, however, limit the outpatients to A risks, and there must be a definite indication and good reason for the patient to be so classified. As compared to ambulatory and hospitalized patients, outpatients are generally a small minority. Therefore, since the techniques described in the discussion on anesthesia for hospitalized patients apply also to outpatients, techniques for outpatients are not discussed separately.

Anesthesia for hospitalized patients

Anesthesia for hospitalized patients will in all instances be dictated by the needs of the individual patient. The vast majority of patients will have been hospitalized because they cannot be treated as ambulatory patients or outpatients. This may be due to the type of surgery required, the patient's general physical condition, or his age.

A hospitalized dental patient should be treated exactly the same as any other patient on the surgical service in that he should be admitted at least 24 hours prior to surgery. He should have a medical evaluation and routine medical care. The preoperative medication and anesthetic procedure should depend on the physical condition and age of the patient, the surgery to be accomplished, and the type of anesthesia to be used.

A patent airway is maintained for practically all hospitalized patients by the insertion of a cuffed nasotracheal tube (Fig. 10-13). Occasionally, however, a very short procedure may be accomplished without employing this type of airway. However, since the introduction of muscle relaxants, intubation has been so simplified that practically all hospitalized patients are maintained with a nasotracheal airway. In my opinion this has in no way prolonged the induction or the recovery but has made the overall procedure more satisfactory.

The anesthesia sequences most commonly employed by us for hospitalized patients are as follows.

Regardless of the technique or anesthesia sequence, all patients are seen the night before surgery and informed about the contemplated procedures and any routines that they are expected to follow. If, for example, the anesthesia and surgery are to take place during the morning hours, the patient is told that he may eat his evening meal but may have no solids thereafter. Liquids, however, are permitted until midnight.

The preanesthetic orders are then written on the chart. Although they will vary from patient to patient, an example for a healthy 20-

to 30-year-old male weighing 70 kilograms and scheduled for surgery at 8 A.M. would be as follows:

Preanesthetic orders for tomorrow, 7/21/67

7/20/67	1. N.P.O. after midnight	
1800	2. Nembutal, 150 mg.	I.M. at 7 A.M.
	3. Vistaril, 75 mg.	
	4. Morphine, 10 mg.	
	5. Scopolamine, 0.5 mg.	

Name ________________ Narcotic no.________

Care should be exercised that all orders be written legibly and clearly, so that they not only can be read but can be understood.

The following morning in the operating room the most frequently used technique is the following sequence:

1. Ultrashort-acting barbiturate (Pentothal, Surital, Brevital) is given intravenously until the lid reflex is absent (approximately 150 to 250 mg.).
2. Muscle relaxant (succinylcholine chloride) is injected intravenously (60 to 100 mg.).
3. Ventilate patient with nitrous oxide (3 L./min.), oxygen (2 L./min.), and halothane (0.5%).
4. When patient is relaxed, insert a cuffed nasotracheal tube (usually 30 or 32 Fr.) by direct laryngoscopy, and inflate the cuff.
5. Attach the nasotracheal tube to the breathing tubes of the anesthetic machine with the proper adapters (Fig. 20-11) and continue to ventilate the patient until spontaneous breathing returns.
6. The patient may be maintained with nitrous oxide and oxygen, or nitrous oxide, oxygen, and halothane. Most often the patient is maintained with nitrous oxide (3 L.), oxygen (2 L.), and halothane (0.5 to 1%).
7. After the surgical procedure is completed, suction the pharynx and oral cavity well. Aspirate through the nasotracheal tube only when indicated, and with a sterile catheter.
8. Insert an oropharyngeal airway.
9. Discontinue the halothane and nitrous oxide. Increase the oxygen and allow the patient to breathe spontaneously for 10 to 12 respirations.
10. Deflate the cuff and remove the nasotracheal tube. If the proper plane of anesthesia has been reached, the patient should not buck, cough, or hold his breath.
11. Place a full face mask on the patient's face, and after 10 to

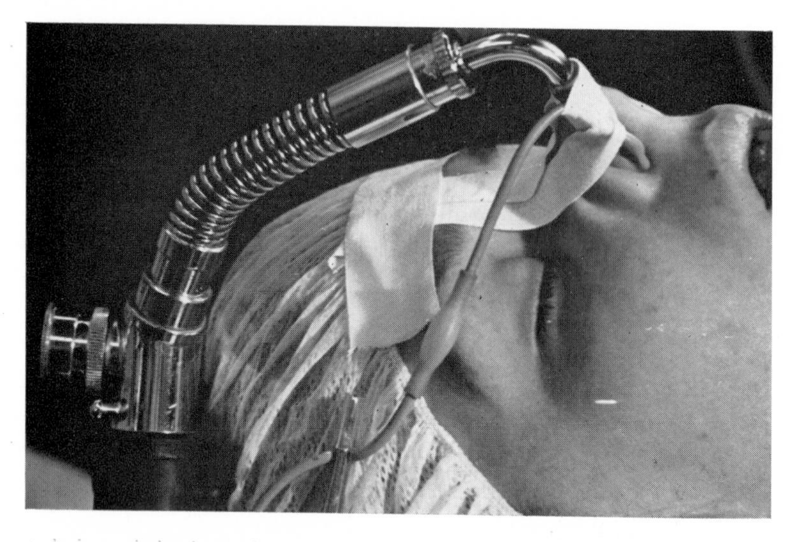

Fig. 20-11. Gooseneck adapter for attaching nasotracheal tube to breathing tubes.

12 breaths remove the mask and transfer the patient to the recovery room.

As a rule the patient will have reacted within a time approximating the surgery time, and he can be discharged from the recovery room to his department.

An increasingly used technique is the following:

1. Induct the patient with nitrous oxide (3 L.), oxygen (2 L.), and halothane (1 to 3%).
2. When a light surgical plane of anesthesia has been attained, a venipuncture is made (in some cases the venipuncture is made before the induction has been started), and 40 to 60 mg. of succinylcholine chloride are injected.
3. The patient is ventilated with nitrous oxide (3 L.), oxygen (2 L.), and halothane (0.5 to 1%).
4. When the relaxation is complete, a cuffed nasotracheal tube is inserted into the trachea by direct laryngoscopy, and the cuff inflated.
5. The patient is ventilated with nitrous oxide (3 L.), oxygen (2 L.), and halothane (0.5 to 1%), until spontaneous breathing occurs.
6. The patient is maintained with the above concentrations.
7. After the surgical procedure is completed, follow steps 7, 8, 9, 10, and 11 of the immediately preceding technique.

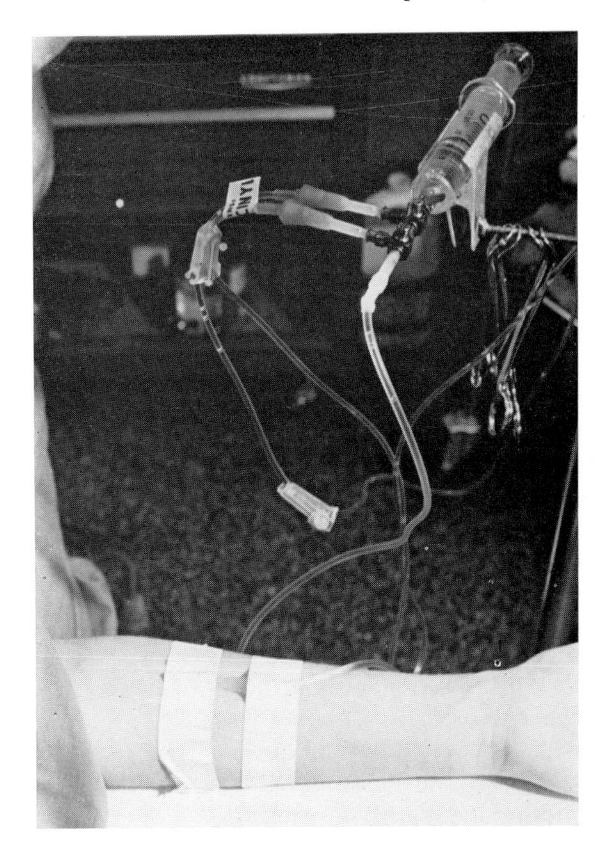

Fig. 20-12. The continuous presence of an intravenous needle or catheter makes possible the administration of intravenous fluids or drugs.

In as many cases as possible the patients are inducted with nitrous oxide, oxygen, and halothane. No intravenous barbiturates are used, and the patients react more quickly with less mental depression and confusion. If the premedication is limited to the belladonna drugs, and the inhalation agents alone are used to induce and maintain anesthesia, the recovery is rapid and complete.

Throughout the procedure an intravenous needle is kept in place. During major cases an intercath or angiocath may be inserted. Five percent dextrose in water or lactated Ringer's solution is administered to keep the intravenous route patent. Narcotics (morphine, 2 mg. per milliliter, and Demerol, 10 mg. per milliliter) are used with increasing frequency. Their use has reduced the amount of anesthetic drugs necessary to maintain a satisfactory level of anesthesia. The intravenous narcotics also permit a more placid arousal. In fact, the narcotics have become an increasingly important ingredient of a general anesthetic.

The previously discussed techniques offer the following advantages:

1. With either the intravenous or inhalation method, the induction is usually rapid, smooth, and pleasant.
2. The use of the muscle relaxants offers ideal conditions for intubation without depressed planes of anesthesia.
3. A satisfactory plane of anesthesia can be maintained easily without hypoxia.
4. The presence of the intravenous needle (Fig. 20-12) or catheter makes possible the administration of narcotics or other drugs when indicated.
5. The intratracheal techniques enable the anesthetist to function free of the operative field.
6. Augmentation or control of ventilation is possible.
7. The tracheobronchial tree is protected by an inflatable cuff.
8. The recovery time is short and uncomplicated.

Open drop techniques. Previously, Vinethine and ether, alone or in combination, were used to produce satisfactory, safe anesthesia for children. However, since the introduction of halothane and the muscle relaxants, the open drop techniques have been used rather infrequently, and mainly for teaching purposes.

Rectal anesthesia. The rectal administration of Avertin, ultrashort-acting barbiturates, and ether is being used less and less frequently. The introduction of the psychosedative drugs, among others, has made it possible to secure excellent sedation by intramuscular injection. Sufficient time should elapse for the drugs to attain their greatest effectiveness. This indicates that the procedure should be planned to allow from 45 minutes to an hour for the intramuscular drugs to obtain the maximum results. As a general rule, psychic depression will be more in evidence than respiratory or circulatory depression. The induction will, of course, be complete with the inhalation or the intravenous agents. The rectal route, as the open drop method, is used mainly for teaching purposes.

The most commonly used rectal drug is Pentothal. Table 20-1 lists suggested basic doses of Pentothal for preanesthetic hypnosis and basal anesthesia. The term basic is used to designate the doses that have proved effective for the majority of patients. It should be stressed that these doses should be varied according to the needs of the individual patient, and the dose should be reduced if the patient is obese, or if an untoward condition exists.

Table 20-1. Suggested basic doses of Pentothal for preanesthetic hypnosis and basal anesthesia

For preanesthetic hypnosis	
In grams of Pentothal	1 Gm./75 lb.; 1 Gm./34.1 kg.
In milligrams of Pentothal	13.3 mg./lb.; 29.3 mg./kg.
In milliliters of 10% solution	0.13 ml./lb.; 0.29 ml./kg.
In milliliters of 3% solution	0.44 ml./lb.; 0.98 ml./kg.
In milliliters of 2% solution	0.67 ml./lb.; 1.47 ml./kg.
For basal anesthesia	
In grams of Pentothal	1 Gm./50 lb.; 1 Gm./22.7 kg.
In milligrams of Pentothal	20.0 mg./lb.; 44.1 mg./kg.
In milliliters of 10% solution	0.20 ml./lb.; 0.44 ml./kg.
In milliliters of 3% solution	0.67 ml./lb.; 1.47 ml./kg.
In milliliters of 2% solution	1.00 ml./lb.; 2.21 ml./kg.

The following formula may be used for calculating the basic dose in milliliters:

$$\frac{W \times P}{10\ N} = \text{number of milliliters in the basic dose}$$

W = body weight
P = milligrams of Pentothal per lb. or kg. of body weight
N = percent of concentration of solution
10 N = milligrams per milliliter

Example:
Patient weighs 20 kg., W = 20
Basal anesthesia desired, P = 44.1
5% solution used, 10 N = 50

$$\text{Basic dose} = \frac{20 \times 44.1}{50} = 17.64 \text{ ml.}$$

SUMMARY

As previously stated, techniques for the administration of anesthesia are many and varied, and each anesthetist develops his own likes and dislikes. For this reason I have discussed the techniques most commonly used by us, with the full realization that they will differ in many respects from those used by many others. It is not my intent to claim superiority for them but only to state that they have proved successful for us. Nevertheless, we constantly vary our procedures, with the hope of improvement.

References

General references

American Medical Association: Fundamentals of anesthesia, ed. 3, Philadelphia, 1954, W. B. Saunders Co.

Burstein, C. L.: Fundamental considerations in anesthesia, ed. 3, Springfield, Ill., 1966, Charles C Thomas, Publisher.

Cecil, R. L., and Loeb, R. F.: A textbook of medicine, ed. 10, Philadelphia, 1959, W. B. Saunders Co.

Clement, F.: Nitrous oxide anesthesia, Philadelphia, 1952, Lea & Febiger.

Collins, V. J.: Principles and practice of anesthesiology, Philadelphia, 1952, Lea & Febiger.

Conference on Neurophysiology in Relation to Anesthesiology, Seattle, May 13-14, 1966, Anesthesiology **28**:1, 1967.

Cullen, S. C.: Anesthesia, ed. 6, Chicago, 1961, Year Book Medical Publishers, Inc.

Dorland's illustrated medical dictionary, ed. 24, Philadelphia, 1965, W. B. Saunders Co.

Dornette, W. H. L.: Anatomy for the anesthesiologist, Springfield, Ill., 1963, Charles C Thomas, Publisher.

Evans, F. T., and Gray, T. C.: General anesthesia, ed. 2, vols. 1 and 2, London, 1965, Butterworth & Co.

Ganong, W. L.: Review of medical physiology, ed. 2, Los Altos, Calif., 1965, Lange Medical Publications.

Lee, J. A.: A synopsis of anesthesia, ed. 4, Baltimore, 1959, The Williams & Wilkins Co.

MacIntoch, R. R., and Pratt-Bannister, F. B.: Essentials of general anesthesia with special reference to dentistry, ed. 5, Oxford, 1952, Blackwell Scientific Publications.

Mackenzie, J. R.: Practical anesthetics, ed. 2, London, 1946, Bailliere, Tindall & Cox.

Powell, W. F.: Comprehensive background for anesthesiologists, Springfield, Ill., 1966, Charles C Thomas, Publisher.

Swartz, C. H., Ngar, S., and Papper, E.: Manual of anesthesiology, Springfield, Ill., 1957, Charles C Thomas, Publisher.
Wright, S.: Applied physiology, ed. 11, London, 1965, Oxford University Press.

Chapters 1 to 4

Ashley, F. L., and Love, H. G.: Fluid and electrolyte therapy, Philadelphia, 1954, J. B. Lippincott Co.
Best, C. H., and Taylor, N. B.: Physiological basis of medical practice, ed. 8, Baltimore, 1966, The Williams & Wilkins Co.
Comroe, J. H., Jr.: The lung, ed. 2, Chicago, 1962, Year Book Medical Publishers, Inc.
Comroe, J. H., Jr.: Physiology of respiration, Chicago, 1965, Year Book Medical Publishers, Inc.
Dale, H. H.: Chemical transmission of effects of nerve impulses (Linacre Lecture), Brit. Med. J. **1**:835, 1934.
DiPalma, J. R., editor: Drill's pharmacology in medicine, ed. 3, New York, 1965, McGraw-Hill Book Co.
Drinker, C. K.: The clinical physiology of the lungs, Springfield, Ill., 1954, Charles C Thomas, Publisher.
Elliott, H. C.: Textbook of the nervous system, ed. 2, Philadelphia, 1954, J. B. Lippincott Co.
Goth, A.: Medical pharmacology, ed. 3, St. Louis, 1966, The C. V. Mosby Co.
Gray, J. S.: Pulmonary ventilation and its physiological regulation. In Pitts, R. F., editor: American lectures in physiology (American Lecture Series), Springfield, Ill., 1950, Charles C Thomas, Publisher.
Guyton, A. C.: Textbook of medical physiology, ed. 3, Philadelphia, 1966, W. B. Saunders Co.
Haussay, B. A.: Human physiology, New York, 1951, McGraw-Hill Book Co.
Kimber, D. C., Grey, C. E., Stackpole, C. E., and Leavitt, L. C.: Textbook of anatomy and physiology, ed. 9, London, 1956, Oxford University Press.
Luchsinger, P. C., and Moser, K. M., editors: Respiration: physiologic principles and their clinical applications, St. Louis, 1960, The C. V. Mosby Co.
MacIntosh, R. R., and Mushin, W. W.: Physics for the anesthetist, Sprinfield, Ill., 1946, Charles C Thomas, Publisher.
Main, R. J., and Richardson, A. W.: Physiology, ed. 2, St. Louis, 1953, The C. V. Mosby Co.
Mendel, B., and Rudney, H.: Studies on cholinesterase: cholinesterase and pseudocholinesterase, Biochem. J. **37**:59, 1943.
Moyer, C. A.: Fluid balance, a clinical manual, Chicago, 1952, Year Book Medical Publishers, Inc.
National Academy of Sciences–National Research Council: Handbook of respiration, Philadelphia, 1958, W. B. Saunders Co.
Price, H. L., and Cohen, P. J.: Effects of anesthetics on the circulation, Springfield, Ill., 1964, Charles C Thomas, Publisher.
Rothlin, E., and Berde, E.: The structure and function of the autonomic nervous system, Aerztl. Mschr. **5**:865, 1949.
Statland, H.: Fluid and electrolytes in practice, ed. 3, Philadelphia, 1963, J. B. Lippincott Co.
Tovey, G. H.: Technique of fluid balance, ed. 2, Springfield, Ill., 1960, Charles C Thomas, Publisher.

White, J. C., Smithwich, R. H., and Simeone, F. A.: The autonomic nervous system, ed. 3, New York, 1952, The Macmillan Co.

Wyburn, G. M.: The nervous system, New York, 1960, Academic Press, Inc.

Youmans, W. B.: Basic medical physiology, Chicago, 1952, Year Book Medical Publishers, Inc.

Chapters 5 to 7

Beecher, H. K.: The physiology of anesthesia, London, 1938, Oxford University Press.

Flagg, P. J.: The art of anesthesia, ed. 7, Philadelphia, 1944, J. B. Lippincott Co.

Guedel, A. E.: Inhalation anesthesia, ed. 2, New York, 1951, The Macmillan Co.

Harris, T. A. B.: The mode of action of anesthetics, Edinburgh, 1951, E. & S. Livingstone, Ltd.

Kemp, W. N.: Elementary anesthesia, Balitomore, 1948, The Williams & Wilkins Co.

Minnitt, R. J., and Gillies, J.: Textbook of anesthetics, ed. 6, Edinburgh, 1945, E. & S. Livingstone, Ltd.

Parry-Price, H.: Practical anesthetics, Baltimore, 1946, The Williams & Wilkins Co.

Plomley, F.: Stages of anesthesia, Lancet **1**:134, 1847.

Snow, J.: On the inhalation of the vapor of ether in surgical operations, London, 1847, J. & A. Churchill, Ltd.

Snow, J.: On chloroform and other anesthetics, London, 1848, J. & A. Churchill, Ltd.

Chapters 8 and 9

Adams, R. C.: Intravenous anesthesia, New York, 1944, Paul B. Hoeber, Inc.

Adriani, J.: The chemistry of anesthesia, Springfield, Ill., 1952, Charles C Thomas, Publisher.

Adriani, J.: The pharmacology of anesthetic drugs, ed. 4, Springfield, Ill., 1960, Charles C Thomas, Publisher.

Artusio, Joseph F., editor: Halogenated anesthetics, clinical anesthesia, Philadelphia, 1963, F. A. Davis Co.

Bergersen, B. S., and Krug, E. E.: Pharmacology in nursing, ed. 10, St. Louis, 1966, The C. V. Mosby Co.

Foldes, F. F.: Muscle relaxants in anesthesiology, Springfield, Ill., 1957, Charles C Thomas, Publisher.

Goodman, L. S., and Gilman, A.: The pharmacological basis of therapeutics, ed. 3, New York, 1965, The Macmillan Co.

Johnstone, M.: The human cardiovascular response to fluothane anesthesia, Brit. J. Anaesth. **28**:392, 1956.

Krantz, J. C., Jr., and Carr, C. J.: The pharmacologic principles of medical practice, ed. 6, Baltimore, 1965, The Williams & Wilkins Co.

Modell, W., editor: Drugs of choice 1968-1969, St. Louis, 1967, The C. V. Mosby Co.

Papper, E. M., and deBeer, E. J., editors: Proceedings of the Conference on the Myoneural Junction, New York, 1955, sponsored by the Department of Anesthesia, Columbia University College of Physicians and Surgeons, and the Burroughs Wellcome Co.

Salter, W. T.: A textbook of pharmacology, Philadelphia, 1952, W. B. Saunders Co.

Selye, H.: Anesthetic effect of steroid hormones, Proc. Soc. Exp. Biol. Med. **46**:116, 1941.
Sollman, T. H.: Manual of pharmacology, ed. 8, Philadelphia, 1957, W. B. Saunders Co.
Symposium on Fluothane, Canad. Anaesth. Soc. J. **4**:183-289, 1957.

Chapter 10

Gillespie, N. A.: Endotracheal anesthesia, ed. 3, Madison, Wis., 1963, University of Wisconsin Press.
Nicholson, M. J.: Technique of endotracheal anesthesia, Surg. Clin. N. Amer. **29**:941, 1949.
Thomas, G. J.: Technique in intubation anesthesia, Anesth. Analg. **17**:301, 1938.
Touffier, T.: Insufflation intratracheale, ses indications, Bull. Soc. Chir. Paris **40**:361, 1914.

Chapters 11 to 14

Adriani, J.: Selection of anesthesia, Springfield, Ill., 1955, Charles C Thomas, Publisher.
Burkett, L. W.: Oral medicine, ed. 5, Philadelphia, 1965, J. B. Lippincott Co.
Comroe, B. I., Collins, L. H., and Crane, M. P.: Internal medicine in dental practice, ed. 4, Philadelphia, 1954, Lea & Febiger.
Dripps, R. D., Eckenhoff, J. E., and Vandam, L. D.: Introduction to anesthesia, ed. 2, Philadelphia, 1961, W. B. Saunders Co.
Hyman, H. T.: Handbook of differential diagnosis, ed. 2, Philadelphia, 1957, J. B. Lippincott Co.
Nicholson, M. J.: Preoperative preparation and premedication, Surg. Clin. N. Amer. **30**:635, 1950.
Prior, J. A., and Silberstein, J. S.: Physical diagnosis, ed. 2, St. Louis, 1963, The C. V. Mosby Co.
Todd, J. C., Sanford, A. H., and Wells, B B.: Clinical diagnosis by laboratory methods, ed. 12, Philadelphia, 1955, W. B. Saunders Co.

Chapter 15

Hosler, R. M.: Emergency treatment of cardiac arrest in surgery. In Hospital topics and buyer's guide, Chicago, 1951, Hospital Topics, Inc.
Hosler, R. M.: Training in resuscitation of the heart, Ohio Med. J. **48**:228, 1952.
Hosler, R. M.: Cardiac arrest from the otolaryngologist's viewpoint, Arch. Otolaryng. **57**:371, 1953.
Hosler, R. M.: Cardiac resuscitation, J. Amer. Geriat. Soc. **1**:459, 1953.
Hosler, R. M.: The emergency treatment of cardiac arrest, J. Int. Coll. Surg. **19**:336, 1953.
Hosler, R. M.: A manual of cardiac resuscitation, ed. 2, Springfield, Ill., 1958, Charles C Thomas, Publisher.
Jacoby, F. F., Hary, J. A., Ziegler, C. H., and Hamelberg, W.: Safety in surgery, Anesth. Analg. **34**:346, 1955.
Keating, V.: Anaesthetic accidents, ed. 2, London, 1961, Lloyd-Luke Medical Books, Ltd.
Monheim, L. M.: Technique for creating an emergency airway in cases of respiratory obstruction, J. Oral Surg. **2**:57, 1953.

Moon, V. H.: Shock and related capillary phenomena, London, 1938, Oxford University Press.

Nataf, H. E., and Lodove, M. S.: Cardiovascular collapse in the operating room, Philadelphia, 1958, J. B. Lippincott Co.

Ruzicka, E. R.: Acute circulatory emergencies, Surg. Clin. N. Amer. **30**:713, 1950.

Zoll, P. M.: Resuscitation of the heart in ventricular standstill by external electrical stimulation, New Eng. J. Med. **247**:768, 1952.

Chapter 16

Album, M. M.: Dental procedures and general anesthesia in cerebral palsy, Dent. Dig. **58**:296, 1952.

Album, M. M.: Dentistry for the handicapped child, Dent. Radiogr. Photogr. **27**:57, 1954.

Album, M. M.: Trichloroethylene anesthesia for operative dentistry on handicapped patients, Oral Surg. **7**:488, 1954.

Album, M. M.: Significance of general anesthesia in operative dentistry, J. Dent. Child. **23**:203, 1956.

Brown, E., and Kopel, H. M.: Procedure of general anesthesia for operative dentistry, J. Dent. Child. **22**:184, 1955.

Buckman, N.: Balanced premedication in pedodontics, J. Dent. Child. **23**:141, 1956.

Gross, G.: General anesthesia for pedodontics, J. Dent. Child. **21**:25, 1954.

Hamilton, W. K., and Eastwood, D. W.: A study of denitrogenation with some inhalation anesthetic systems, Anesthesiology **16**:861, 1955.

Hunt, K. H.: Resistance in valves and canisters, Anesthesiology **16**:190, 1955.

Jackson, E. B.: Treatment of the young child in the hospital, Amer. J. Orthopsychiat. **12**:56, 1942.

Kaye, R.: Patient work-up at hospital admittance, J. Dent. Child. **23**:200, 1956.

Leigh, M. D., and Belton, M. K.: Pediatric anesthesia, New York, 1948, The Macmillan Co.

Levy, D. M.: Psychic trauma of operations in children, Amer. J. Dis. Child. **69**:7, 1945.

Lewis, G.: Nonrebreathing valve, Anaesthesia **17**:618, 1956.

Pender, J. W.: Endotracheal anesthesia in children; advantages and disadvantages, Anesthesiology **15**:495, 1954.

Prugh, D. G.: Investigations dealing with the reactions of children and families to hospitalization and illness: problems and potentialities. In Caplan, G., editor: Emotional problems of early childhood, New York, 1955, Basic Books, Inc.

Report of a Working Party on Anesthetic Explosions, London, 1956, Her Majesty's Stationary Office.

Severinghaus, J. W.: The rate of uptake of nitrous oxide in man, J. Clin. Invest. **33**:1183, 1954.

Slater, H. M., and Stephen, C. R.: Anesthesia for infants and children: nonrebreathing technique, Arch. Surg. **62**:251, 1951.

Stephen, C. R., and Slater, H. M.: A nonresisting, nonrebreathing valve, Anesthesiology **9**:550, 1948.

Stephen, C. R., and Slater, H. M.: A nonrebreathing mask, Anesthesiology **13**:226, 1952.

Chapter 18

Gordon, I., Turner, R., and Price, T. W.: Medical jurisprudence, ed. 3, Edinburgh and London, 1953, E. & S. Livingstone, Ltd., chap. 18, p. 510.

State v. Borah, 51 Ariz. 318, 115 Am. Law Rep. 254.

21 Rule, Case Law 386.

Vigneault v. Dr. Hewson Dental Co., 15 N. E. (2d) 185.

Moscicki v. Shor, 107 Pa. Supreme Court 192.

69 Am. Law Rep. 1145; 129 Am. Law Rep. 107.

26 Am. Law Rep. 1037; 53 Am. Law Rep. 1056.

Wolfe v. Feldman, 158 Misc. 656, 286 N. Y. Supp. 118.

Dawson v. Allen, 191 Ill. Appellate Court 399.

Knocker, D.: Accidents in their medico-legal aspect, London, 1910, Butterworth & Co., Ltd., and Ballière, Tindall & Cox, Ltd., p. 74.

Loudon v. Scott, 58 Mont. 645, 194 P. 488, 12 Am. Law Rep. 1487.

12 Am. Law Rep. 1494, 1495.

41 Am. Juris. 208, sec. 90.

59 Am. Law Rep. 1074.

Coleman v. Wilson, 85 N.J.L. 203.

Turner v. Sanders, 247 Ky. 90, 56 S.W. (2d) 718.

Nelson v. Sandell, 202 Iowa 109, 209, N.W. 440.

48 Corpus Juris. 1145, sec. 155; 41 Am. Juris. 238, sec. 128.

Mayer v. Hipke, 183 Wisc. 382, 197 N.W. 333.

De Groot v. Winter, 265 Mich. 274, 251 N.W. 425.

Chubb v. Holmes, 111 Conn. 482.

Dolan v. O'Rourke, 56 N.D. 416, 217 N.W. 666.

Donoho v. Rawleigh, 230 Ky. 11, 18 S.W. (2d) 311.

Regan, L. J.: The doctor and patient and the law, ed. 2, St. Louis, 1949, The C. V. Mosby Co., p. 386.

Chapter 20

Monheim, L. M., and Tessler, K.: The rebirth of nitrous oxide, Oral Surg. **8**:1146, 1955.

Peiffer, G. W., and Monheim, L. M.: Preliminary report on chemanesia combined with analgesia for the ambulatory dental patient, Oral Surg. **10**:504, 1957.

Appendix

Conversion tables

Temperature			
F.	***C.***	***C.***	***F.***
0	−17.8	0	32.0
95	35.0	35.0	95.0
96	35.6	35.5	95.9
97	36.1	36.0	96.8
98	36.7	36.5	97.7
99	37.2	37.0	98.6
100	37.8	37.5	99.5
101	38.3	38.0	100.4
102	38.9	38.5	101.3
103	39.4	39.0	102.2
104	40.0	39.5	103.1
105	40.5	40.0	104.0
106	41.1	40.5	104.9
107	41.7	41.0	105.8
108	42.2	41.5	106.7
109	42.8	42.0	107.6
110	43.3	100.0	212.0

F. to C.: 5/9 (F. − 32)
C. to F.: (9/5 × C.) + 32

Conversion tables—cont'd

***Weight* (*1 lb. = 0.454 kg.; 1 kg. = 2.204 lb.*)**			
lb.	***kg.***	***kg.***	***lb.***
1	0.5	1	2.2
2	0.9	2	4.4
4	1.8	3	6.6
6	2.7	4	8.8
8	3.6	5	11.0
10	4.5	6	13.2
20	9.1	8	17.6
30	13.6	10	22.0
40	18.2	20	44.0
50	22.7	30	66.0
60	27.3	40	88.0
70	31.8	50	110.0
80	36.4	60	132.0
90	40.9	70	154.0
100	45.4	80	176.0
150	68.2	90	198.0
200	91.0	100	220.0

***Length* (*1 in. = 2.54 cm.; 1 cm. = 0.3936 in.*)**			
in.	***cm.***	***cm.***	***in.***
1	2.5	1	0.4
2	5.1	2	0.8
4	10.2	3	1.2
6	15.2	4	1.6
8	20.3	5	2.0
12	30.5	6	2.4
18	46.0	8	3.1
24	61.0	10	3.9
30	76.0	20	7.9
36	91.0	30	11.8
42	107.0	40	15.7
48	122.0	50	19.7
54	137.0	60	23.6
60	152.0	70	27.6
66	168.0	80	31.5
72	183.0	90	35.4
78	198.0	100	39.4

Approximate dose equivalents for grains and grams

Grains	Grams (Gm.)	Milligrams (mg.)
1/600	0.0001	0.1
1/500	0.00012	0.12
1/400	0.00015	0.15
1/300	0.0002	0.2
1/250	0.00025	0.25
1/200	0.0003	0.3
1/150	0.0004	0.4
1/120	0.0005	0.5
1/100	0.0006	0.6
1/80	0.0008	0.8
1/60	0.001	1
1/30	0.002	2
1/20	0.003	3
1/15	0.004	4
1/12	0.005	5
1/10	0.006	6
1/8	0.088	8
1/6	0.010	10
1/4	0.015	15
1/3	0.020	20
3/8	0.025	25
1/2	0.032	32
3/4	0.050	50
1	0.065	65
1½	0.100	
2	0.130	
2½	0.150	
3	0.200	
4	0.250	
5	0.325	
7½	0.500	
10	0.650	
15	1	
30	2	
45	3	
60	4	

Metric equivalents

Volume	
1 minim (water)	0.066 ml.
1 fl. dr.	3.70 ml.
1 fl. oz.	29.5737 ml.
1 apothecary oz. (water)	31.1035 ml.
1 pt.	0.4732 liters
1 qt.	0.9464 liters
1 gal. (U.S.)	3.7854 liters
1 cu. in.	16.387 ml.
1 ml.	16.23 minims (water)
1 ml.	0.2702 fl. dr.
1 ml.	0.0338 fl. oz.
1 liter	1.0567 qt.
1 liter	0.2642 gal.
1 liter	33.84 fl. oz.
liter ÷ 3.78	gal. (231 cu. in.)
1 ml.	0.061 cu. in.
ml. ÷ 16.387	cu. in.
ml. ÷ 3.697	fl. dr.
ml. ÷ 29.57	fl. oz.

Solutions	
0.1% solution	1 mg. per ml.
0.2% solution	2 mg. per ml.
0.5% solution	5 mg. per ml.
1 % solution	10 mg. per ml.
2 % solution	20 mg. per ml.
5 % solution	50 mg. per ml.
10 % solution	100 mg. per ml.
20 % solution	200 mg. per ml.
50 % solution	500 mg. per ml.
100 % solution	1000 mg. per ml.

Gram-ionic weights and gram-equivalent weights for the most important ions present in the body

Ion	Ionic weight (gram)	Equivalent weight (gram)	Conversion factors	
			mEq./L.	*mg. %*
Na+	23.0	23.0	mg. % × 0.435	mEq./L. × 2.30
K+	39.1	39.1	mg. % × 0.256	mEq./L. × 3.91
Ca++	40.1	20.0	mg. % × 0.498	mEq./L. × 2.00
Mg++	24.3	12.2	mg. % × 0.823	mEq./L. × 1.21
Cl^-	35.5	35.5	mg. % × 0.282	mEq./L. × 3.55
HCO_3–	61.0	61.0	vol. % (CO_2) × 0.450	mEq./L. × 2.22 (vol. %)
HPO_4–	96.0	48.0*	mg. % (P) × 0.580	mEq./L. × 1.72 (P)
SO_4–	96.1	48.0	mg. % (S) × 0.613	mEq./L. × 1.60 (S)

*At the normal pH of body fluids, 20% of the phosphate radical is combined with 1 equivalent of base as BH_2PO_4 and 80% with 2 equivalents of base as B_2HPO_4. Under these conditions, base equivalence per unit of HPO_4 is therefore $0.2 + (0.8 \times 2) = 1.8$, and the equivalent weight of 53.3 is obtained by dividing the ionic weight by 1.8 instead of by 2.

Abbreviations for weights and measures

gr.	grain or grains	ʒ i̇ss	1½ drams
ggt.	drop		
ggts.	drops	ʒ ïi	2 drams
♏	minim		
℈	scruple	℥ i̇	1 ounce
ʒ	dram		
℥	ounce	℥ s̄s̄	½ ounce
O	pint		
C	gallon	℥ i̇ss	1½ ounces
āā	equal parts	℥ ïi	2 ounces
s̄s̄	one half	ml.	milliliter
ʒ i̇	1 dram	Gm.	gram
ʒ s̄s̄	½ dram	mg.	milligram

Normal blood values

Hematocrit: men, 45% (38–54%); women, 40% (36–47%)
Hemoglobin: men, 14–18 grams %; women, 12–16 grams %; children, 12–14 grams %

Blood counts	Per cubic millimeter	Percentage
Erythrocytes		
Men	$5.0(4.5\text{–}6.0) \times 10^6$	
Women	$4.5(4.3\text{–}5.5) \times 10^6$	
Reticulocytes		0–1
Leukocytes, total	5000–10,000	100
Myelocytes	0	0
Juvenile neutrophils	0–100	0–1
Band neutrophils	0–500	0–5
Segmented neutrophils	2500–6000	40–60
Lymphocytes	1000–4000	20–40
Eosinophils	50–300	1–3
Basophils	0–100	0–1
Monocytes	200–800	4–8
Platelets	200,000–500,000	

Bleeding time	1–3 min. (Duke)
Coagulation time (venous)	6–10 min. (Lee and White) 10–30 min. (Howell)
Prothrombin time	10–20 sec. (Quick)
Circulation time, arm to tongue (sodium dehydrocholate)	9–16 sec.
Sedimentation rate	
Men	0– 9 mm. per hr. (Wintrobe)
Women	0–20 mm. per hr. (Wintrobe)
Total blood volume	5000–6000 ml. (78–85 ml./kg.)
Oxygen capacity	18–22 volumes %
Oxygen content (arterial)	17–21 volumes %
Oxygen content (venous)	10–16 volumes %
Oxygen % saturation, arterial	94–96 volumes %
Oxygen % saturation, venous	60–85 volumes %
pH	7.3–7.4
Albumin, serum	4.0–5.2 grams/100 ml.
Amylase, serum	less than 50 units/100 ml.
Base, total, serum	0.1–0.8 mg./100 ml.
Calcium, serum	9–11 mg./100 ml.
Carbon dioxide–combining power, serum	50–65 volumes %
Chlorides, serum (as Cl)	100–106 mEq./L.
Cholesterol, total, serum	120–260 mg./100 ml.
Potassium, serum	4.0–5.0 mEq./L.
Proteins, total, serum	6.5–8.0 grams/100 ml.
Sodium, serum	137–143 mEq./L.
Glucose	80.0–120.0 mg. per 100 ml.

Continued on next page.

Normal blood values—cont'd

Electrolytes		
Element	***mEq./L.***	***mg./100 ml.***
Calcium	4.5–5.5	9–11
Chlorides (as Cl)	96–107	340–380
Phosphates (inorganic P)	1.65–2.5	3–4.5
Potassium	3.5–5	13.5–19.5
Sodium	135–145	310–335
Magnesium	1.5–3	1.25–2.5

Table of tests

Kidney function tests

Phenolsulfonphthalein test **(*PSP test*)**

Inject intramuscularly or intravenously a solution of phenolsulfonphthalein, a drug that is eliminated only by the kidneys. The amount of this drug in the urine is estimated by colorimetric methods.

Normal value: total excretion in 2 hours of 60 to 80% of the amount injected.

Concentration test **(*Fishberg method*)**

The first sample of urine voided in the morning is saved. The patient should rest in bed 1 hour after awaking, and a second sample of urine should be collected in a separate container. If possible, the patient should arise and, after 1 hour's activity, a third sample of urine should be collected in another container. All 3 samples are examined at about 10 A.M. If the renal function is unimpaired, the specific gravity of at least 1 sample of urine will be between 1.022 and 1.032. If there is very severe impairment, the specific gravity may be as low as 1.010, and in intermediary conditions it will be between 1.010 and 1.020.

Total nonprotein nitrogen

The nitrogen retention may be taken as an index of the degree of disability of the kidneys.

Normal values: total nonprotein nitrogen, 25 to 30 mg. per 100 ml. of blood; urea nitrogen, 12 to 15 mg. per 100 ml. of blood; uric acid, 2 to 3 mg. per 100 ml. of blood; creatinine, 1 to 2 mg. per 100 ml. of blood.

Liver function tests

Bromsulphalein test **(*BSP retention*)**

Not used for patients with jaundice. 5 mg. of dye for each kilogram of body weight are injected into vein. Determination of dye retention is made at the end of 45 minutes after intravenous administration.

Normal: 5% or less

Thymol turbidity reaction of serum

Normal values vary from 0 to 5 units.

Cephalin-cholesterol flocculation test

Normal value is from negative to 1+.

Urinalysis (normal values)

Specific gravity, 1.003–1.030
pH, 6 (4.7–8.0)
Volume, 1200 (600–2500) ml./24 hrs.
Sugar, none
Albumin, negative (up to 20 mg. normal)
Acetone, negative
Red blood count, none
White blood count, none

Dosage for children

$$\text{Clark's rule: } \frac{\text{Weight of child in pounds}}{150} \times \text{Adult dose}$$

$$\text{Young's rule: } \frac{\text{Age of child in years}}{\text{Age} + 12} \times \text{Adult dose}$$

$$\text{Cowling's rule: } \frac{\text{Age of child next birthday}}{24} \times \text{Adult dose}$$

Physiological information

Temperature of the body

The normal oral temperature of adults is 98.6° F.; of the aged, 98.8°; of children, the rectal temperature is 1 degree higher and the axillary temperature is 1 degree lower than the oral temperature. The daily variation is from 1 degree to 1.5 degrees, the maximum temperature being reached between 5 and 7 P.M.

Relation of pulse and temperature

A variation of 1 degree of temperature above 98° F. is approximately equivalent to a difference of 10 beats in the pulse—thus:

Temperature of 98° F. corresponds with pulse of 60
Temperature of 99° F. corresponds with pulse of 70
Temperature of 100° F. corresponds with pulse of 80
Temperature of 101° F. corresponds with pulse of 90
Temperature of 102° F. corresponds with pulse of 100
Temperature of 103° F. corresponds with pulse of 110
Temperature of 104° F. corresponds with pulse of 120
Temperature of 105° F. corresponds with pulse of 130
Temperature of 106° F. corresponds with pulse of 140

Physiological information—cont'd

Average frequency of pulse at different ages in health		
Age	***Bears per minute (Carpenter)***	***Other authorities***
In fetus in utero	Between 150–140	
Newborn infants	Between 140–130	150–130
1 yr.	From 130–115	130–108
2 yr.	From 115–100	108– 90
3 yr.	From 105– 95	90– 80
7 to 14 yr.	From 90– 80	80– 72
14 to 21 yr.	From 85– 75	85– 80
21 to 60 yr.	From 75– 80	av. 72
In old age	Between 75– 80	av. 67

The pulse is generally more rapid: in females by 10 to 14 beats per minute; during and after exertion unless long continued; during digestion or mental excitement; and occurs more frequently in the morning.

Respiration at various ages	
Age	***Number of respirations per minute***
First year	25–35
At puberty	20–25
Adult age	16–18

Average normal blood pressure			
Age	***Systolic***	***Diastolic***	***Pulse***
10 yr.	103	70	33
15 yr.	113	75	38
20 yr.	120	80	40
25 yr.	122	81	40
30 yr.	123	82	41
35 yr.	124	83	41
40 yr.	126	84	42
45 yr.	128	85	43
50 yr.	130	86	44
55 yr.	132	87	45
60 yr.	135	89	46

Abbreviations for preoperative and postoperative orders

Term	*Latin or Greek*	*Translation*
a.c.	ante cibum	before eating
b.i.d.	bis in die	twice a day
b.o.r.		before time of operation
c.b.c.		complete blood count
det.	detur	let be given
dil.	dilue	dilute
d.t.d.	dentur tales doses	let such doses be given
enem.	enema	an enema
et.	et	and
garg.	gargarisma	gargle
h.	hora	hour
h.s.	hora somni	at bedtime
in d.	in dies	from day to day
liq.	liquor	a solution
M.	misce	mix (thou)
m. dict.	modo dictu	as directed
mollis		soft
N.B.	nota bene	note well
N.F.		National Formulary
non rep.	non repetatur	do not repeat
n.s.q.		not sufficient quantity
o.d.	omne die	once a day
o.m.	omne mane	each morning
omn. hor.	omni hora	every hour
o.n.	omne nocte	each night
p.c.	post cibum	after eating
p.o.	per os	by mouth
p.r.n.	pro re nata	when required
q.2h.	quaque secunda hora	every 2 hours
q.i.d.	quater in die	4 times a day
q.s.	quantum sufficit	a sufficient quantity
S.O.S.	si opus sit	if necessary
ss.	semis	a half
Stat.	statim	at once
tab.	tablet	a tablet
Tbsp.		tablespoon
t.i.d.	ter in die	3 times a day

Drug used for premedication*

Drug	*Dosage*	*Mode of administration*
Barbiturates		
Pentobarbital (Nembutal)	1½–3 grains (100–200 mg.)	Oral; I.V.; I.M.; rectal
Secobarbital (Seconal)	1½–3 grains (100–200 mg.)	Oral; I.V.; I.M.; rectal
Amobarbital (Amytal)	1½–3 grains (100–200 mg.)	Oral
Phenobarbital (Luminal)	1½–3 grains (100–200 mg.)	Oral
Nonbarbiturate		
Ethinamate (Valmid)	500–1000 mg.	Oral
Narcotics		
Opiates		
Morphine	1/8, 1/6, 1/4 grain (8, 10, 15 mg.)	I.M.; I.V.
Pantopon	1/3 grain (30 mg.)	I.M.
Dihydromorphinone (Dilaudid)	1/20–1/30 grain (3–2 mg.)	Oral; subcutaneously
Codeine	1/4, 1/2, 1 grain (15–65) mg.)	Oral; subcutaneously
Opioids		
Meperidine (Demerol)	3/4–1½ grains (50–100 mg.)	Oral; I.V.; I.M.
Alphaprodine (Nisentil)	1/3–1 grain (20–60 mg.)	I.V.; subcutaneously
Anileridine (Leritine)	1/30–1/20 grain (2–3 mg.)	Oral; subcutaneously
Antagonist for overdose or depression by narcotics		
Nalorphine (Nalline)	5–10 mg. (in severe cases larger doses may be used)	I.V.; I.M.; subcutaneously
Levallorphan (Lorfan)	1 mg. for 1 or 2 doses (0.5 mg. for additional doses)	I.V.
Nalorphine and levallorphan are not effective against depression by barbiturates.		
Belladonna alkaloids		
Atropine	1/100–1/150 grain (0.6–0.4 mg.)	I.M.; I.V.
Scopolamine	1/100–1/150 grain (0.6–0.4 mg.)	I.M.; I.V.
Ataraxic drugs for potentiation		
Promethazine (Phenergan)	12.5–50 mg.	Oral; I.M.; I.V.

*Average adult doses.

Glossary

absorption the passage of a substance into the interior of another by solution or penetration.

acapnia diminished carbon dioxide in the blood.

acid a chemical substance which in aqueous solution undergoes dissociation with the formation of hydrogen ions (pH) which ranges from 0 to 6.9.

acid salt a salt containing one or more replaceable hydrogen ions.

acidemia a decreased pH of the blood, irrespective of changes in the blood bicarbonate.

acidosis a clinical term commonly used to indicate acidemia or lowered blood bicarbonate with a tendency toward acidemia.

adrenergic activated or transmitted by epinephrine. A term applied to the nerve fibers that liberate sympathin at a synapse when a nerve impulse passes. Postganglionic sympathetic fibers.

adrenergic blocking agent a drug that blocks the action of neurohormone sympathin or of adrenergic drugs at sympathetic neuroeffectors.

adrenocortical steroid a hormone extracted from the adrenal cortex or a synthetic substance similar in chemical structure and biological activity to such hormones.

adrenolytic an adrenergic blocking agent, especially one more effective in blocking the actions of circulating adrenergic substances than those of actual sympathetic nervous impulses.

adsorption a process believed to be physical in nature in which molecules of a gas or liquid condense or adhere on the surface of another substance.

afferent conveying from the periphery to the center.

afferent impulse an impulse that arises in the periphery and is carried into the central nervous system. An afferent nerve conducts the impulse from the site of origin to the central nervous system.

airway a clear passageway for air into and out of the lungs. A device for securing unobstructed respiration during general anesthesia or in states of unconsciousness.

alkali a strong water-soluble base.

alkaline reserve one of the buffer systems of the blood that can neutralize the acid valences formed in the body; it is made up by the base of weak acid salts and usually measured by determining the bicarbonate concentration of the plasma.

alkalosis a chemical term commonly used to indicate alkalemia or increased blood bicarbonate with a tendency toward alkalemia.

allergen purified protein substance used to test a patient's sensitivity to food, pollens, etc.

allergy an antigen-antibody reaction that results in a condition of unusual or exaggerated specific susceptibility to a substance that is harmless in similar amounts for the majority of the members of the same species.

alveolar ventilation the process of supplying alveoli with air or oxygen.

alveolus an air sac of the lungs formed by terminal dilations of the bronchioles.

analeptic an agent that acts to overcome depression of the central nervous system.

analgesia loss of all pain sensations due to the administration of a drug, but without loss of consciousness.

analgesic the ability of a drug to raise the pain threshold.

anatomical dead space the actual capacity of the respiratory passages, which extend from the nostrils to and including the terminal bronchioles.

anemic hypoxia hypoxia brought about by the result of the reduction of the oxygen-carrying capacity of the blood due to decrease of the complete blood counts or alteration of the hemoglobin constituents.

anesthesia, basal a state of narcosis prior to the administration of a general anesthetic that permits production of states of surgical anesthesia, with greatly reduced amounts of general anesthetic agents.

anesthesia, general irregular, reversible depression of the cells of the higher centers of the central nervous system which makes the patient unconscious and insensible to pain.

anesthetic agent any drug capable of producing anesthesia.

anesthetic, local a drug which when injected into the tissues has little or no irritating effects and when absorbed into the nerve will temporarily interrupt its property of conduction.

anoxia a condition of total oxygen lack; frequently misused as a synonym for hypoxia.

anoxic hypoxia hypoxia due to inadequate oxygen in inspired air or to interference with gaseous exchange in the lungs.

anticholinergic a drug that acts to block the effects of the neurohormone acetylcholine or of cholinergic drugs at postganglionic cholinergic neuroeffectors. A cholinergic blocking agent.

anticholinesterase a drug that inhibits the enzyme cholinesterase, resulting in stimulation of organs innervated by cholinergic fibers.

antiemetic a drug used to prevent or relieve nausea and vomiting.

antihistaminic a drug that acts to prevent or antagonize the pharmacological effects of histamine and allergic symptoms stemming from histamine released in the tissues.

antisialogogue a drug that reduces salivation.

antispasmodic a drug that relieves muscle spasm.

apnea a temporary cessation of respiratory movements.

armamentarium the outfit of a practitioner or institution, including books, medicines, and surgical supplies.

arrhythmia any variation from the normal rhythm of the heart.

asphyxia a condition of suffocation due to restriction of oxygen intake plus interference with elimination of carbon dioxide.

asthma a disease marked by recurrent attacks of paroxymal dyspnea, with wheezing, coughing, and a sense of constriction due to the spasmotic contraction of the bronchi. It may result from direct irritation of the bronchial mucous membrane or from reflex irritation.

ataractic capable of producing ataraxia.

ataraxia calmness and complete peace of mind.

ataraxic a drug that produces calmness; a tranquilizer.

atelectasis complete collapse of a lung.

augmentation assistance to respiration by the application of intermittent pressure on inspiration.

base a solution that yields hydroxyl ions and neutralization in acid to form a salt and water. It is capable of combining with a protein. A base turns red litmus paper blue and has a pH higher than 7.

basal metabolic rate the heat production of a person at the lowest level of cell activity, or the minimal amount of cell activity necessary for the continuous function of respiration, circulation, and secretion.

basic salt a salt containing replaceable or hydroxyl groups.

blood pressure the pressure of the blood on the walls of the arteries, which depends on the energy of the heart action, the elasticity of the walls of the arteries, the resistance in the capillaries, and the volume and viscosity of the blood.

boiling point the temperature at which the vapor pressure within a liquid equals atmospheric pressure.

bradycardia abnormal slowness of the heart (under 60 beats per minute) as evidenced by slowing of the pulse.

bradypnea abnormal slowness of breathing.

bronchiectasis dilation of the bronchi, either local or general.

bronchodilator a drug that dilates or expands the size of the lumina of the air passages of the lungs by relaxing the muscular walls.

bronchospasm spasmodic contraction of the muscular coat of the bronchial tubes, such as occurs in asthma.

buffer any substance in a fluid which tends to lessen the change in hydrogen ion concentration, which otherwise would be produced by adding acids or alkalis.

carbon dioxide absorber a device that removes carbon dioxide from a mixture of gases.

chemanesia reversible amnesia produced by a chemical or drug (author's original word).

chemoreceptors a receptor adapted for excitation by chemical substances. Carotid body or aortic (supracardiac) bodies.

Cheyne-Stokes respiration a type of breathing characterized by rhythmical variations in intensity that occurs in cycles.

cholinergic blocking agent a drug that inhibits the action of acetylcholine or cholinergic drugs at postganglionic cholinergic neuroeffectors. An anticholinergic agent.

cholinergic drug a drug that mimics the effects of neurohormone acetylcholine.

cholinesterase inhibitors chemicals that interfere with the activity of the enzyme cholinesterase.

compensated acidosis a condition in which the blood bicarbonate is usually lower than normal, but the compensatory mechanisms have kept the pH within normal range.

compensated alkalosis a condition in which the blood bicarbonate is usually higher than normal, but the compensatory mechanisms have kept the pH within normal range.

complemental air *see* inspiratory reserve volume.

compound a substance that consists of two or more chemical elements in union.

conjugation in chemistry the joining of two compounds to produce another compound, such as the combination of a toxic product with some substance in the body to form a detoxified product, which is then eliminated.

controlled respiration maintenance of adequate pulmonary ventilation in apneic patients.

cough a sudden noisy expulsion of air from the lungs.

cyanosis a bluish tint to the skin.

degradation the reduction of a chemical compound to one less complex, as when one or more groups are split off.

depression decrease of functional activity.

derivative the resultant of a chemical reaction.

detoxify (detoxicate) to remove the toxic quality of a substance.

dextrorotatory rotating to the right.

dialysis diffusion through a membrane.

diffusion the process of becoming widely spread, such as gases from a small jet that spread throughout a room. In liquids, the velocity of the molecules of two solutions will cause them to diffuse, the diffusion varying in rate according to their molecular weight and temperature.

dose, lethal the amount of a drug that would prove fatal to the majority of persons.

dose, minimal lethal (***MLD_{50}***) the amount of a drug fatal to 50% of the animals in controlled experimental conditions.

dose, therapeutic the amount of a drug required to achieve the desired result. The amount will vary between minimal and maximal amounts.

dose, toxic the amount of a drug that causes untoward symptoms in the majority of persons.

drug a chemical agent that affects living protoplasm.

dyspnea difficult, labored, or gasping respiration; inspiration, expiration, or both may be involved.

efferent conveying impulses away from a nerve center toward the periphery.

element a simple substance that cannot be decomposed by chemical means and that is made up of atoms which are alike in their peripheral electronic configuration and chemical properties, but differ in their nuclei, atomic weight, and radioactive properties.

emetic a drug that induces vomiting.

emphysema the presence of air in the intra-alveolar tissue of the lungs due to distention or rupture of the pulmonary alveoli with air. It may be interstitial (interlobular) when due to the escape of air from the lungs into the interstitial tissue between the alveoli, or vesicular (alveolar) when due to distention of the alveoli with air.

endotracheal inhalation inhalation of an anesthetic mixture into the lungs through an endotracheal catheter at low or atmospheric pressure.

endotracheal insufflation forcing of an anesthetic mixture into the lungs through an endotracheal catheter under pressure.

enzyme a substance elaborated by living cells and possessing catalytic properties.

ester any compound formed from alcohol and an acid.

esterase an enzyme that splits off an ester.

eudaemonic applied to a drug that brings about a feeling of normal well-being in a previously depressed patient.

euphoric a substance that produces an exaggerated sense of well-being.

eupnea easy or normal respiration.

exhalation valves a vale that permits escape of exhaled gases into the atmosphere and prevents them from being rebreathed.

expiratory reserve volume the maximal volume that can be expired from the resting expiratory level.

external respiration ventilation of the lungs and oxygenation of the blood.

full face mask a device used in anesthesia that confines the gas delivered into the mask into the respiratory tract through the nose or mouth.

functional residual air *see* functional residual capacity.

functional residual capacity the volume of gas in the lungs at resting expiratory level.

ganglionic blocking agent a drug that prevents passage of nerve impulses at the synapse between preganglionic and postganglionic neurons.

gram a weight in the metric system that equals 1,000 mg. or 15.437+ grains troy weight.

hematinic an agent that tends to increase the hemoglobin content of the blood.

Hering-Breuer reflex the nervous mechanism that tends to limit the respiratory excursions. Stimuli from the sensory endings in the lungs and perhaps in other parts passing up the vagi tend to limit both inspiration and expiration during ordinary breathing.

hiccup an involuntary spasmodic contraction of the diaphragm, which causes a beginning inspiration that is suddenly checked by closure of the glottis, thus producing a characteristic sound.

hippus tremor of the iris that produces rapid, spasmodic alteration of the pupil.

histotoxic hypoxia hypoxia that is the result of the inability of the tissue cells to use the oxygen that may be present in normal amount and tension.

hydrogenation the process of adding hydrogen to an unsaturated compound.

hydrolysis reaction between the ions of a salt and those of water to form an acid and a base, one or both of which are only slightly dissociated. A process whereby a large molecule is split up by the addition of water. The end products divide the water, the hydroxyl group being attached to one and the hydrogen ion to the other.

hydroxyl the univalent radical which, in combination with other radicals, forms hydroxides.

hypalgesia diminished sensation to pain that results from a raised pain threshold.

hyperalgesia a greater-than-normal pain sensation that may be due to a painful stimulus or a lowered pain threshold.

hypercapnea the presence of more than the normal amount of carbon dioxide in the blood tissues due to either an increase of carbon dioxide in the inspired air or a decrease in elimination.

hyperpnea an increased respiratory volume, the result of increased rate and depth of breathing.

hypertension abnormally high blood pressure.

hypertonic a solution having a greater osmotic pressure than blood serum.

hypnotic a drug that induces sleep or depresses the central nervous system at a cortical level.

hypocapnia a deficiency of carbon dioxide in the blood that stimulates respiration.

hypopnea abnormally shallow and rapid respirations.

hypotension abnormally low tension, especially low blood pressure.

hypotensive a drug that reduces blood pressure, used in the treatment of hypertension.

hypoxemia deficient oxygenation of the blood.

hypoxia low oxygen content or tension.

idiosyncrasy abnormal or unusual response to a drug when an extremely small dose has been given. The reaction is similar to a toxic overdose.

impulse an uncontrollable wave of excitation transmitted along a nerve fiber due to a stimulus.

injection the act of introducing a liquid into a part, such as the bloodstream or tissues.

insertion the act of implanting or, as it refers to regional analgesia, of introducing the needle into the tissues.

inspiratory reserve volume the maximum volume that can be inspired from end of tidal inspiration.

internal respiration mechanism of gaseous exchange between blood and tissues.

intrapleural pressure pressure within the pleura.

intrapulmonic pressure in the substance of the lungs.

ion the product formed by the electrolytic dissociation of a molecule; carries one or more positive or negative charges.

irritant an agent that causes irritation or stimulation.

levorotatory rotating to the left.

lipophilic showing marked attraction or solubility in lipids.

margin of safety margin between lethal and toxic doses.

metabolism the sum of chemical changes involved in the function of nutrition. There are two phases—anabolism, constructive or assimilative changes, and catabolistm, destructive or retrograde changes.

minimal air volume of air in the air sacs themselves (part of the residual air).

miotic a drug that constricts the pupil.

molecular weight the sum of atomic weights of all the atoms in molecules.

molecule a chemical composition of two or more atoms that form a specific chemical substance.

mydriatic a drug that dilates the pupil.

myoneural blocking agent a drug that prevents transmission of nerve impulses at the junction of the nerve and the muscle.

narcotic a drug that raises the pain threshold and depresses the cerebral cortex. It can induce euphoria.

narcotic antagonist a narcotic drug that acts specifically to reverse depression of the central nervous system.

nasal inhaler a device that is placed over the nose and that permits inhalation of anesthetic agents.

neutral solution a solution that has a pH of 7. Equal numbers of hydrogen and hydroxyl ions are formed on dissociation.

nicotinic an agent that mimics the effects of nicotine, especially at autonomic ganglia and at myoneural junctions in skeletal muscle.

normal capacity *see* functional residual capacity.

orthopnea inability to breathe except in an upright position.

oxidization the combination of oxygen with other elements to form oxides. The process in which an element gains electrons.

paralysis cessation of cell function.

parasympatholytic drug a drug that blocks nerve impulses passing from parasympathetic nerve fibers to postganglionic neuroeffectors.

parasympathomimetic drug a drug that has an effect similar to that produced when the parasympathetic nerves are stimulated.

parenteral solution a sterile solution or substance prepared for injection.

partial pressure the pressure exerted by each of the constituents of a mixture of gases.

pH concentration of hydrogen ions expressed as the negative logarithm of base 10.

phase any one of the varying aspects or stages through which an anesthetic or process may pass.

physiological dead space the air passages up to, but not including, the alveoli of the lungs, equal to about 150 ml.

pneumothorax an accumulation of air or gas in the pleural cavity. The air enters by an external wound, by a lung perforation, from burrowing abscess, or from the rupture of a superficial lung cavity. Pneumothorax is accompanied by sudden, severe pain and rapidly increasing dyspnea.

polypnea a rapid or panting respiration.

potentiation increase in the action of a drug by the addition of another drug that does not necessarily possess similar properties.

precipitate an insoluble solid substance that forms from chemical reactions between solutions.

pressor a drug that causes a rise in blood pressure.

propagation the reproduction or the continuance of an impulse along a nerve fiber in an afferent or efferent direction.

psychomotor stimulant a drug that increases psychic activity, alertness, and motor activity.

psychosomatic pertaining to the mind-body relationship and producing bodily symptoms of a mental origin.

pulse pressure the difference between the systolic and diastolic pressures.

racemic acid a mixture of equal parts of dextrolevo compound.

radical a group of atoms that act as single elements when in chemical reactions.

reduction removal of oxygen; addition of hydrogen; gain of electrons.

relaxant an antispasmodic; a drug that relaxes spasm of smooth or skeletal muscle.

reserve air *see* expiratory reserve volume.

residual air *see* residual volume.

residual capacity *see* residual volume.

residual volume volume of air in the lungs at end of maximal inspiration.

respiration the gaseous exchange between the cells of the body and its environment.

respiratory acidosis acidemia produced by hypoventilation, which results in an increase in plasma carbonic acid and plasma bicarbonte.

respiratory alkalosis alkalemia produced by hyperventilation; as a result the plasma carbonic acid decreases and there is an excretion of bicarbonate in the urine to restore the carbonic acid–sodium bicarbonate ratio and prevent a change in pH. Plasma bicarbonate is therefore decreased in respiratory alkalosis but raised in metabolic alkalosis.

salt a compound of a base and an acid; a compound of an acid some of whose replaceable hydrogen atoms have been substituted.

sedative a remedy that allays excitement and slows down the basal metabolic rate without impairing the cerebral cortex.

sialogogue a substance that increases the flow of saliva.

sneeze an involuntary, sudden, violent expulsion of air through the mouth and nose; may be elicited during Pentothal anesthesia by corneal stimulation.

soporific a sleep-producing drug.

spasmolytic a drug that reduces spasm in smooth or skeletal muscle.

stable a term applied to a substance that has no tendency to decompose spontaneously. As applied to chemical compounds, it denotes their ability to resist chemical alterations.

stage a period or distinct phase in the course of an anesthetic.

stagnant hypoxia hypoxia due to decreased circulation in an area.

sternutator a sneeze-inducing substance.

stertorous respiration snoring.

stimulant an agent that causes an increase in functional activity, usually of the central nervous system.

stimulation increased function of protoplasm induced by some extracellular substance or agent.

stimulus a chemical, thermal, electrical, or mechanical influence that changes the normal environment of irritable tissue and creates an impulse.

stridorous respiration a high-pitched sound during respiration due to adduction of the vocal cords.

strong acid an acid that is completely ionized in aqueous solution.

supplemental air *see* expiratory reserve volume.

supplemental volume *see* expiratory reserve volume.

sympatholytic a drug that blocks the effects of stimulation of the sympathetic nervous system. An adrenergic blocking agent.

sympathomimetic resembles the effect produced by stimulation of the sympathetic nervous system.

synergism the ability of two drugs to increase the action of each other to an extent greater than the action of each when used alone.

tachycardia excessively rapid action of the heart; the pulse rate is usually above 100 beats per minute.

tachyphlaxis a decreasing response that follows consecutive injections at short intervals.

tachypnea excessively rapid respiration. A respiratory neurosis marked by quick, shallow breathing.

tidal air *see* tidal volume.

tidal volume the volume of gas inspirated or expired during each respiratory cycle.

total lung capacity the volume of air in the lungs at the end of maximal inspiration.

tranquilizer a calming agent that reduces anxiety and tension without depressing mental or motor functions.

uncompensated acidosis acidemia usually accompanied by lowered blood bicarbonate, as after the ingestion of hydrochloric acid or in terminal nephritis. (In uncompensated carbon dioxide acidosis, the bicarbonate may be normal.)

uncompensated alkalosis alkalemia, usually accompanied by an increased blood bicarbonate, as after ingestion of sodium bicarbonate or after vomiting with the resultant loss of hydrochloric acid. (In uncompensated carbon dioxide alkalosis the bicarbonate may be normal.)

vagomimetic a drug with actions similar to those produced by stimulation of the vagus nerve.

vagovagal reflex a reflex in which the afferent and efferent impulses travel via the vagus nerve. The afferent impulses travel centrally via the sensory nucleus of the vagus. The efferent impulses travel via the motor fibers of the vagus.

vasoconstrictor (vasopressor) causes a rise in blood pressure by constriction of the blood vessels. In local areas, constriction of thet arterioles and capillaries.

vasodilator a drug that relaxes the smooth muscle walls of the blood vessels and increases their diameter.

vasopressor *see* vasoconstrictor.

vital capacity the maximal volume of air that can be expired after maximal inspiration.

weak acid an acid that is only slightly ionized in aqueous solution.

Index*

*The term "anesthesia" signifies general anesthesia unless otherwise stated.